Comprehensive Atlas of Practical Pediatric Urodynamics

Subhasis Saha • Poonam Guha Vaze
Editors

Comprehensive Atlas of Practical Pediatric Urodynamics

Techniques, Interpretation and Troubleshooting

Springer

Editors
Subhasis Saha
Clinincal Lead
Department of Pediatric Surgery
Manipal Hospitals
Kolkata, India

Poonam Guha Vaze
Neotia Bhagirathi Woman and Child Care Centre
Newtown, Kolkata, India

Department of Pediatric Surgery
Nilratan Sircar Medical College and Hospital
Kolkata, India

ISBN 978-981-95-2708-3 ISBN 978-981-95-2709-0 (eBook)
https://doi.org/10.1007/978-981-95-2709-0

This Springer imprint is published by the registered company Springer Nature Singapore Pte Ltd.
The registered company address is: 152 Beach Road, #21-01/04 Gateway East, Singapore 189721, Singapore

Foreword

I have a great pleasure in writing a foreword for this excellent collection of Pediatric Urodynamic studies. The editors, Dr. Subhasis Saha and Dr. Poonam Guha Vaze, have illustrated important urological issues in various common diseases of the lower urinary tract, both structural, such as posterior urethral valve and exstrophy bladder, and functional, as in neurogenic bladder. They have also wisely included children with behavioral issues, cerebral palsy, and Down's syndrome in whom the bladder problems are often neglected by the treating physician, which yet can have serious consequences on the kidneys. Closer to home (for a Pediatric surgeon), anorectal malformations can also present with an array of abnormal bladder functions, which have also been included in this collection.

Urodynamic studies need patience, both from the patient and the treating team. All facts of the case have to be put together, such as history and radiological studies to make a coherent diagnosis. The authors have included these in the case description, without which an isolated urodynamic study is of poor value. For the readers, they do need to sit down and meticulously read all the relevant information given in the case illustration to understand and gain from this collection. A quick reading is just not possible. It is well to remember the proverb "Patience is the mother of all virtues" when doing and interpreting urodynamics.

As a senior teacher and surgeon, who has dedicated a lifetime of work to children with bladder disorders, I convey my blessings to this publication of urodynamic studies by Dr. Saha and Dr. Poonam.

Sudipta Sen

Professor and Senior Consultant
Department of Pediatric Surgery
PSG IMS&R
Coimbatore, Tamil Nadu, India

Retd. Professor and HOD
Department of Pediatric Surgery
CMC Vellore
Vellore, Tamil Nadu, India

Foreword

Shaping the Understanding of Pediatric Urodynamics—"From that Spark to this Atlas"!

It is a privilege to write the foreword for this landmark volume on Pediatric Urodynamic Study (UDS). Pediatric Urology continues to evolve rapidly, and UDS has emerged as one of its most powerful tools, offering objective insights into bladder physiology and dysfunction that guide us toward safer, evidence-based, and child-centered care.

Spearheaded by Dr. Subhasis Saha, the journey of UDS in India owes much to Dr. Poonam Guha, whose vision and energy as a young pediatric surgeon and urologist ignited the first spark for this field nationally. Her pioneering efforts found a steadfast mentor in Dr. Subhasis Saha, whose profound expertise in video-urodynamics and commitment to teaching have provided the discipline with strong academic and clinical foundations. Together, they have nurtured a culture of curiosity, precision, and collaboration that continues to inspire the next generation.

This multiauthored book, supported by the Atlas of Pediatric Urodynamics, beautifully reflects that spirit. It is at once a scholarly reference and a practical guide, designed to empower both trainees and seasoned practitioners to integrate UDS meaningfully into clinical practice.

On behalf of the Indian Association of Pediatric Surgeons (IAPS), I congratulate the editors and contributors for this timely contribution. I am confident it will illuminate the path for pediatric surgeons and urologists across the country and world, ensuring that our children receive care that is both scientifically robust and deeply compassionate.

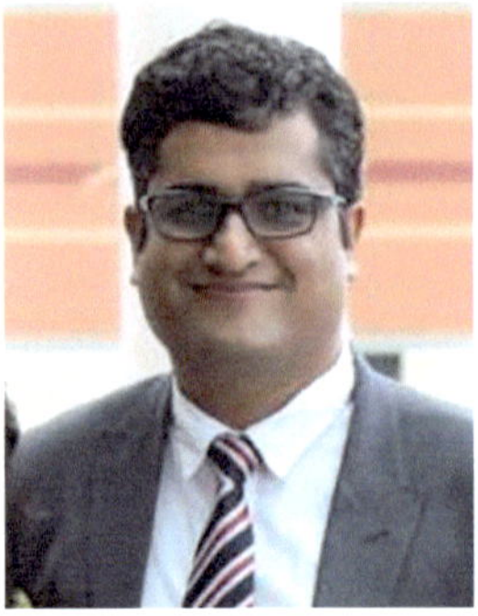

Vikesh Agrawal

Professor and Head, Department of Pediatric Surgery,
NSC Bose Government Medical College
Jabalpur, India

Preface

In the fall of 2003, at the end of my fellowship in Pediatric Surgery, I had the good fortune to be allowed a month's observership at the department of Pediatric Surgery, All India Institute of Medical Sciences, New Delhi, thanks to the then Prof and Head, Dr D.K. Gupta. Besides observing the stalwarts in the discipline, Dr V. Bhatnagar and Dr Minu Bajpai from close quarters, Mr. Grover taught me the technical aspects of performing urodynamic studies in children. When I came back to Kolkata, I planned to start performing Pediatric UDS in collaboration with a leading adult Urologist in town. But our thoughts did not match often. Then I realized the need for a standalone Pediatric UDS setup.

Fast forward to 2013—prodded by my colleague Ped Nephrologist Dr Rajiv Sinha to start a Pediatric Bladder clinic, we visited CMC Vellore and spent some time under the tutelage of Dr Sudipta Sen who made the difficult interpretations simple as usual and instilled in us the courage to set up our own Pediatric UDS unit. We started our exclusive Pediatric UDS facility soon after—the first such initiative in Eastern part of our country. That was the beginning. The machine was a discarded refurbished machine which gave way to a new machine a few years later. Our efforts got a fillip when Dr Poonam joined our unit infusing fresh energy and an immense zeal to delve into the details of Urodynamic assessment. For the first time we had someone in our team who loved the subject. The next few years saw many babies and children at our bladder clinic in whom we found our Urodynamic findings profoundly influencing the management and recovery of their ailments. Our first publication on this subject in the *Journal of Pediatric Urology* followed soon after. In the various meetings and conferences across the country, we found more and more inquisitive young minds who questioned us and the quest kindling in us the desire to go further. We developed a Pediatric bladder online group in 2021. We were also profoundly influenced by Dr Israel Franco from Washington and his thoughts. In May 2022, we held the first online ICCS international meet, which surpassed our expectations. We realized it was time to document our humble understanding of the Pediatric bladder functioning. Most of the available books and literature on Urodynamics are based on adult experience. So we tried to summarize our experience with kids and this atlas is a culmination of this effort. We sincerely hope that our efforts encourage many young surgeons to take up this not so costly evaluation under their close supervision. It is possible that in the days to come, their endeavour may open up new avenues to diagnose and manage bladder ailments in children and throw some light on the yet unanswered questions.

Kolkata, West Bengal, India Subhasis Saha

Preface

This book is the outcome of a dream project conceptualized by Dr Saha and myself, with the aim of consolidating our observations on pediatric urodynamic studies and sharing them with the wider medical community.

At the 'Pediatric Bladder Clinic', we encountered a wide spectrum of voiding dysfunctions in children—functional, anatomical, and neurological. In the early days, management was often uncertain, but urodynamics (UDS) provided crucial answers. Guided by its findings, we observed varied patterns and encouraging clinical responses, which inspired us to adopt newer modalities such as EMG and Video-UDS. Challenging cases pushed us further, leading us to perform UDS even in very small children and in the presence of gross vesicoureteric reflux (VUR), with gratifying results in many instances.

In children with posterior urethral valves (PUV) or bladder outflow obstruction (BOO) and persistent bladder dysfunction, guidance from our adult urology colleagues helped us interpret voiding parameters to differentiate residual obstruction from poor bladder contractility. The use of Qmax and PdetQmax during pressure-flow studies proved so valuable that it has become an essential part of our routine practice.

This book seeks to reshape the application of urodynamics in children by challenging long-held beliefs—such as its limitations in infants or in the presence of VUR. It introduces new approaches to assess voiding parameters and manage neurogenic bladder. The book emphasizes on asking the right 'UDS question', performing the study appropriately, and interpreting results to gain deeper insights into bladder function and treatment.

Each chapter has been carefully structured, with concepts illustrated through real case scenarios to highlight both understanding and application. The book presents our experiences and observations in a concise, practical manner, enabling readers to apply this knowledge effectively and, most importantly, improve patient outcomes through the wider adoption of these concepts.

With limited resources, I have established a small Urodynamics laboratory and have conducted more than 300 cases annually. Drawing on this experience, we have included practical guidance on setting up and running a Urodynamics lab, so that others may benefit from and build upon our journey.

It is worth highlighting that many clinicians who do not routinely perform UDS often cite the reason as limited availability of such facilities. Yet, paradoxically, they have access to far more advanced and expensive technologies such as robotic surgical systems. When the significant investment needed to establish robotic infrastructure—with only marginal advantages over conventional minimally invasive surgery—is weighed against the comparatively modest resources required for a UDS setup and its indispensable value as a diagnostic tool, the disparity becomes apparent. 'Non-availability of UDS' is more a mindset than a reality. What is truly needed is a change in perspective and a genuine passion for the subject—because with the right outlook, setup and training can be established in no time.

Kolkata, West Bengal, India Poonam Guha Vaze

Acknowledgements

This atlas is the culmination of a dream since the days we started a dedicated Pediatric Bladder clinic way back in 2013 on a suggestion from my friend and Pediatric Nephrologist Dr Rajiv Sinha. I would like to thank both Dr Rajiv and Dr Sushmita Banerjee—Pediatric Nephrologists in town for their faith in us since 2003, and subsequently, we healed and improved the lives of so many kids with nephrological and urological problems together.

I sincerely thank my co-editor Dr Poonam Guha Vaze for mooting the idea of summing up our experience in the form of a book/atlas, and it is her perseverance that encouraged me throughout to contribute, and finally our work is about to see the light of the day.

I owe a great debt to Dr Israel Franco, Dr Aniruddh Deshpande, Dr Anne Wright and all our other co-authors for sparing their valuable time and enriching our publication.

I am grateful to Dr Sudipta Sen, Dr V. Sripathy, Dr Minu Bajpai, Dr Ramesh Babu and Dr Sujit Chowdhary for introducing us to the need to appreciate UDS as an important tool in Pediatric Urological practice and illustrating the importance of the same in innumerable talks since our student days. I am indebted to my friend Dr V.V.S. Chandrasekharam for his encouragement throughout, especially in continuing our monthly Pediatric Bladder group meetings and his positive inputs for our UDS teaching. I also thank all my senior Pediatric surgeons and urologists across the country for their support. Dr U.S. Chatterjee, senior Urologist and Pediatric Surgeon from Kolkata, had been very supportive since our team started performing UDS in children.

We are grateful to the parents who smilingly provided us the consent for the study on their children and had full faith on us. Indrani Chatterjee showed indomitable courage and commitment in single handedly handling the technical part of the procedure and effortlessly maintained the children in good humour during the study. Indebted to the management of erstwhile AMRI Hospitals Mukundapur for installing the machine.

Contributing to this book has been meaningful and cherishing because of the kind and loving support I have received from my wife, Shyamasree, and daughter, Suchetana.

The publishing team from Springer has been supportive and co-operative at all stages. Without their valuable guidance it would not have been possible for us to publish this atlas.

Subhasis Saha

I extend my deepest gratitude to Dr Subhasis Saha, a pioneer in pediatric urodynamics in Kolkata, whose vision and openness to innovation have been truly inspiring. I was privileged to join him and Dr Rajiv Sinha in 2018 at the 'Bladder Clinic', the first of its kind in Eastern India and through the 'Bladder Clinic'.

I remain indebted to Dr Rajiv Sinha for his dedication to patient care and his efforts in advocating for UDS facilities within corporate hospital, which laid the foundation for this book.

I am thankful to Dr Indrani Subramanian for establishing a pediatric UDS laboratory at Neotia Bhagirathi Hospital, Newtown, and for making these services accessible to underprivileged children—an initiative that benefitted countless patients while enriching our clinical experience.

I warmly acknowledge my mentor, Dr Sirish Yande, for the invaluable experience gained at his lab and for his meticulous and passionate approach to urodynamics. My heartfelt appreciation also goes to Dr Israel Franco, whose guidance opened new perspectives on bladder function and dysfunction, and whose gracious acceptance to be a co-author of this book is an honour.

I am also grateful to Dr Vikesh Agarwal for the opportunity to conduct a UDS workshop at SPUCON 2022, an experience that ultimately inspired us to compile this book as a ready reference.

Special thanks to my team—Zulekha Husmat, Firdaus Khatun, Indrani Chatterjee and our radiology technicians—for their patience and dedication in working with children; together, we grew through this journey of learning and care.

I am equally indebted to Dr Sumantra Raut, Dr Sushmita Banerjee, Dr Amitava Pahari, Dr Jyoti Sharma and all our pediatric nephrology and pediatrician colleagues, for their trust and acceptance of UDS-based treatment approaches.

I gratefully acknowledge the support of our pediatric surgical colleagues, whose referrals allowed us to work with patients from diverse backgrounds—an experience that has greatly enriched both our practice and the data presented in this book. Special thanks to Dr Rupa and Dr Saibal for constant sources of support and ready reference in hours of need.

I would like to acknowledge the constant support of Prakash and Kundan from the Hospimedica group, who have always addressed technical issues with the machine promptly and efficiently.

Finally, I must thank the most important people in my life—my parents, my son, Aprameya, and my friend, Archana—whose love, support, and patience gave me the strength to persevere through the long hours of work. This book is as much theirs as it is mine.

Poonam Guha Vaze

Contents

Abbreviations

ALPP	Abdominal leak point pressure
APD	Anteroposterior diameter
BBD	Bladder bowel dysfunction
BCI	Bladder contractility index
BNI	Bladder neck incision
BOO	Bladder outlet obstruction
BOOI	Bladder outlet obstruction index
CIC	Clean intermittent catheterization
CP	Cerebral palsy
CP	Cerebral palsy
DLPP	Detrusor leak point pressure
DO	Detrusor overactivity
DO-LPP	Detrusor overactivity leak point pressure
DSD	Detrusor sphincter dyssynergia
DV	Dysfunctional voiding
EDOF	Extraordinary daytime only frequency
EMG	Electromyograph
FUC	Follow-up case
HDN	Hydronephrosis
HDUN	Hydroureteroneohrosis
ICCS	International Children's Continence Society
ICS	International Continence Society
i-UDS	Invasive UDS
LSMMC	Lubosacral meningo-myelocele
LUT	Lower urinary tract
MMC	Meningomyelocele
NB	Neurogenic bladder
NGT	Nasogastric tube
NNNB	Non-neurogenic-neurogenic bladder
OAB	Overactive bladder
Pabd	Abdominal pressure
Pdet max	Maximum detrusor pressure during voiding
Pdet Qmax	Detrusor pressures at point of maximum flow
Pdet	Detrusor pressure

PUV	Posterior urethral valve
Pves	Vesical pressure
PVR	Post-void residue
Qmax	Maximum flow rate
UB	Urinary bladder
UDS	Urodynamic study
UTI	Urinary tract infection
VD	Voiding diary
VUR	Vesicourteric reflux

1 What Is Urodynamics?

Subhasis Saha and Poonam Guha Vaze

The urinary bladder is the only organ of our body which is conditioned to stay relaxed while it is being filled by the efflux of urine from the kidneys via the ureters by active recruitment of neurotransmitters and adrenergic nerve fibres. This continues till a level of optimal filling occurs, when the person gets a full bladder sensation. Thereafter, the process of micturition takes over which though initiated voluntarily is involuntary and involves complete relaxation of outlet resistance and gradually increasing and then waning flow of urine usually to completion of bladder emptying. There is a complex interaction of bladder sensation, intact neurological network, cortical inputs, optimal detrusor function and an intact outlet with no outflow obstruction for a coordinated voiding cycle. So a multitude of diseases might require urodynamic assessment.

The urodynamic assessment pathway includes the complete/holistic assessment of lower urinary tract (LUT) function; it allows us to assess whether there is any dysfunction, identifying the dysfunction, quantifying its severity and planning the management strategy. It includes pretesting clinical assessments and urodynamic instrumented tests; the latter is classically referred to as urodynamics (UDS). Whereas pretesting clinical assessments are employed in all patients presenting with or suspected as having LUT dysfunction, the choice of 'instrumented tests' of type of UDS investigation is tailored to each individual patient.

S. Saha (✉)
Department of Pediatric Surgery, Manipal Hospitals, Kolkata, India

P. G. Vaze
Neotia Bhagirathi Woman and Child Care Centre, Newtown, Kolkata, India

Department of Pediatric Surgery, Nilratan Sircar Medical College and Hospital, Kolkata, India

S. Saha, P. Guha Vaze (eds.), *Comprehensive Atlas of Practical Pediatric Urodynamics*, https://doi.org/10.1007/978-981-95-2709-0_1

Complete Urodynamic Assessment Armamentarium

- *Clinical pretesting information*
  - History
  - Questionnaires
  - Physical examination
  - Voiding charts
- *Urodynamics (UDS)*
  - ICS defines UDS as 'the general term to describe all the measurements that assess the function and dysfunction of the lower urinary tract (LUT) by any appropriate method. Urodynamics allows direct assessment of LUT function by the measurement of relevant physiological parameters'.
  - The various components of UDS include:

    Non-invasive
    - Uroflowmetry

    Invasive
    - Cystometry
    - Pressure flow studies
    - Cystometry with EMG/videofluoroscopy
    - Urethral pressure assessment
    - Ambulatory UDS

In clinical parlance, urodynamic study involves in-depth study of the lower urinary tract functions.

Urodynamic assessment starts from a well-maintained *voiding diary*. A voiding diary for 48 hours is a basic tool which gives us an idea about the functional bladder volume, urinary frequency and symptoms of leakage, pain, dribbling and bedwetting. In a non-toilet-trained baby, this may be substituted by a 4-hour voiding chart, which tells us the frequency of voiding and a gross estimate of the volume.

Uroflowmetry with or without EMG is a non-invasive procedure which may be done as an outpatient procedure and, if properly done, often obviates the need for an invasive cystometry.

Invasive cystometry needs insertion of a catheter into the bladder, is an uncomfortable procedure for the patients and is indicated in certain specific situations. Cystometry and pressure flow studies provide information about the functioning of the bladder in the filling and voiding phase which include the bladder capacity, sensations, detrusor pressures, cause of leak, state of the outflow tract, voiding strength of the bladder, etc. and help plan further management. If one wants to visualise the anatomy of the lower urinary tract alongside the assessment of its function, this urodynamic basic study is complemented by fluoroscopic imaging of the bladder and the urethra—*videourodynamic study*. Some patients may not manifest any abnormal bladder function during the short span of the performance of the invasive cystometry and may benefit from a more prolonged assessment of bladder function. So the one-time lab investigation is modified to *ambulatory urodynamics* and *natural fill cystometry*—which is the same assessment under natural bladder filling scenario.

Proper reporting of a urodynamic study needs a lot of commitment on the part of the investigator, who needs to carry on conversation with the child/person during the investigation so that proper correlation of the pressure changes with the relevant symptoms may be done.

So when should a urodynamic assessment be advised? This is summarised as the 'urodynamic question'. Urodynamics benefits personnel managing posterior urethral valve (PUV), neurogenic bladder (NB), non-neurogenic-neurogenic bladder (NNNB) including bowel bladder disorders (BBD) and young children in various stages of chronic kidney disease, to differentiate between primary and secondary VUR; investigating a child with non-monosymptomatic enuresis; and assessing a child prior to renal transplantation.

Urodynamics gives us a glimpse of the potential of renal damage in neurogenic bladder patients. Not all neurogenic bladder patients are similarly affected as far as bladder pathology is concerned and hence if we can tailor the anticholinergic medications or any other bladder intervention depending on the urodynamic status. Most children with spina bifida are born with normal kidneys but a section of them ends up in renal failure to various extent. Both the schools of therapy—the proactive one and the symptom-based one—need a urodynamic assessment to comprehend and document the potential for renal compromise. Early initiation and lifetime clean intermittent catheterisation often save the kidneys.

A child with PUV has a diseased bladder with various degree of loss of elasticity and compliance. PUV patients form a spectrum and the specific plan beyond fulguration or incision of the valve depends to a large extent on the bladder assessment. UDS gives us an idea about the compliance, overactivity and outlet hindrance, thereby giving us an approximate idea about the possible continuing upper tract damage. Further therapy can be planned based on the findings.

A greater role of urodynamics lies in assessing the bladder of chronic renal compromise patients prior to renal transplantation lest the implanted kidney also may suffer the same fate.

There are several misconceptions regarding the need/utility of UDS. Some urologists believe that observing a child passing urine is an alternative to a tempered uroflowmetry. The fallacy lies in the fact that a good flow in the face of subtle outflow obstruction may be produced by generating a very high voiding pressure which has potential to affect the renal function. Some surgeons also believe that imaging modalities like USG and MCUG may predict the necessity of a pressure study. If the contour looks normal on both, a UDS may be done away with. But we have seen children with almost normal-looking MCUG and minimal changes on ultrasound with undue overactivity and high voiding pressure which were corrected after intervention.

To conclude, urodynamics is a part and parcel of office practice of pediatric urology. Any physician with a basic understanding of the normal physiology of voiding and the pathological spectrum should be able to successfully run a urodynamics clinic. We encourage parents to stay alongside, and there are plenty of ways to divert the attention of children and mobile phones have a great role here. The urinary infection rate following the procedure in our experience is less than 2% if proper precautions are followed. Though the urinary bladder behaviour continues to mature for more than a year after birth, there are instances where even in infants, UDS can be helpful and we have dedicated a special chapter on that.

Declarations

Competing Interests The author(s) has no competing interests to declare that are relevant to the content of this manuscript.

Ethics Approval The author(s) declares that this manuscript does not include primary research with human participants.

The author(s) declares that this manuscript does not include primary studies involving animals.

Suggested Reading

1. Mario P. Noninvasive urodynamics and flowmetry in children, adolescents, and young adults. In: Mosiello G, et al., editors. Clinical urodynamics in childhood and adolescence, Urodynamics, neurourology and pelvic floor dysfunctions; 2018.
2. Rosier PFWM, Schaefer W, Lose G, Goldman HB, Guralnick M, Eustice S, Dickinson T, Hashim H. International continence society good urodynamic practices and terms 2016: urodynamics, uroflowmetry, cystometry, and pressure-flow study. Neurourol Urodyn. 2017;36(5):1243–60. https://doi.org/10.1002/nau.23124. Epub 2016 Dec 5.
3. Bauer SB, Nijman RJ, Drzewiecki BA, Sillen U, Hoebeke P. International children's continence society standardization subcommittee. International children's continence society standardization report on urodynamic studies of the lower urinary tract in children. Neurourol Urodyn. 2015;34(7):640–7. https://doi.org/10.1002/nau.22783. Epub 2015 May 21.

Urodynamics Hardware

2

Poonam Guha Vaze and Subhasis Saha

UDS Machine

UDS machines are available in two basic varieties (Fig. 2.1a, b):

- Trolley based—Desktop based; dedicated trolley with pump system and pressure transducers; difficult to move around
- Pole based—Laptop based; pump and pressure transducer on a pole; easy to move around

P. G. Vaze (✉)
Neotia Bhagirathi Woman and Child Care Centre, Newtown, Kolkata, India

Department of Pediatric Surgery, Nilratan Sircar Medical College and Hospital, Kolkata, India

S. Saha
Department of Pediatric Surgery, Manipal Hospitals, Kolkata, India

S. Saha, P. Guha Vaze (eds.), *Comprehensive Atlas of Practical Pediatric Urodynamics*, https://doi.org/10.1007/978-981-95-2709-0_2

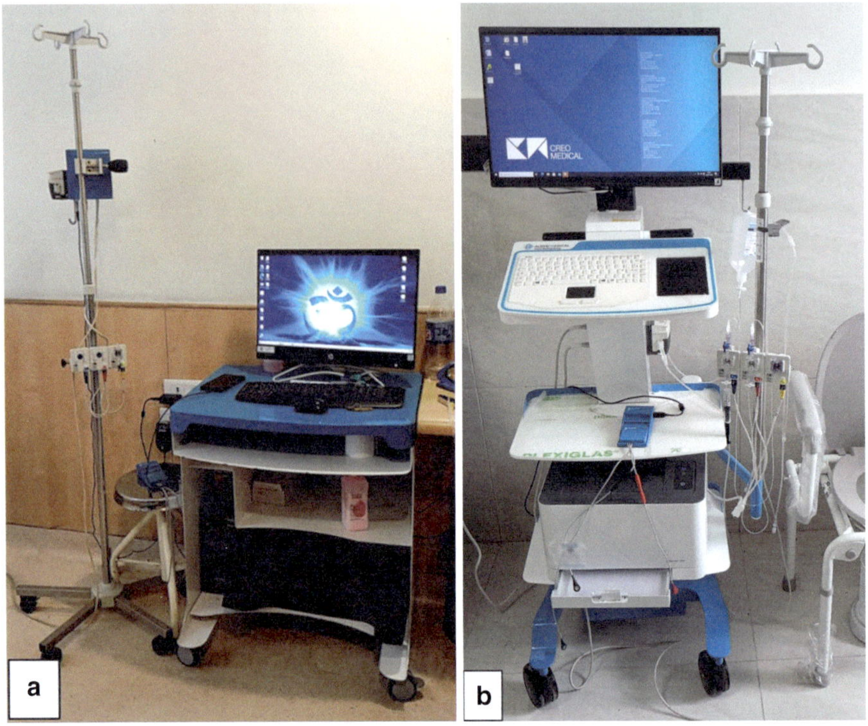

Fig. 2.1 Pole-based (**a**) and trolley-based (image courtesy: Hospimedica Group) (**b**) UDS systems

Parts of the Machine (Fig. 2.2)

- Desktop/laptop
- Pump
- Pressure transducers (dome)
- Uroflowmeter
- Seat—X-ray-compatible UDS chair/customised bed/commode chair with reducer seat cover

  There are options of various add-ons with the basic machine

- EMG—Preferably double channel—perineal and abdominal
- Video UDS—X-ray-compatible couch with C-arm
- Biofeedback
- Puller for UPP

Catheters Several choices of catheters are available.

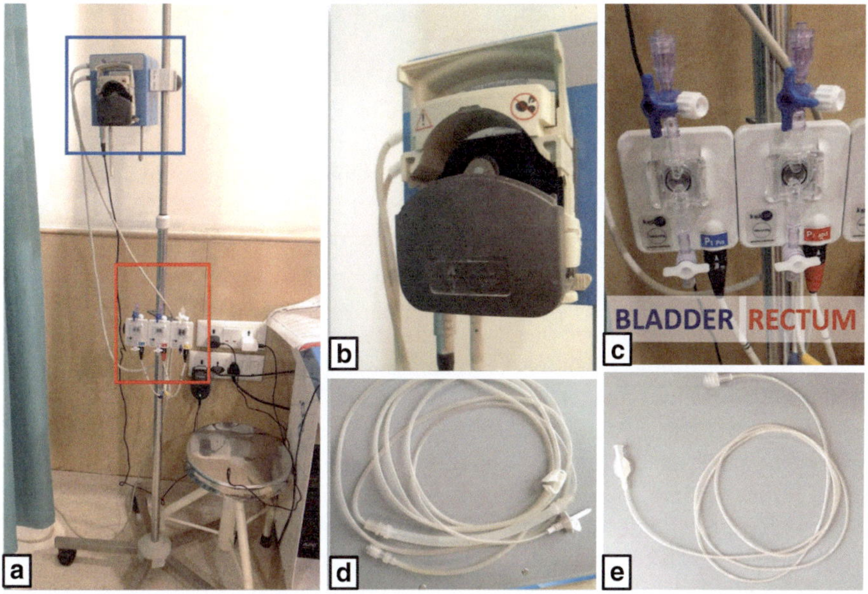

Fig. 2.2 Working pole of a UDS machine (**a**) with the pump (blue square) and the pressure transducers (red square). The enlarged images of the pump and the transducer are shown in images (**b**) and (**c**), respectively. Pump tubing and pressure monitoring tubing are shown in (**d**) and (**e**), respectively

Fig. 2.3 6 and 8 Fr double-lumen urethral catheters

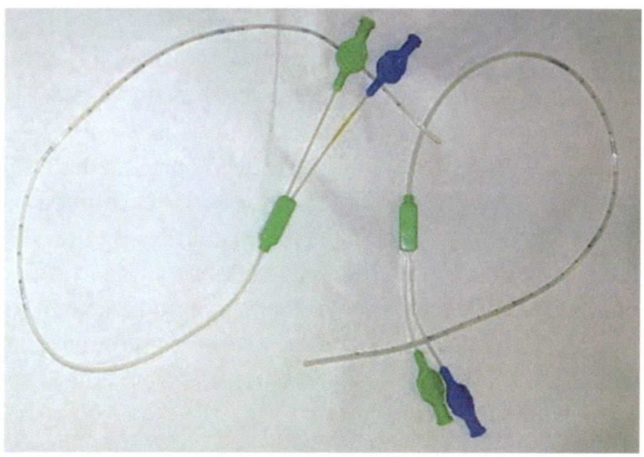

Urethral Catheters

Double-lumen urethral catheters

Water filled, 6 Fr, 8 Fr—Most commonly used (Fig. 2.3). Meant to be disposable, but these are reused after proper sterilisation in most of the centres across India. The transducer is in the machine outside the patient. It reads pressure across a continuous column of fluid from the transducer up to the bladder/rectum. It gets dampened by presence of microbubbles in the column and shows significant artefacts if the tube is shaken.

Transducer tip/air charged—5 Fr. In the case of air-charged catheters, the transducers are placed at the tip of the catheter and lie within the body cavity. These are single-use/disposable catheters. Pressure readings of these catheters are not affected by presence of air bubbles, but these are less sensitive to rapid pressure changes like coughing. The pressure recordings of fluid-filled systems and air-charged systems do not match and there are no guidelines/nomograms for pressures obtained with air-charged systems.

Two 5Fr IFTs—Urethra in children beyond 1 year of age usually admits two 5 Fr IFTs simultaneously, one of which is used for monitoring pressures and the other one is used for filling. If voiding is to be assessed, the catheter used for filling is removed before child is asked to void. Many centres in India use this technique, but we have moved away from this technique as it has several limitations: insertion of two feeding tubes in the urethra is painful for the child; removal of one of the catheters before voiding causes significant urethral irritation so that it becomes very difficult for the child to void. We have had one experience where the vesical ends of both the catheters recoiled and entered the urethral lumen while voiding; thus, there were four channels within the urethra which got impacted and had to be removed under general anaesthesia.

Rectal Catheters

Different types of rectal catheters are available. The usual principle involves a fluid-filled catheter which senses rectal pressure with a barrier at the tip so that the catheter does not get occluded by fecal matter. The commercially available rectal catheters may have a perforated balloon at the tip (Fig. 2.4a). These are rather difficult to clean as fecal matter tends to enter the balloon and should ideally be used as single-use system. Catheters with non-perforated balloons at the tip (Fig. 2.4b) have a three-way connector. Before connecting the catheter to the patient, the catheter can be charged with saline and then the 3-way stopcock opened to let the excess fluid out. After connecting to the patient, whenever the catheter is flushed, the three way has to be opened so that no excess fluid remains in the balloon which can artefactually elevate the rectal pressure tracing. We find these catheters to be very stiff and uncomfortable for young kids.

We routinely use indigenously prepared rectal catheter using a 5 or 8 Fr IFT and a cut finger of a latex glove which has been slit near the tip (Fig. 2.4c, d). It provides excellent traces and works out to be very cheap and hygienic as a new set can be used for each patient.

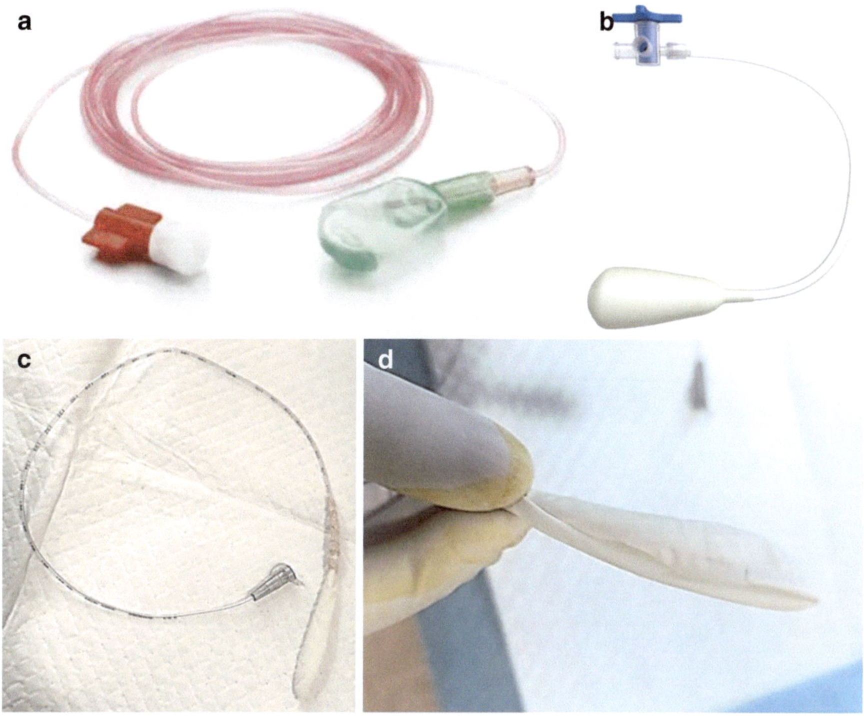

Fig. 2.4 (**a–d**) Different types of rectal catheters.

Seating Options

Seating options classically include C-arm-compatible UDS chair (Fig. 2.5a) wherein patient can be made to lie down for catheterisation and then made to sit up for the studies and commode seat with a funnel (Fig. 2.5b) which can be used when video UDS is not being used and study is to be done in sitting position. Several centres, where video UDS is not performed, use customised beds with reclining facility (Fig. 2.5c, d).

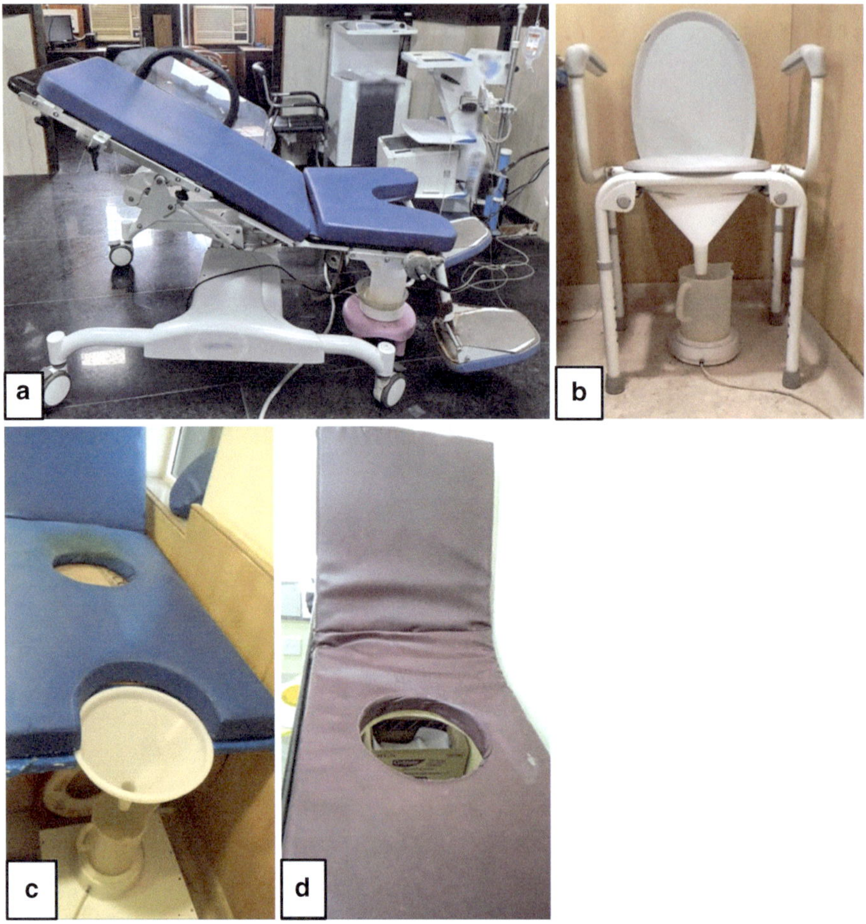

Fig. 2.5 (**a**–**d**) Seating options. (Image courtesy (**a**): Prof. Debansu Sarkar, HOD, Department of Urology, SSKM Hospital, Kolkata. Image courtesy (**d**): Dr. Sirish Yande, Consultant Urologist, Crystal Centre, MMF- Ratna Memorial Hospital, Pune 411053)

Declarations

Competing Interests The author(s) has no competing interests to declare that are relevant to the content of this manuscript.

Ethics Approval The author(s) declares that this manuscript does not include primary research with human participants.

The author(s) declares that this manuscript does not include primary studies involving animals.

Setting Up a Pediatric UDS Lab

3

Poonam Guha Vaze and Subhasis Saha

UDS lab is a prerequisite for any centre dealing with pediatric urological patients. Setting up a UDS lab is rather easy; it just needs a thought process as to its utility, the clientele (Figs. 3.1, 3.2, and 3.3).

Infrastructural requirements

1. Adequate- sized room—Specially for performing pediatric UDS as children may feel uncomfortable in small- sized rooms/cramped-up spaces. Also, parents are usually made to stay with the child, so number of people present in the room increases.

   Provision should be made for more space if the setup is being planned in a teaching institute for allowing observers to stand comfortably.

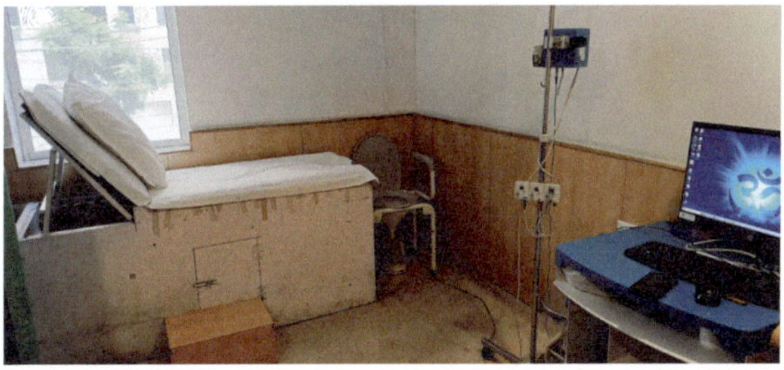

Fig. 3.1 Basic UDS setup with a customised bed and desktop-based 'pole' type of UDS machine in a 10 ft × 10 ft room

P. G. Vaze (✉)
Neotia Bhagirathi Woman and Child Care Centre, Newtown, Kolkata, India

Department of Pediatric Surgery, Nilratan Sircar Medical College and Hospital, Kolkata, India

S. Saha
Department of Pediatric Surgery, Manipal Hospitals, Kolkata, India

S. Saha, P. Guha Vaze (eds.), *Comprehensive Atlas of Practical Pediatric Urodynamics*, https://doi.org/10.1007/978-981-95-2709-0_3

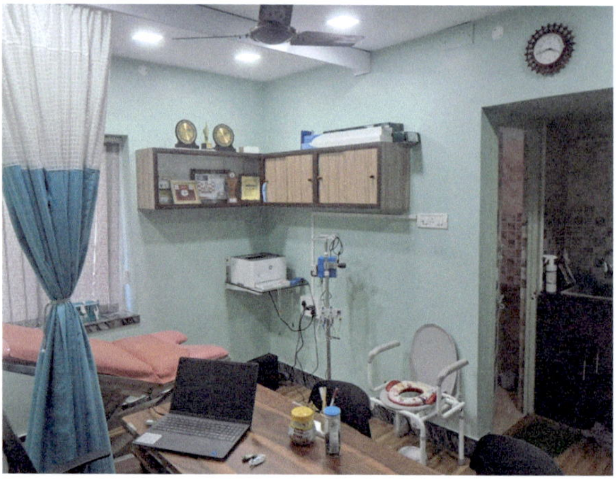

Fig. 3.2 Basic UDS setup in a 10 ft × 12 ft room with an attached toilet and wash basin, height adjustable reclining bed, commode chair laptop and pole-based UDS system

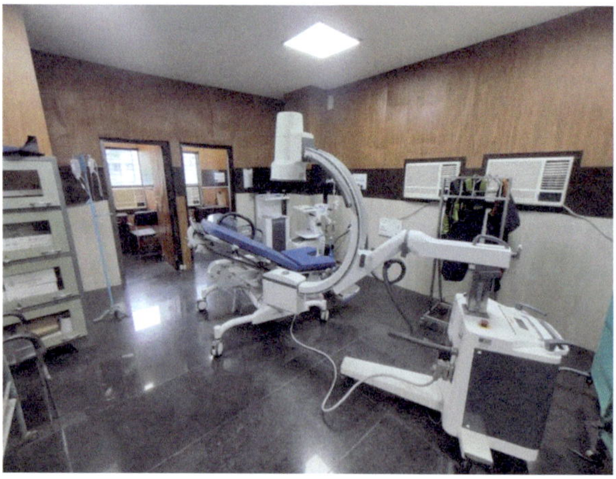

Fig. 3.3 Video UDS lab setup with UDS trolley, C-arm-compatible bed and C-arm. (Courtesy: Prof Debanshu Sarkar, HOD, Dept of Urology, SSKM Hospital, Kolkata)

2. Wash basin inside the cabin and attached washroom
3. Provision for change of clothes for the patients
4. Good lighting
5. Storage space for storing consumables
6. Should be fully accessible for wheelchair-bound patients
7. Interesting wallpapers for children (themed on comic characters, aquarium, nature, etc.) with soothing wall colours (Fig. 3.4)
8. USG facility in a neighbouring room is helpful as we can tag simple OPD procedures like uroflowmetry and PVR assessment through USG.

Facilities/equipments required
1. Access to sterilisation facilities
2. Access to biomedical waste disposal
3. Resuscitation trolley

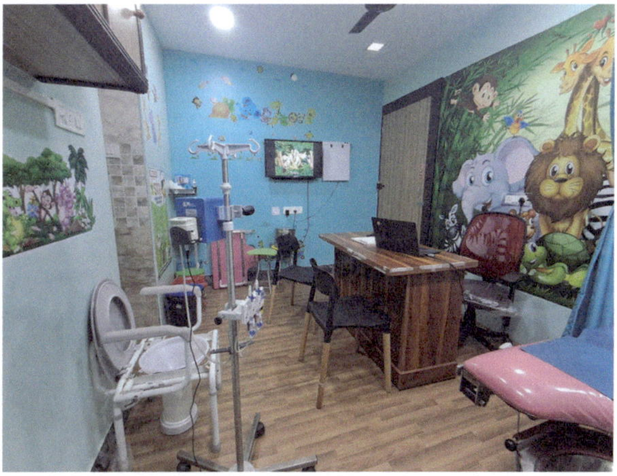

Fig. 3.4 Child-friendly lab setup with soothing wall colours, cartoon wallpapers and television for playing videos

4. Seating arrangements for different age group of patients
   - Reclining bed with Gyne Cut-out (preferably with adjustable height)
   - Commode chair with adaptors for children
   - Stool/footrest
5. Proper arrangement of UDS bed/commode chair/UDS trolley and examiner's table so that the examiner can observe the patient during the test
6. Provision of curtains for privacy of elder children when seated/lying down
7. Provisions to keep children engaged
   - Television for cartoon videos
   - Sweetmeats/stickers/toys
8. Recording system—The laptop or the computer where the software is downloaded should have a cloud storage attached to store all files. In most hospitals, EMR of the patients are available and the physician supervising the UDS can have access to all records of the patient. It is always a good practice to document a brief history including previous surgical interventions and medical therapy in a nutshell before correlating the imaging and lab reports and finally report the uroflowmetry and UDS curve in this perspective.

Additional requirements for video UDS

- Larger room—Preferably 15 ft × 20 ft; minimum 15 ft × 15 ft
- C-arm-compatible patient bed should be placed at the centre of the room so that the C-arm can be positioned on either side of the bed.
- UDS trolly should be placed on the left side of the bed.
- Proper radiation screening facilities (fortification of the walls using barium or lead) should be taken care of to minimise radiation hazards.

Personnel

- Technician +/– (If the doctor himself/ herself performs the test, technician may not be needed)
- Trained nurse
- Housekeeping

Running cost

- *Consumables used per patient*:
  - Gloves, syringes, normal saline, lubricating jelly, betadine, gauze, feeding tube (for rectal catheter), adhesive tape, ECG electrodes, waterproof adhesive
- *Items which can be reused with proper sterilisation*
  - Catheters
  - Pressure monitoring tubings
  - Pump tubings
- *Items which need replacement due to wear and tear*
  - Transducer dome
  - Double-lumen catheters (after certain number of usage)—Last longer if contrast is not given (video UDS not simultaneously done); also need replacement.

Declarations

Competing Interests The author(s) has no competing interests to declare that are relevant to the content of this manuscript.

Ethics Approval The author(s) declares that this manuscript does not include primary research with human participants.

The author(s) declares that this manuscript does not include primary studies involving animals.

Voiding Diary

4

Poonam Guha Vaze and Subhasis Saha

Voiding diary (VD) includes depiction of fluid intake, voiding frequency, voided volumes and any other symptoms in the form of a table which is maintained by the parents at home. This is a simple, cost-effective real-time indirect assessment of bladder function in natural settings and comfort of home. Being non-invasive, it adds simplicity to this basic evaluation tool. This is also referred to as frequency/volume chart. Frequency volume chart in toilet-trained children is different from that in infants or younger children.

Voiding Diary (VD) in Toilet-Trained Children

Points to Be Recorded in a VD (Fig. 4.1)

1. Each episode of fluid intake—time and amount
2. Each passage of urine—time and amount
3. Any episode of leak with time—approximate amount (1 rupee coin, bigger blotch, underpants + pants, dripping down)
4. Any special event like urgency, posturing, dysuria, straining while passing urine, urine stream (interrupted/continuous)

P. G. Vaze (✉)
Neotia Bhagirathi Woman and Child Care Centre, Newtown, Kolkata, India

Department of Pediatric Surgery, Nilratan Sircar Medical College and Hospital, Kolkata, India

S. Saha
Department of Pediatric Surgery, Manipal Hospitals, Kolkata, India

S. Saha, P. Guha Vaze (eds.), *Comprehensive Atlas of Practical Pediatric Urodynamics*, https://doi.org/10.1007/978-981-95-2709-0_4

Name: ______________________________ Date: ________________________

Went to bed at: _____________________ Woke up at: ____________________

Time	Amount of fluid drunk	Amount of urine passed	Urgency	Leakage	Comments

Only fill this out if your child wets the bed:

First time waking up about 2 hours after going to bed	Second time waking up about 5 hours after going to bed	Morning urine
Amount (ml): _____	Amount (ml): _____	Amount (ml): _____
Time:	Time:	Time:
Bed wet: yes ☐ no ☐	Bed wet: yes ☐ no ☐	Bed wet: yes ☐ no ☐

As an alternative: Weigh nappies

- Let your child go to the washroom whenever he/ she wants; don't 'ask him' to go
- After each void mention if he had (***) severe urgency and could not wait, (**) urgency but could wait, (*) no urgency
- If there are episodes of urinary leakage mention (*) for dampness of undergarments, (**) –trousers becoming wet, (***) large amount of urine leaked out wetting trousers/ spilling on floor/ feet
- Mention any other events like pain/ having to strain during passing urine/ had to wait and took time to start urine flow etc. in the comments column.
- If your child wakes up at night to pass urine, it should also be measured
- If you perform CIC to empty your child's bladder, note down the CIC volume and mention CIC

Fig. 4.1 Sample proforma for voiding diary—day 1

Technical Points

- ICCS recommends performing a voiding diary for 2 days (48 hours) which may not be successive. Each day starts with the second void of the morning and incorporates the first void of the next day.
- Child is made to drink from a measured container whenever he/she is thirsty.
- Child passes urine whenever he/she has an urge to pass urine. He/she is not supposed to be coaxed to.
- The child is asked to pass urine into a graduated container. More often, such graduated containers are not available for pediatric size. We usually ask the parents to make the child pass urine in any container and then measure it with the help of a 10- or 20-ml syringe which is easily available and an accurate measurement is possible. This is easily applicable for illiterate patients as well as they just note the number of syringes measured.
- Few children become very excited during the test and rush to pass urine repeatedly which does not match with their usual voiding behaviour. In such cases, we ask the VD to be maintained for 3–4 days. The child's excitement usually dies off after the initial 1–2 days and rest of the recordings are reliable.
- If a child passes urine without informing on a few occasions, we ask the parents to mark the events with a 'tick' along with the time so that we get the true frequency.
- If the child bed-wets on those days, it has to be marked in the chart. The number of times child is passing urine when asleep, approximate time when the child is wetting the bed, diaper weight measurement (if possible) or approximate amount of leak (wetting of pants/complete passage of urine) has to be recorded.
- In patients with clean intermittent catheterization (CIC diary should replace VD), it should note volumes of urine emptied with CIC and any episodes of self-voids/leaks in between.
- Usually, a VD is solicited along with a stool diary for 7 days (Bristol stool chart or other charts) to rule out a concomitant bladder bowel dysfunction (Fig. 4.2).
- Occasionally, we find that children with overactive bladders tend to avoid drinking water and show a very small fluid intake on the VD. In such children, increased frequency may be masked. They pass urine in small volumes but we cannot differentiate whether small urine volumes are due to reduced fluid intake or small bladder capacity. In such cases, we ask to repeat the VD with adequate water intake as per age when features of increased frequency and small-volume void gets unmasked.
- A thorough explanation to the parents and child about importance of a proper VD and the procedure of maintaining it is of paramount importance. Active participation of the child involves the child in the treatment process which is very important for success of any urotherapy programme.

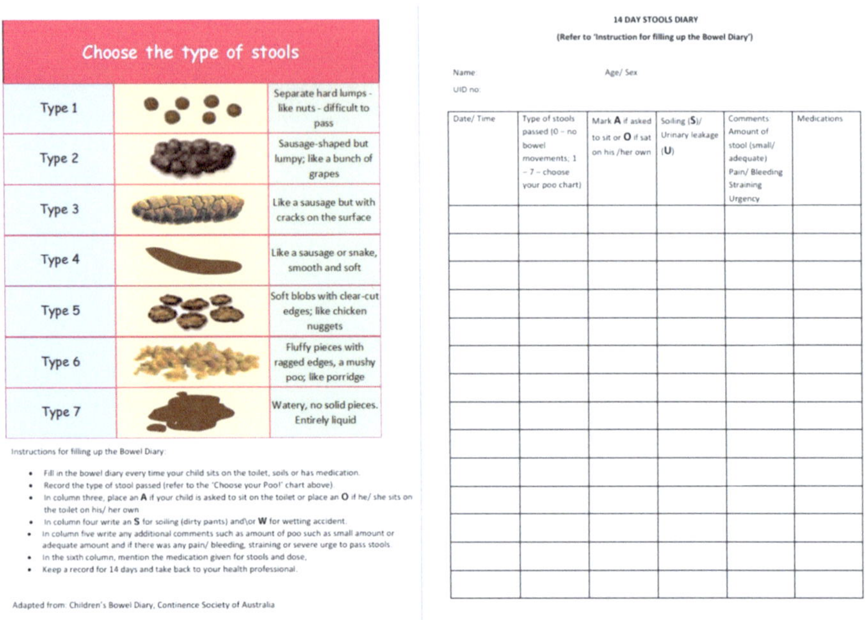

Choose the type of stools

Type 1		Separate hard lumps - like nuts - difficult to pass
Type 2		Sausage-shaped but lumpy; like a bunch of grapes
Type 3		Like a sausage but with cracks on the surface
Type 4		Like a sausage or snake, smooth and soft
Type 5		Soft blobs with clear-cut edges; like chicken nuggets
Type 6		Fluffy pieces with ragged edges, a mushy poo; like porridge
Type 7		Watery, no solid pieces. Entirely liquid

Instructions for filling up the Bowel Diary:

- Fill in the bowel diary every time your child sits on the toilet, soils or has medication.
- Record the type of stool passed (refer to the 'Choose your Poo!' chart above)
- In column three, place an **A** if your child is asked to sit on the toilet or place an **O** if he/ she sits on the toilet on his/ her own
- In column four write an **S** for soiling (dirty pants) and\or **W** for wetting accident.
- In column five write any additional comments such as amount of poo such as small amount or adequate amount and if there was any pain/ bleeding, straining or severe urge to pass stools.
- In the sixth column, mention the medication given for stools and dose,
- Keep a record for 14 days and take back to your health professional.

Adapted from: Children's Bowel Diary, Continence Society of Australia

14 DAY STOOLS DIARY

(Refer to 'Instruction for filling up the Bowel Diary')

Name: Age/ Sex

UID no:

Date/ Time	Type of stools passed (0 – no bowel movements; 1 – 7 – choose your poo chart)	Mark **A** if asked to sit or **O** if sat on his /her own	Soiling (**S**)/ Urinary leakage (**U**)	Comments: Amount of stool (small/ adequate) Pain/ Bleeding Straining Urgency	Medications

Fig. 4.2 Sample proforma for stool diary using the Bristol stool chart

ICCS Definitions and Normative Values

MVV (maximum voided volume)—The largest voided volume, exclusive of the first morning micturition (inclusion of morning voided volume makes the value highly variable)

MVV, excluding the first morning void, is considered small or large if found to be < 65% or > 150% of EBC, respectively.

The term expected bladder capacity (EBC) is used as a reference or standard for comparison. The EBC is defined by the formula: (30 × [age in yrs + 1] ml) (for children > 2 years old).

Children are said to have increased daytime urinary if they void >= 8 times per day and decreased daytime urinary frequency if they void <= 3 times per day.

Polyuria is defined as voided urine volumes of >40 ml/kg body weight during 24 hours or > 2.8 L urine for a child or adolescent weighing >= 70 kg.

Nocturnal polyuria is relevant in children suffering from enuresis and is defined in this cohort as a nocturnal urine output exceeding 130% of EBC for age.

Enuresis and daytime urinary incontinence are considered significant if it occurs > 1 episode per month and a frequency of 3 episodes over 3 months. The significance of enuresis may be classified as frequent (> 4 per week) or infrequent (< 4 times per week).

Practical Applications of VD

VD is a window to assess basic bladder function. It tells us what is the maximum bladder volume and what is the functional bladder capacity.

- Most of the functional bladder dysfunctions can be diagnosed solely on the basis of VD:
    1. Overactive bladder—high-frequency, small-volume voids with urgency +/– urge incontinence (Fig. 4.3)
    2. Pollakiuria—extraordinarily high frequency during daytime only; no night-time symptoms (Fig. 4.4)
    3. Voiding postponement—large-volume infrequent voids (Fig. 4.5)
- VD is a simple tool to diagnose increased frequency of micturition due to excess water intake either due to compulsive water intake or due to diabetes insipidus/mellitus (Fig. 4.6).
- CIC diary gives us the usual bladder volumes when CIC is done (Fig. 4.7a). This tells us about the bladder capacity in the child. If the child leaks/voids in between the CICs, we have to determine the cause of leak by an invasive UDS. If the leak is due to outlet weakness, bladder neck procedure may be needed. But if the leak is due to overactivity or poor compliance, anticholinergics have to be added to

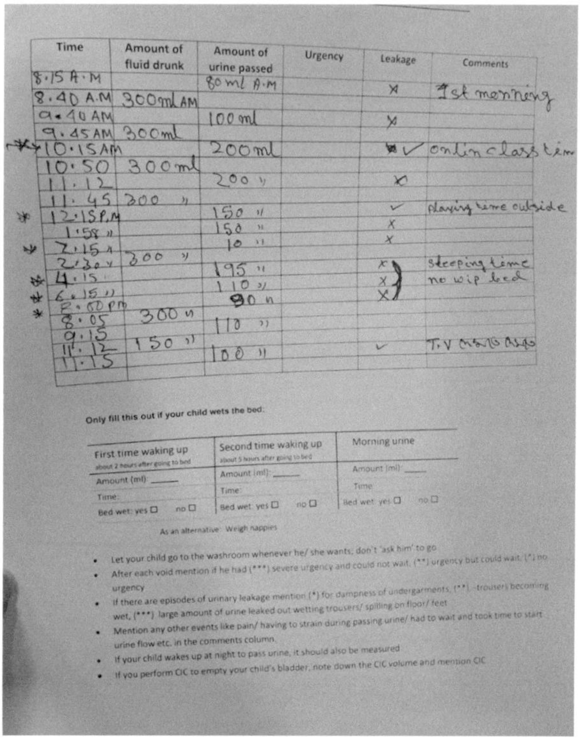

Time	Amount of fluid drunk	Amount of urine passed	Urgency	Leakage	Comments
8.15 A.M		80 ml A.M		X	1st morning
8.40 A.M	300ml AM				
9.40 AM		100 ml		X	
9.45 AM	300ml				
* 10.15 AM		200ml		✓	onlin class tim
10.50	300 ml				
11.12		200 "		X	
11.45	300 "				
* 12.15 P.M		150 "		✓	playing time outside
1.58 "		150 "		X	
* 2.15 "		10 "		X	
2.30 "	300 "				
* 4.15		195 "		X	sleeping time
* 6.15 "		110 "		X	no wip bed
* 8.00 pm		90 "		X	
8.05	300 "				
9.15		110 "			
11.12	150 "			✓	T.V [illegible]
11.15		100 "			

Only fill this out if your child wets the bed:

First time waking up (about 2 hours after going to bed)	Second time waking up (about 5 hours after going to bed)	Morning urine
Amount (ml): ______	Amount (ml): ______	Amount (ml): ______
Time:	Time:	Time:
Bed wet: yes ☐ no ☐	Bed wet: yes ☐ no ☐	Bed wet: yes ☐ no ☐

As an alternative: Weigh nappies

- Let your child go to the washroom whenever he/ she wants; don't 'ask him' to go
- After each void mention if he had (***) severe urgency and could not wait, (**) urgency but could wait, (*) no urgency
- If there are episodes of urinary leakage mention (*) for dampness of undergarments, (**) -trousers becoming wet, (***) large amount of urine leaked out wetting trousers/ spilling on floor/ feet
- Mention any other events like pain/ having to strain during passing urine/ had to wait and took time to start urine flow etc. in the comments column.
- If your child wakes up at night to pass urine, it should also be measured
- If you perform CIC to empty your child's bladder, note down the CIC volume and mention CIC

Fig. 4.3 A 24-hour observation in a 10-year-old girl with history of urinary incontinence, repeated episodes of UTI, and constipation (bladder-bowel dysfunction). VD shows MVV to be 200 ml (EBC—330), increased-frequency, small-volume voids along with three episodes of leak. The parents have not marked the column for urgency. The VD suggests overactive bladder

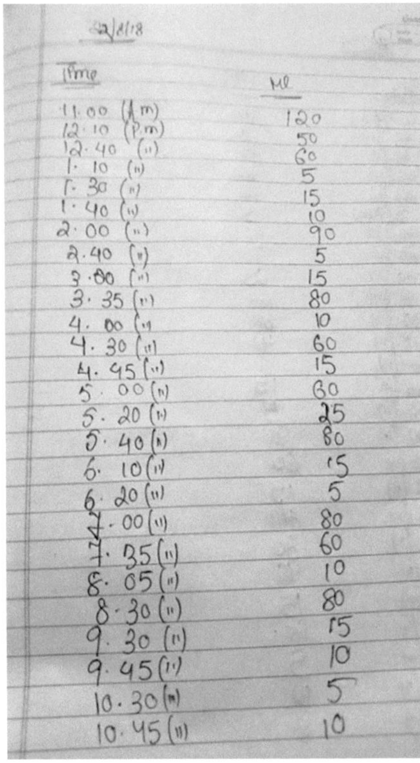

Time	ml
11.00 (Am)	120
12.10 (P.m)	50
12.40 (")	60
1.10 (")	5
1.30 (")	15
1.40 (")	10
2.00 (")	90
2.40 (")	5
3.00 (")	15
3.35 (")	80
4.00 (")	10
4.30 (")	60
4.45 (")	15
5.00 (")	60
5.20 (")	25
5.40 (")	80
6.10 (")	15
6.20 (")	5
7.00 (")	80
7.35 (")	60
8.05 (")	10
8.30 (")	80
9.30 (")	15
9.45 (")	10
10.30 (")	5
10.45 (")	10

Fig. 4.4 A 12-hour observation in a 5-year-old child with extraordinary daytime-only frequency (EDOF). The child did not have any episodes of incontinence or night-time symptoms and USG KUB was normal

Fig. 4.5 A 24-hour observation in a 10-year-old girl with repeated episodes of UTI. VD shows reduced frequency of micturition with large voided volumes s/o voiding postponement

Time	Urine (ml)
9am	1000
4 pm	600
10pm	575
7am	900

stabilize the bladder. Follow-up of CIC diary with reduction of episodes of leak an help assess treatment response. We usually aim to abolish self-voids/leaks by adjusting dose of anticholinergics to keep the bladder pressures in safe range (Fig. 4.7b).

- Maintenance of VD in a follow-up case of PUV gives us evidence of small-capacity bladder/overactivity, etc., and may prompt further invasive investigations (Fig. 4.8).

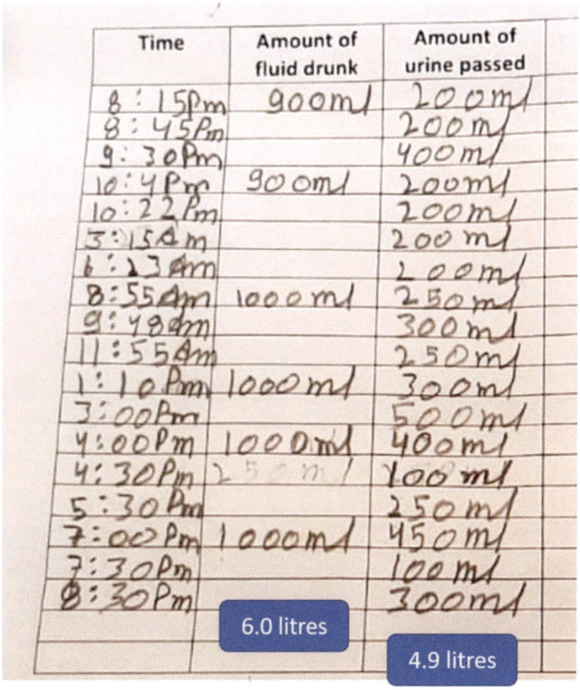

Time	Amount of fluid drunk	Amount of urine passed
8:15Pm	900ml	200ml
8:45Pm		200ml
9:30Pm		400ml
10:4Pm	900ml	200ml
10:22Pm		200ml
3:15Am		200ml
6:23Am		200ml
8:55Am	1000ml	250ml
9:48Am		300ml
11:55Am		250ml
1:10Pm	1000ml	300ml
3:00Pm		500ml
4:00Pm	1000ml	400ml
4:30Pm		100ml
5:30Pm		250ml
7:00Pm	1000ml	450ml
7:30Pm		100ml
8:30Pm		300ml
	6.0 litres	4.9 litres

Fig. 4.6 A 10-year-old boy presented with increased urinary frequency; found to have compulsive excess water intake resulting in polyuria

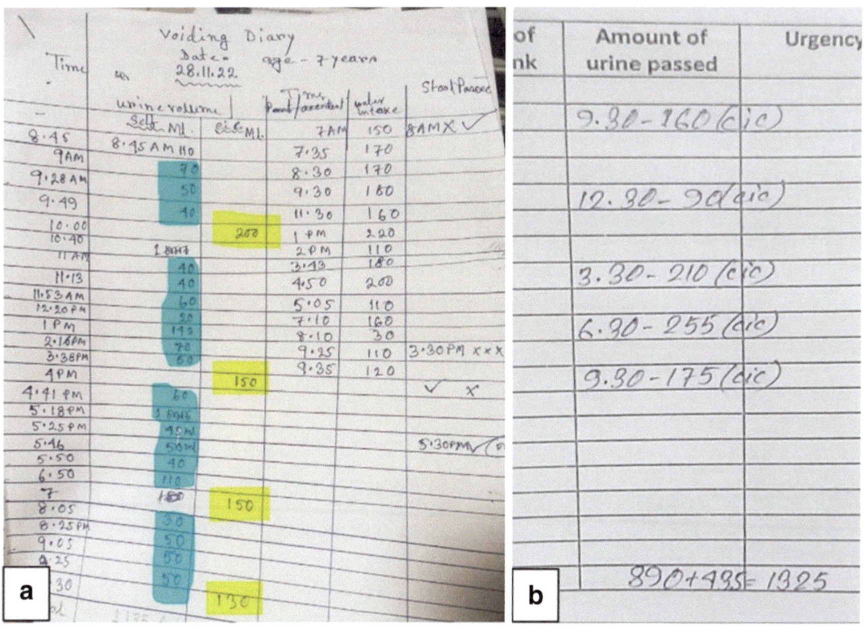

Fig. 4.7 CIC and self-void record of a 7-year-old girl with neurogenic bladder at baseline (**a**). CIC voids marked in yellow and self-voids marked in blue. UDS showed she had urge to self-void at Pdet of 30–40 cm H_2O so she was started on anticholinergics. Repeat CIC diary after 6 months (**b**) showed increase in CIC volumes and disappearance of 'self'-voids

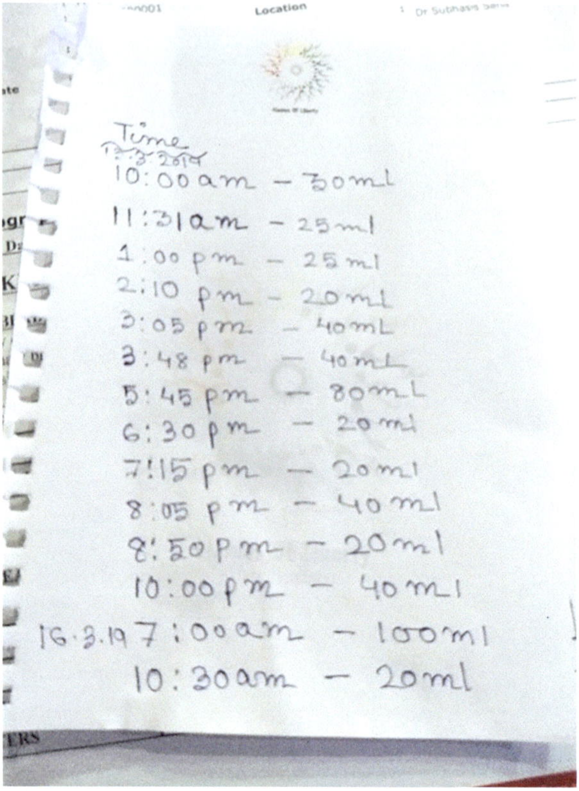

Fig. 4.8 A 24-hour observation in a 6-year-old boy with PUV showing small frequent voided volumes prompting further investigations

- Most of the children with functional bladder problems need long-term lifestyle changes for management. If the family comes back with a properly maintained VD, it signifies that the parents understand the importance of the VD and are dedicated enough to manage the problem.
- Serial VDs are excellent tools to assess treatment response (Fig. 4.9a and b).
- Small-volume voids may also be caused due to scanty fluid intake and needs to be differentiated from small volume due to detrusor overactivity. Total urine output during the day gives idea about total fluid intake. The test needs to be repeated with adequate fluid intake (Fig. 4.10).

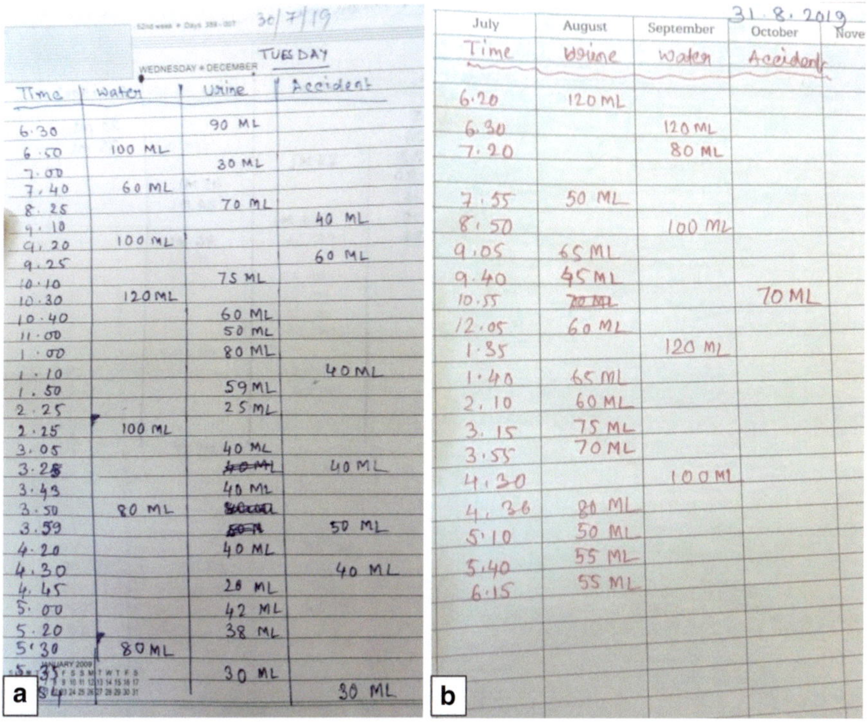

a

30/7/19 TUES DAY

Time	Water	Urine	Accident
6.30		90 ML	
6.50	100 ML		
7.00		30 ML	
7.40	60 ML		
8.25		70 ML	
9.10			40 ML
9.20	100 ML		
9.25			60 ML
10.10		75 ML	
10.30	120 ML		
10.40		60 ML	
11.00		50 ML	
1.00		80 ML	
1.10			40 ML
1.50		59 ML	
2.25		25 ML	
2.25	100 ML		
3.05		40 ML	
3.28		[illegible]	40 ML
3.43		40 ML	
3.50	80 ML	[illegible]	
3.59		[illegible]	50 ML
4.20		40 ML	
4.30			40 ML
4.45		20 ML	
5.00		42 ML	
5.20		38 ML	
5.30	80 ML		
5.35		30 ML	
5.40			30 ML

b

31.8.2019

Time	Urine	Water	Accident
6.20	120 ML		
6.30		120 ML	
7.20		80 ML	
7.55	50 ML		
8.50		100 ML	
9.05	65 ML		
9.40	45 ML		
10.55	~~70 ML~~		70 ML
12.05	60 ML		
1.35		120 ML	
1.40	65 ML		
2.10	60 ML		
3.15	75 ML		
3.55	70 ML		
4.30		100 ML	
4.36	80 ML		
5.10	50 ML		
5.40	55 ML		
6.15	55 ML		

Fig. 4.9 A 24-hour voiding observation in a 6-year-old boy with cerebral palsy (**a**). The child passed urine on cues in a urine pot when the amount was measured directly and several times in between in the diaper which was measured by diaper weight (marked as accidents). The chart shows high-frequency, small-volume voids with several episodes of leaks (mentioned as accidents), suggesting a small-capacity bladder (probable overactivity). As there was no PVR on USG, and constipation had been managed, he was started on anticholinergics. One month later (**b**), the voided volumes have increased marginally, but the leaks/accidents have reduced significantly

Day 1		Day 2	
Time	Urine (ml)	Time	Urine (ml)
6.20am	320	6.30 am	250
7.35 am	stool	7.00 am	stool
11.20 am	100	8.35 am	20
12.00 noo	stool	12.40 pm	25
2.20 pm	25	3.40pm	100
4.45 pm	100	8.45 pm	200
7.40 pm	stool	9.30 pm	150
10.20 pm	150	9.40 pm	stool

Fig. 4.10 An 8-year-old boy, follow-up case of primary bladder diverticulum excision, otherwise asymptomatic with normal USG findings. Voiding diary shows small-volume voids. But voiding frequency is not increased. Total voided volume in 24 hours is only around 700–800 ml denoting reduced fluid intake. Thus, the finding of small voided volumes is due to reduced intake rather than an overactive detrusor

4-Hour Voiding Observation

Non-invasive assessment of bladder behaviour in non-toilet-trained children can be made by observing voiding behaviour over a period of 4 hours. It can be assessed as early as 3 months of age.

Observations are made as children perform activities that are consistent with their daily routine. A dry diaper with a colour-change, vibratory or alarm indicator is placed at the outset which signals when it is wet. The diaper is weighed (against its dry weight) and sonographic PVR is obtained to calculate bladder capacity. If no wetness indicator is available, the child is checked frequently to accurately assess when voiding occurred so that measurements can be taken.

Interrupted voiding is considered when two or three voidings occur over a 10-minute interval.

Voiding pattern in different ages and disease states have been observed in different studies and have been enumerated below:

- Preterm neonates: One void per hour; voids at 53% bladder capacity, 58% interrupted voids. At least one void during 4 hours should show no PVR.
- Infants and toddlers: Voiding frequency decreases slowly from five to two voiding episodes per 4 hours from ages 3 months to 3 years. Interrupted voiding may be recorded in 33% of subjects at age 3 months, but this condition is rare after age 2 years. Bladder capacity increases from a median of 52 to 67, 68 and 123 ml during years 1 to 3, respectively. At ages 3 months, 1 year, 2 years and 3 years, median post-void residual urine volume is 4, 5.5, 3.5 and 0 ml (mean 6, 7, 7 and 3), respectively.

Name Sex

Age Date of birth

(4 hours each day X 3 days)

	Date:					
Time	Urine/ Amount	Stream	Straining	No of instalments	Feeds	Sleeping time

Fig. 4.11 Sample proforma for obtaining 4-hour observation in absence of direct observation/ USG facilities

- PUV—Within 3 months of valve incision, voiding frequency is on an average 6 times in 4 hours, but with a large variability of 2–12 times. Bladder capacity is large in 33% and small in 6%. Median PVR is 9 ml with great variability (0–121 ml).
- Neurogenic bladder—Some children with spinal dysraphism have frequent small voids/leakages and low bladder volumes while few have infrequent voiding and high volumes. Leakage during bladder provocation test and not voiding with a stream are not seen in healthy neonates but are common in newborns with spinal dysraphism.
- Anorectal malformation (pre-PSARP and post-PSARP bladder dysfunction)—In children with neurogenic element, large number of voiding episodes, a large number of interrupted voiding, small bladder capacity, increased post-void residual urine and leakage between voiding episodes are identified. It is difficult to diagnose bladder dysfunction due to tethered cord in small children. Post-PSARP peripheral denervation damage is often accompanied by greater bladder capacity and incomplete emptying.

We do not have the facility to keep babies under observation and perform USG after every void. We ask the parents to maintain a 4-hour voiding observation at home (Figs. 4.11 and 4.12) mentioning the time of void, estimate of the amount (good amount/small amount/few drops), any abnormality noticed during voiding and visual observation of the stream (good, poor, continuous/interrupted).

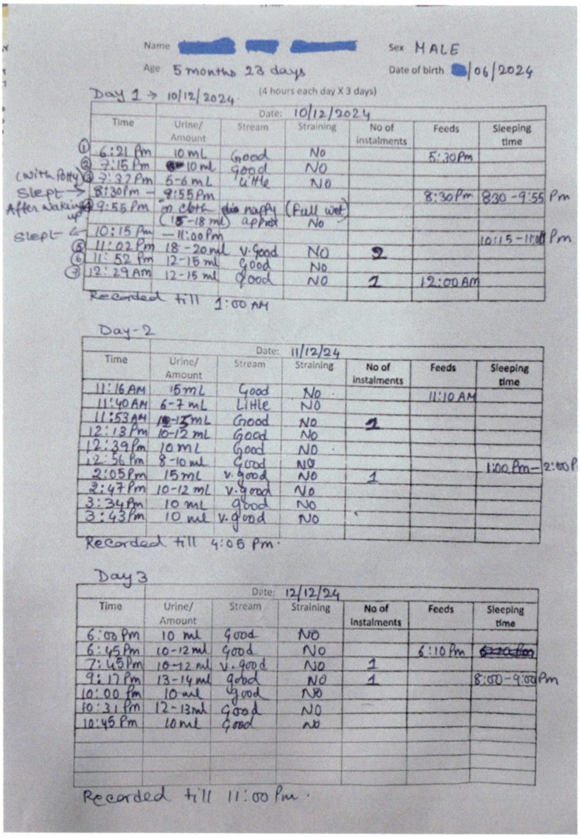

Name [redacted] Sex MALE

Age 5 months 23 days Date of birth [redacted]/06/2024

Day 1 → 10/12/2024. (4 hours each day X 3 days)

Date: 10/12/2024

Time	Urine/ Amount	Stream	Straining	No of instalments	Feeds	Sleeping time
① 6:21 Pm	10 mL	Good	No		5:30 Pm	
② 7:15 Pm	10 ml	good	NO			
(with Potty) ③ 7:37 Pm	5-6 mL	little	NO			
Slept → 8:30 Pm –	9:55 Pm				8:30 Pm	8:30 - 9:55 Pm
After waking up ④ 9:55 Pm	on cloth (15-18 ml)	nappy approx	(Full wet) No			
Slept ← 10:15 Pm	– 11:00 Pm					10:15 - 11:00 Pm
⑤ 11:02 Pm	18 - 20 ml	V. Good	NO	2		
⑥ 11:52 Pm	12-15 ml	Good	No			
⑦ 12:29 AM	12-15 ml	Good	NO	1	12:00 AM	

Recorded till 1:00 AM

Day-2

Date: 11/12/24

Time	Urine/ Amount	Stream	Straining	No of instalments	Feeds	Sleeping time
11:16 AM	15 mL	Good	No		11:10 AM	
11:40 AM	6-7 mL	Little	NO			
11:53 AM	10-12 mL	Good	NO	1		
12:13 Pm	10-12 mL	Good	No			
12:39 Pm	10 mL	Good	NO			
12:56 Pm	8-10 ml	Good	NO			1:00 Pm – 2:00 Pm
2:05 Pm	15 mL	v. good	NO	1		
2:47 Pm	10-12 mL	v. good	No			
3:34 Pm	10 mL	good	NO			
3:43 Pm	10 ml	v. good	NO			

Recorded till 4:05 Pm.

Day 3

Date: 12/12/24

Time	Urine/ Amount	Stream	Straining	No of instalments	Feeds	Sleeping time
6:00 Pm	10 ml	Good	NO			
6:45 Pm	10-12 ml	Good	No		6:10 Pm	~~6:10 Pm~~
7:45 Pm	10-12 ml	v. good	NO	1		
9:17 Pm	13-14 ml	good	NO	1		8:00 - 9:00 Pm
10:00 Pm	10 ml	good	NO			
10:31 Pm	12-13 ml	Good	NO			
10:45 Pm	10 ml	Good	no			

Recorded till 11:00 Pm.

Fig. 4.12 A 4-hour observation for a 6-month-old boy with two episodes of UTI showing small-volume voids 7–10 times in 4 hours. This child passed urine in few drops each time before the actual stream began. The mother was vigilant enough and could measure all the voided volumes

Declarations

Competing Interests The author(s) has no competing interests to declare that are relevant to the content of this manuscript.

Ethics Approval The author(s) declares that this manuscript does not include primary research with human participants.

The author(s) declares that this manuscript does not include primary studies involving animals.

Suggested Reading

1. Austin PF, Bauer SB, Bower W, Chase J, Franco I, Hoebeke P, Rittig S, Walle JV, von Gontard A, Wright A, Yang SS, Nevéus T. The standardization of terminology of lower urinary tract function in children and adolescents: update report from the standardization committee of the International Children's Continence Society. Neurourol Urodyn. 2016;35(4):471–81. https://doi.org/10.1002/nau.22751. Epub 2015 Mar 14.
2. Bauer SB, Nijman RJ, Drzewiecki BA, Sillen U, Hoebeke P, International Children's Continence Society Standardization Subcommittee. International Children's Continence Society standardization report on urodynamic studies of the lower urinary tract in children. Neurourol Urodyn. 2015;34(7):640–7. https://doi.org/10.1002/nau.22783. Epub 2015 May 21.

3. Borg H, Sillén U, Doroszkiewicz M, Holmdahl G, Sjöström S, Abrahamsson K. Four-hour voiding observations detect neurogenic lower urinary tract dysfunction in neonates with anorectal malformation. J Pediatr Urol. 2021;17(1):76.e1–9. https://doi.org/10.1016/j.jpurol.2020.10.016. Epub 2020 Oct 16.
4. Ibrahim S, Prodromou K, Mishra P, Wright A, Clothier J, Garriboli M. Four hour voiding observation study in infants with posterior urethral valves. J Pediatr Urol. 2024;20(4):729.e1–7. https://doi.org/10.1016/j.jpurol.2024.04.003. Epub 2024 Apr 20. PMID: 38719686.
5. Jansson UB, Hanson M, Hanson E, Hellström AL, Sillén U. Voiding pattern in healthy children 0 to 3 years old: a longitudinal study. J Urol. 2000;164(6):2050–4.
6. Sillén U, Sölsnes E, Hellström AL, Sandberg K. The voiding pattern of healthy preterm neonates. J Urol. 2000;163(1):278–81. https://doi.org/10.1016/s0022-5347(05)68036-6. PMID: 10604376.
7. Wide P, Duchén K, Mattsson S, Glad MG. Four-hour voiding observation with provocation test reveals significant abnormalities of bladder function in newborns with spinal dysraphism. J Pediatr Urol. 2020;16(4):491.e1–7. https://doi.org/10.1016/j.jpurol.2020.06.022. Epub 2020 Jun 20.

Uroflowmetry I: The Conventional Approach

5

Poonam Guha Vaze and Subhasis Saha

Uroflowmetry is the assessment of the speed and pattern of flow of urine.

The speed of flow/pattern is determined by the force which is pushing the urine out and the diameter of the outflow tract. If the force of detrusor contraction is inadequate or there is significant narrowing proximally in the outflow tract, the flow will be poor. On the other hand, if the detrusor contraction is very strong, the stream may be very strong and short-lived. If there is mild obstruction in the distal part of the urethra, the stream may be forceful but thin, goes a long distance but takes a long time (e.g., meatal stenosis).

'Visible' Uroflowmetry

The easiest and the most inexpensive way to assess uroflowmetry is to watch the child or the baby pee. Often, we ask the parents to share with us the videos of micturition which gives us an idea of the approximate flow rate, time, intermittency, degree of straining and post-void dribble.

Visible uroflowmetry relies on the 'speed' of the jet of urine which comes out and its visible thickness.

There are fallacies of visual estimation of flow: A 'visibly good' stream in an operated patient of hypospadias may not be reliable as although the urine is coming out in jet, the neourethra may not be sufficiently distensible. The effect will be

P. G. Vaze (✉)
Neotia Bhagirathi Woman and Child Care Centre, Newtown, Kolkata, India

Department of Pediatric Surgery, Nilratan Sircar Medical College and Hospital, Kolkata, India

S. Saha
Department of Pediatric Surgery, Manipal Hospitals, Kolkata, India

S. Saha, P. Guha Vaze (eds.), *Comprehensive Atlas of Practical Pediatric Urodynamics*, https://doi.org/10.1007/978-981-95-2709-0_5

similar to keeping a finger in front of a water hose which makes the water jet go to a farther distance. Any mild urethral stricture or significant phimosis can have similar effect and the flow will appear to be 'good'. This can only be picked up by quantitatively by assessment of Qmax in uroflowmetry.

'Machine' Uroflowmetry

The only way to objectively record the flow parameters is a 'free uroflowmetry'. The child is asked to pass urine into a funnel through which the urine flows into a jar which rests on the sensor. The sensor senses the weight of the urine falling on it and plots it against time.

Sensors use various technologies to sense the weight of urine. Various types of equipment to record the uroflow are:

1. Rotating disc flowmeter
2. Weight transducer flowmeter
3. Capacitance type of flowmeter

Prerequisites

While performing a uroflowmetry, the following factors are taken into consideration:

- Uroflowmetry is performed in the privacy of the urodynamic study suite which is secluded, if necessary, with a curtain so that the child does not have eye contact with the investigator.
- The child should be allowed to void in a posture in which he/she is habituated to.
- The child should have a usual desire to void. Bladder over-distention with bladder capacity {voided volume (VV) + post-void residue (PVR)} of more than 115% of expected bladder capacity (EBC), or VV of more than 100% of EBC, may be associated with high rates of abnormal uroflow patterns and elevated PVRs.
- The investigator should be able to observe the child when he/she is voiding to notice any straining/delay between voiding command and initiation of flow/any urine falling outside the jar/kick to the flowmeter.
- When the voiding command is given, it should be simultaneously marked on the graph. In the absence of EMG, the delay between command to void and initiation of flow can give indirect idea about hesitancy.
- For any value of maximum flow rate (Qmax) to be regarded as significant, it should persist for > = 2 s. Any spike of shorter duration may be an artefact and should be ignored (Fig. 5.1).

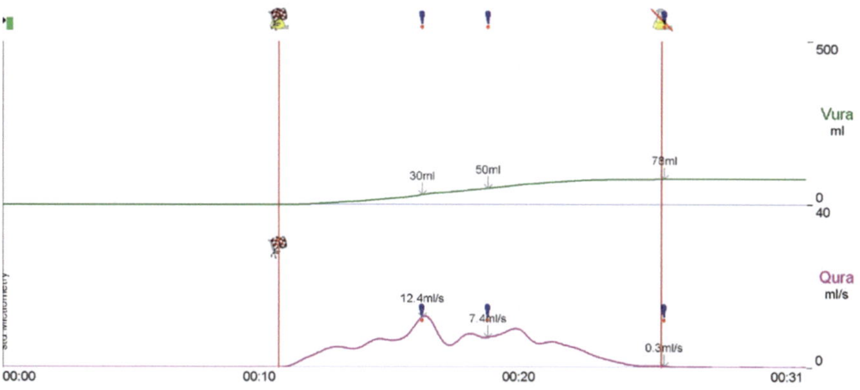

Fig. 5.1 Uroflow with a spike. The spike of 12.4 ml/sec is to be ignored as the spike is of <2 sec. The corrected Qmax should be around 7–8 ml/sec

- For children, the voided volume must be at least 50% of EBC. For adults, a minimum volume of 150 ml is required.
- A bladder diary/voiding diary is very helpful before the uroflowmetry is done. It gives us an assessment of usual voided volumes. The voided volume (VV) during the study must be close to the maximum voided volume in voiding diary for it to be valid. If a 9-year-old child has a usual daytime volume of 100 ml of urine in his bladder diary, we should not expect a void of 200 ml for him. In such a flow with a small VV, if we get an abnormal uroflow showing a tower- or plateau-shaped curve, it may be representative of the underlying pathology, whereas a bell-shaped curve may be fallacious and should be disregarded.
- It is better to record two voids as the child may be apprehensive/excited during the first void, and the flow pattern may be abnormal (Fig. 5.2a, b).
- It should be confirmed from the parents whether the pattern observed during the study matches the usual voiding behaviour at home. A very apprehensive/shy child may produce a very weak stream with significant PVR in office conditions, whereas the stream may be robust at home. Thus, the observed uroflowmetry cannot be relied upon.
- Measurement of post-void residue (PVR)—The PVR is estimated with ultrasound or invasively by inserting a catheter at the end of free uroflowmetry. PVR may be used to estimate the efficiency of bladder emptying (bladder voiding efficiency) by using the formula BE = VV/(VV + PVR).
- The scale of the printing should be adjusted in order to make the curve easily visible. Scaling of the printout has been suggested as follows: 1 mm can equal 1 s on the x-axis and 1 mL/s and 10 mL VV on the y-axis, but the trace must be clearly readable whatever scale is used. Any changes in the scale in the print report can make the shape of the curve distorted. See the chapter on artefacts.

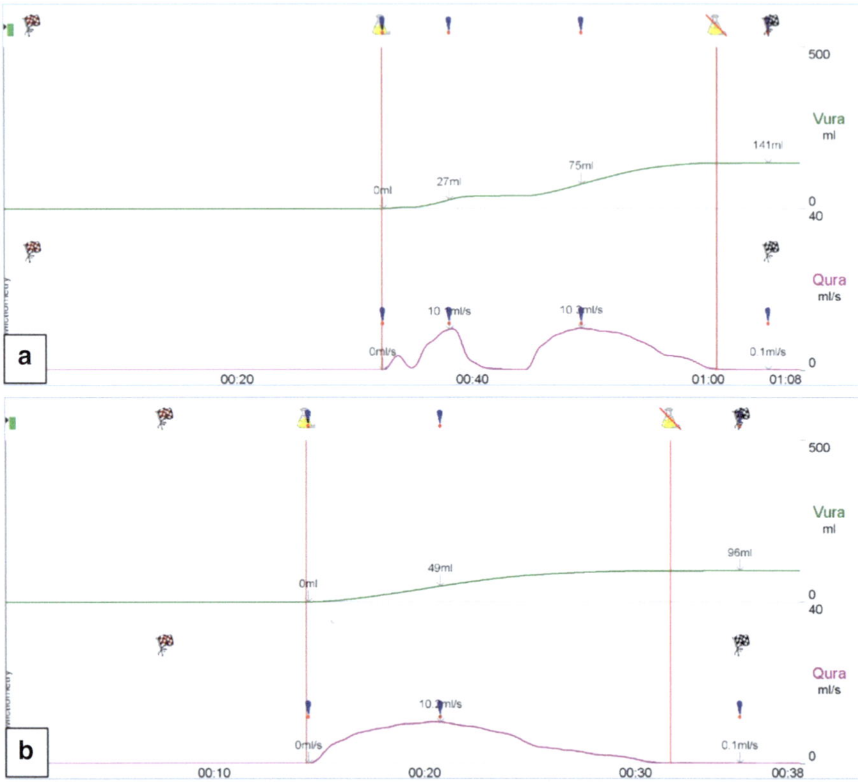

Fig. 5.2 Importance of performing two studies. Two urine flows recorded in a 5-year-old boy with Down syndrome. The first flow (**a**) shows an interrupted flow whereas the second flow (**b**) shows a bell-shaped curve

The Uroflowmetry Curve

The uroflowmetry curve is a graphical representation of weight of urine coming out per sec vs time (Fig. 5.3).

The following parameters are noted in a uroflowmetry curve

1. Voiding time (total duration of the act of micturition—in seconds)
2. Flow time (the time during which flow of urine was recorded—in seconds)
3. Time to maximum flow (time taken from starting of the flow to reaching maximum flow rate—in seconds)
4. Delay time (time from the command for micturition and the actual onset of flow)
5. Lag time—When uroflowmetry is done with simultaneous EMG monitoring, lag time is the time between the start of pelvic floor relaxation and the beginning of urine flow. A proper lag time denotes optimal detrusor sphincter coordination.

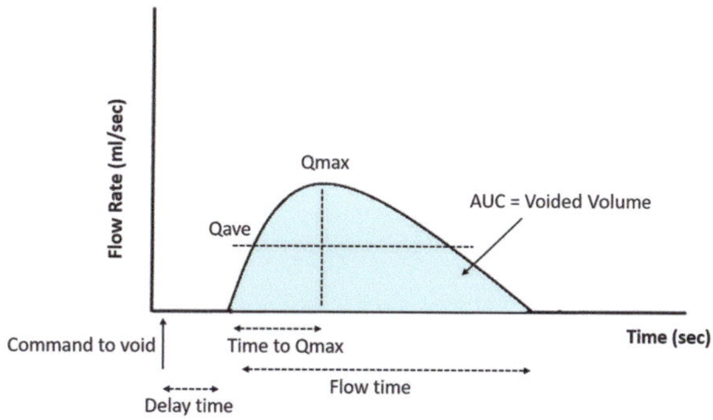

Fig. 5.3 Schematic diagram of a normal bell-shaped uroflowmetry curve

6. Maximum flow rate (Qmax—in ml/seconds)—depicted by the highest point in the uroflowmetry curve
7. Average flow rate (Qav—in ml/seconds)
8. Volume at maximum flow (the total volume of urine passed by the time maximum flow rate is reached)
9. Voided volume (VV)
10. Residual volume (RV) and the method used for measurement of PVR (USG, bladder scanner or catheterisation)

Types of Uroflowmetry Curves

Based on the pathology, there are various shapes of the curve

1. *Bell-shaped curve*—Normal (starts promptly, rapidly rises to a climax Qmax and then comes down at a slope slightly lesser than the ascent) (Fig. 5.4).

   Qmax is reached in the first 30% of VV and within 3 to 10 s from the flow start. If the square of the maximum flow rate ($Qmax^2$) equals or exceeds the VV (ml), the recorded Qmax is most probably normal.
2. *Tower curve*—This is a sudden, high-amplitude curve of short duration that suggests an overactive bladder produced by an explosive voiding contraction. A very high Qmax is reached within first 1–3 s followed by a rapid fall (Fig. 5.5). Tower curves are steeper than bell curves. A_Qmax of a main curve $\geqq 80°$ may be used as an objective parameter to identify tower curves (Fig. 5.6a, b).
3. *Plateau curve*—This is a flattened, low-amplitude prolonged flow curve. Yang defined it as 'an even flow curve with a Qmax/flow time < 0.5 without bladder over-distension', which may be better for practical use. It signifies either a fixed bladder outflow obstruction or poor detrusor contractility (Figs. 5.7 and 5.8). The only way to differentiate between the two causes of plateau curve is to assess the detrusor pressures during voiding which can be demonstrated in an invasive urodynamics.

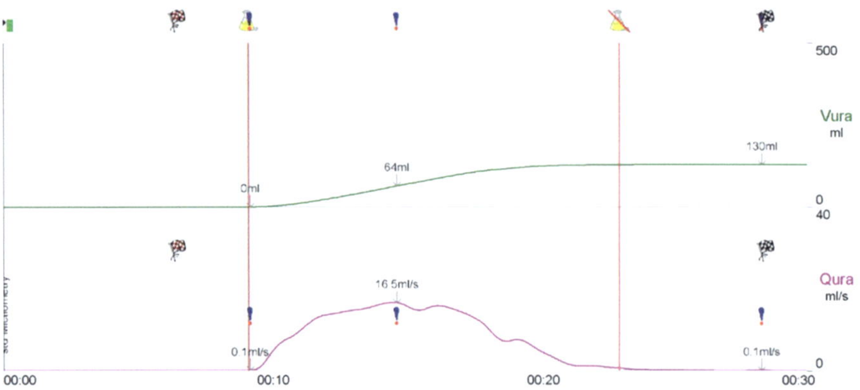

Fig. 5.4 A normal bell-shaped uroflowmetry curve

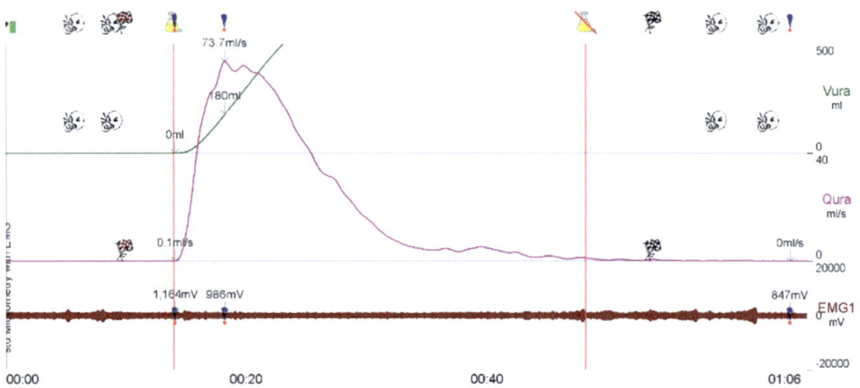

Fig. 5.5 Tower-shaped uroflowmetry curve. A 12-year-old female with primary enuresis, daytime urgency and recurrent UTI. Tower-shaped curve denotes overactive bladder. She was started on bladder relaxants after adequate management of constipation after which her symptoms resolved

4. *Staccato curve*—A series of curves without the trough touching the baseline in between. The fluctuations should be larger than the square root of the Qmax. It can be seen in cases with dysfunctional voiding or underactive detrusor with some element of Valsalva voiding.

   Staccato curve with otherwise good flow rates suggests dysfunctional voiding which corroborates with spin top appearance of urethra on MCU (Fig. 5.9).

   Staccato curve with poor flow rates and straining during voiding suggests detrusor underactivity (Fig. 5.10).

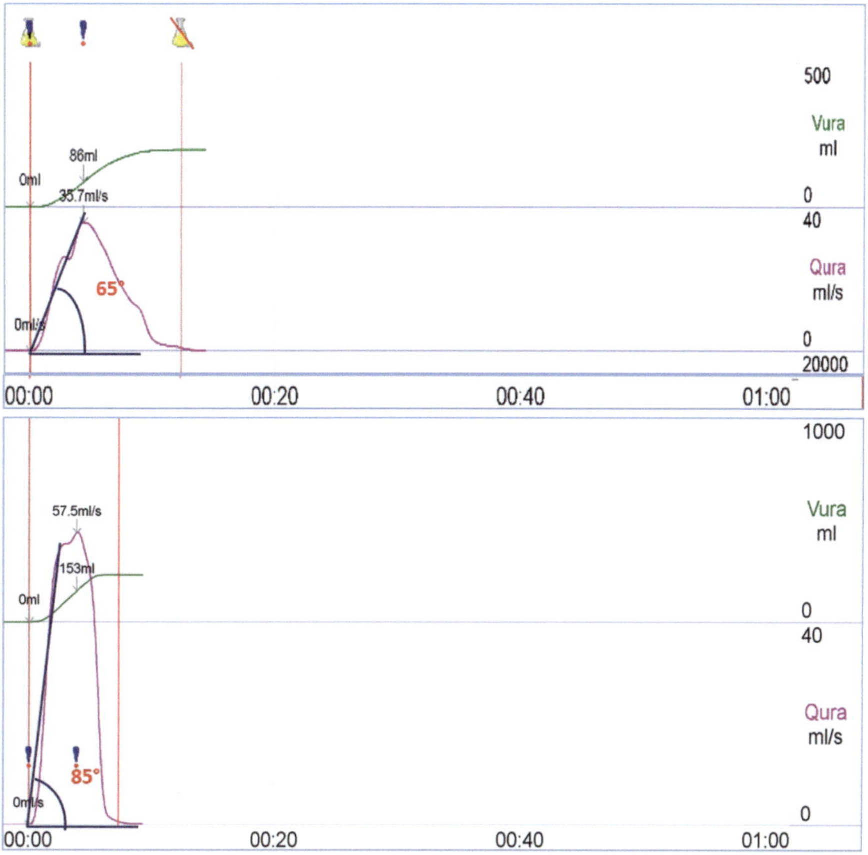

Fig. 5.6 Angle_Qmax in bell-shaped (**a**) and tower-shaped (**b**) curves. (Adapted from: Yang et al. [8])

5. *Interrupted flow curve*—A series of crests and troughs touching the baseline in between. Detrusor underactivity with voiding primarily by abdominal compresses/Valsalva results in interrupted flow (Figs. 5.11 and 5.12).
6. There may be a *combination* of one or more types.

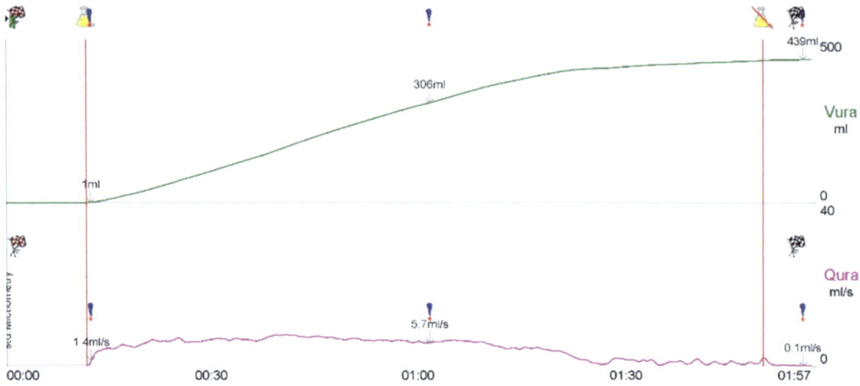

Fig. 5.7 Plateau-shaped uroflowmetry curve. A 12-year-old male child underwent urethroplasty for distal penile hypospadias at 6 years of age. Presently complaining of intermittent post-void dribbling. Visible stream is good, goes far, but thin. After the uroflowmetry, he was found to have meatal stenosis, for which meatoplasty was done

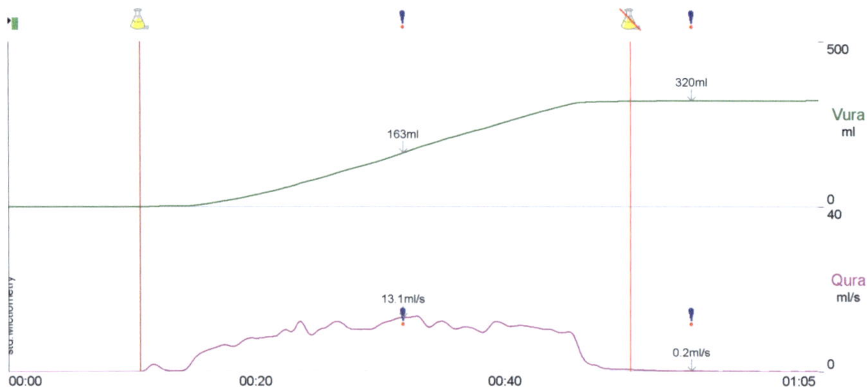

Fig. 5.8 Plateau-shaped curve in an 8-year-old boy with a large voided volume. He had history of voiding postponement infrequent voids, constipation and one episode of UTI. USG showed bilateral mild hydroureter with normal bladder and insignificant PVR. Findings suggest probable early myogenic failure in a 'lazy' bladder

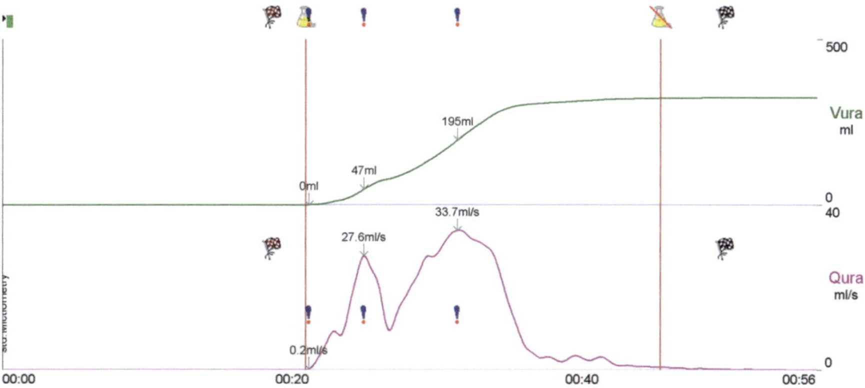

Fig. 5.9 Staccato curve. A 12-year-old girl with recurrent episodes of UTI, habit of postponing micturition/stools; urgency +, urge incontinence +; occasional holding maneuvers +; no enuresis; constipation ++

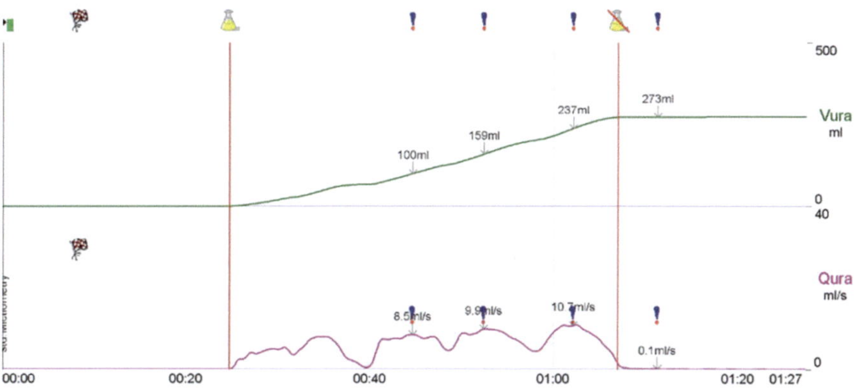

Fig. 5.10 Staccato curve with visible straining (Valsalva voiding) during the void suggestive of detrusor underactivity. Follow-up case of ARM, underwent colostomy followed by abdominoperineal pull through at 2 years age. Had h/o recurrent UTI before pull through—improved after surgery. He passed urine in relatively poor stream; informed before passing urine; occasional straining while passing urine; occasional dribbling while playing. USG showed normal upper tracts with bladder wall thickness of 2.8 mm—probable neurogenic detrusor underactivity

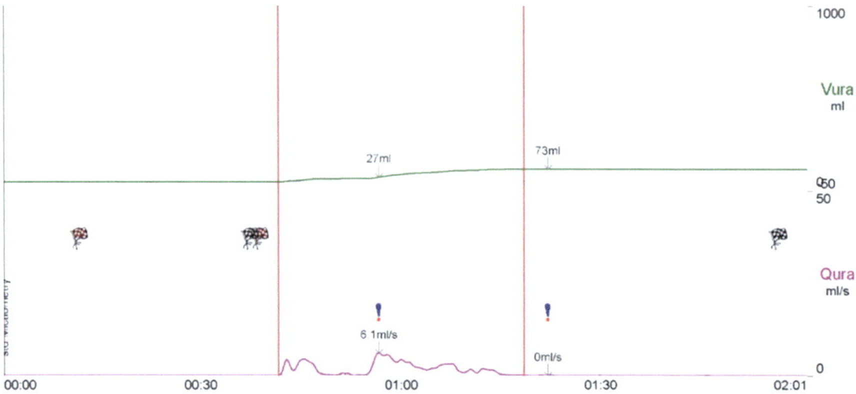

Fig. 5.11 Interrupted stream in a 5-year-old child of trisomy 21. He had h/o significant straining while passing urine with a visibly poor stream. USG showed thick-walled UB with right HDUN. Cystoscopy revealed a prominent bladder neck with very prominent sphincteric impression—probable dysfunctional voiding associated with trisomy 21

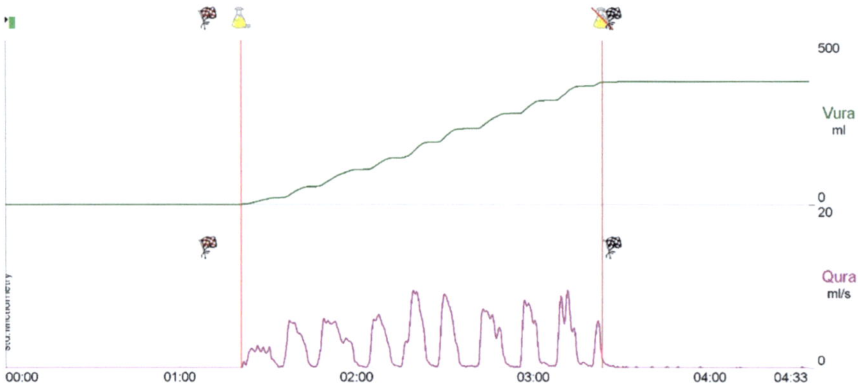

Fig. 5.12 Interrupted stream in a 12-year-old boy—Valsalva voiding in a case of neurogenic bladder with a significant PVR of 400 ml

Pitfalls of Uroflowmetry

Variability in Curves and Interpretation

It has been well documented that there is a lot of variability between two uroflowmetries from a single child as well as inter- and intra-observer variability in interpretation of the same curve. Several alternative systems including the Franco Yang Flow Index and SPU guideline system have been proposed to objectively classify uroflow curve but none have been proven to be valid enough.

Fallacies of Weight-Based Uroflowmetry

The stream in case of meatal stenosis or significant phimosis may be thin but goes very far, whereas the stream in case of PUV may be relatively thick but falls very close. In both the cases, volume/weight of the urine coming out per second may be same, and thus, weight-based uroflowmetry produces the same type of plateau-shaped curve in both the situations. Thus, direct observation by the investigator is very important. There are experimental models which assess the 'speed' or velocity of the stream which is coming out of the urethra in mm/sec. Such an assessment can differentiate the two situations objectively.

Fallacies of Normal Bell-Shaped Flow

A bell-shaped flow does not guarantee a normal contractility/outflow parameters. As the good contractility of pediatric detrusor can overcome outlet resistance, the peak flow rate might not be a good parameter for monitoring voiding function. Also, bell-shaped curve can be generated in the presence of underactive detrusor with strong abdominal contraction. This error may be obviated by the use of two sets of EMG electrodes (perineal + abdominal) and direct observation by the observer.

Fallacies of PVR

Most of the parents initiate lots of fluid intake preceding the study, and hence, if the post-void assessment is delayed for a while, the resultant diuresis may lead to erroneously high PVR. Thus, the PVR needs to be assessed within 5 minutes of voiding. Secondly, in children with high-grade VUR (vesicoureteral reflux), even if the voiding is efficient, in a short while, the upper tract contents empty into the bladder with a high estimated PVR. In such a situation, true PVR can only be estimated if bladder volume is estimated immediately at the end of voiding by a handheld device or observation under fluoroscopy during MCUG or video-UDS.

Declarations
Competing Interests The author(s) has no competing interests to declare that are relevant to the content of this manuscript.

Ethics Approval The author(s) declares that this manuscript does not include primary research with human participants.

The author(s) declares that this manuscript does not include primary studies involving animals.

Suggested Reading

1. Austin PF, Bauer SB, Bower W, Chase J, Franco I, Hoebeke P, Rittig S, Walle JV, von Gontard A, Wright A, Yang SS, Nevéus T. The standardization of terminology of lower urinary tract function in children and adolescents: update report from the standardization committee of the International Children's Continence Society. Neurourol Urodyn. 2016;35(4):471–81. https://doi.org/10.1002/nau.22751. Epub 2015 Mar 14.
2. Brucker BM, Nitti VW. Urodynamic studies: types and indications. In: Rovner Eric S, Koski Michelle E, editors. Rapid and practical interpretation of urodynamics. Springer; 2015. p. 6.
3. Chang SJ, Yang SS. Inter-observer and intra-observer agreement on interpretation of uroflowmetry curves of kindergarten children. J Pediatr Urol. 2008;4:422–6.
4. Drach GW, Layton TN, Binard WJ. Male peak urinary flow rate: relationships to volume voided and age. J Urol. 1979;122:210–4.
5. Tarcan T, Acar O, Agarwal M, Rubilotta E, De Nunzio C, Rosier P. ICS educational module: the practice of uroflowmetry in adults. Continence. 2024;9:101065. https://doi.org/10.1016/j.cont.2023.101065.
6. Van Batavia JP, Pohl HG, Farhat WA, Chiang G, BaniHani A, Collett-Gardere T, Franco I. Is it time to reconsider how we document pediatric uroflow studies?: a study from the SPU voiding dysfunction task force. J Pediatr Urol. 2023;19(5):546–54. https://doi.org/10.1016/j.jpurol.2023.04.018. Epub 2023 May 12.
7. Yang S, Chang S-J. Practical urodynamics in children, part 2: normal uroflowmetry curve is not a guarantee of normal voiding function. Urol Sci. 2012;23:55–7. https://doi.org/10.1016/j.urols.2012.04.002.
8. Yang SS-D, Chang S-J. Differentiating tower from bell curves in smooth continuous uroflowmetry curves of healthy adolescents. Urol Sci. 2019;30(4):74–8. https://doi.org/10.4103/UROS.UROS_100_18.

Uroflowmetry: An Alternative View Using a Quantitative Approach

6

Israel Franco

Uroflowmetry is a noninvasive means of measuring bladder function. This involves measuring the rate of flow of urine as it exits the urethra. There are numerous ways of measuring flow rate ranging from visual observation, listening, air displacement, casting distance, height of ascent, timing, gravimetry, induction, drop spectrometry, ultrasonic volumetry, and rotating disc. Irrespective of the method of measuring the flow rate, the principle behind flow rate is dictated by the contraction velocity of the bladder, the volume in the bladder, and the shape and resistive forces of the urethra.

Our first attempt at approaching uroflowmetry from a quantitative approach stems back to 2015 where we built a foundation for this methodology by developing the concept of an idealized voider in our publication "A quantitative approach to the interpretation of uroflowmetry in children" [2]. The concept of an idealized voider is critical to developing a foundation for what is expected from the perfect voider. The definition of normal is variable depending on the population it is being developed for, and therefore, there is significant variability with this definition. Similarly, the use of the term asymptomatic or identifying asymptomatic patients does not mean that the patient is voiding appropriately; it just means they have no symptoms or are not aware that they do not void according to the norms. Many nomograms have been built utilizing an aggregation of asymptomatic or normal patients in which there is a broad spectrum of flow rates and flow types, but in the end, to build a foundation to judge voids, one needs to have an ideal void to work off.

I. Franco (✉)
Urology and Pediatrics, University of Tennessee- Chattanooga, School of Health Sciences, Chattanooga, TN, USA

Urology, Yale School of Medicine, New Haven, CT, USA

Pediatric Urology, Children's Hospital at Erlanger, Chattanooga, TN, USA
e-mail: Israel.Franco@yale.edu; Israel.Franco@erlanger.org

S. Saha, P. Guha Vaze (eds.), *Comprehensive Atlas of Practical Pediatric Urodynamics*, https://doi.org/10.1007/978-981-95-2709-0_6

Ideal Voider Concept

The idealized voider is a person who voids, with a continuous void, who does not exceed 115% of estimated bladder capacity, has a post void residual of less than 20 cc, and voids with a bell curve [2]. Herein lies the conundrum in this model. What is a bell curve? We have no standardized definition of a bell curve at the present time [3]. We have decided to take what was expert opinion and develop an ideal voider [2] from which we can model a perfect flow equation, which can be used to predict an estimated flow rate. This would then allow for a flow index (actual Q/estimated Q). Once we have achieved this, we can then put to practical use the concept of the flow index based on the ideal voider.

It is essential to the idea of creating a flow index that the estimated Q be calculated from the volume in the bladder at the time that voiding is initiated and not just simply the voided volume (VV). Unfortunately, many attempts have been made to use VV for this purpose and they have been ineffective [4]. If we utilize the following fundamental laws of physics, it is possible to prove that the volume in the bladder at the time of voiding is critical to improve of flow predictions. The laws of conservation of mass, conservation of energy, and the second law of thermodynamics will lead to the continuity equation $Q = C_{\text{vol}}{}^{0.667}V_c)$ [5], where Vol is the instantaneous bladder volume, V_c is the bladder wall contraction velocity, and C is a shape-dependent constant which in the case of a sphere is equal to 0.7697 [6]. The fundamental characteristic that determines the ability to calculate flow rates accurately from bladder volumes is that bladder volume is the voided volume plus the post void residual, in other words the total volume in the bladder [2]. A quantitative approach to uroflowmetry utilizes this concept to achieve the correct estimated Q's where we can create an index by comparing the actual void to the ideal void.

Flow Index

The concept of the flow index is not new and dates back to the early work of Von Garrelts [7] where he described a curvilinear relation between Q (flow) and VV (voided volume):

$$cQ = Q / \sqrt{\text{VV}} \tag{6.1}$$

Expanding on this concept, he produced the indexes for average flow and maximum flow:

$$\text{VQI}_{\text{max}} = \frac{Q_{\text{max}}}{\sqrt{\text{VV}}} \tag{6.2}$$

$$\text{VQI}_{\text{avg}} = \frac{Q_{\text{avg}}}{\sqrt{\text{VV}}} \tag{6.3}$$

The concept of using the $\frac{Q_{\text{max}}}{\sqrt{\text{VV}}}$ has persisted and is the foundation for the use of $\sqrt{\text{VV}}$ as the proxy for an adequate void. Griffiths et al. [8] later produced an index in the form of the actual flow rate/bladder volume $^{0.66}$. The Griffiths equation never caught on and there are numerous publications that show that $\sqrt{vv}$ is not the optimal equation to model flow on, but it continues to persist in the literature [9]. Mattsson in 1994 [9] used it to create their volume-corrected nomograms. This concept allows for the ability of each void to be normalized to voided volume. They used voided volume and exponents of 0.3 for Q_{max} ($vv^{0.3}$) and 0.42 for Q_{avg} ($vv^{0.42}$). These indexes rely on estimates for flow rates that exhibit exponential growth or power equations that do not take into account the true nature of voiding which is that there is a decrease in Q_{max} as the bladder is overdistended. To appropriately model voiding and to create reliable indexes, we need to identify the ideal situation and then create models from those situations.

Ideal Voider Equations

Q actual/Q idealized voider is the index that has been developed. For normal voiders, this index will approach unity at 1. Prior work by Agarwal [10] on utilizing a flow index based on Q actual/$\sqrt{\text{total bladder capacity}}$ has yielded very good predictive ability to identify abnormal voiders by cutting off abnormal voiders at one standard deviation from the norm [10]. This modification of the original von Garrelts equation leads to greater accuracy than the original which was confined to using voided volume. In an in-depth analysis on this, we found that the error rate increases in patients that void with abnormal flow and elevated residuals when the $Q_{max}/\sqrt{vv}$ is used [4].

Q actual/Q idealized voider is the closest we can get to a standard definition to what a normal bell curve voider should void like. The perfect bell curve would have an FI = 1. Recognizing that flow rates can be modeled with quadratic equations more reliably than with power or exponential equations, we have utilized the original dataset from the Zhou Chi study by Yang and Chang to develop equations for children aged 4–12 [11]. Utilizing a separate dataset of patients composed of 12–21 yo males and females compiled by J. Netto and myself who had bell curves with no evidence of EMG activity during voiding, we modeled their flows to create a group of equations (Table 6.1) for these older normal voiders. Since an adolescent has attained adult-size bladder but is not encumbered by the enlarged prostates and other factors that may interfere with normal voiding in both males and females, these equations could be used as proxies for normal adult males and females. The equations have been created in two forms: known total bladder volume (VV and PVR) and VV only. The former equation will undoubtably be more accurate since it is based on the principles previously espoused in the last section. The VV only equations should only be used with patients known to have low post void residuals. Otherwise, patients with elevated residual more than 100 cc will have marked changes in the expected flow rates and the values will be inaccurate. All these equations begin to have greater error at larger volumes since the original dataset was constrained by limited datapoints when volumes exceeded 450 cc. Therefore, we recommend that patients be asked to void at volumes below 450 cc which will increase the accuracy and predictability of the equations.

Table 6.1 Formulas for calculating estimated flow values (FEV) for Q_{avg} and Q_{max} and objective values to identify the flow curve pattern

Ideal voider equations		
Voided volume (VV) with no PVR available	Q_{avg}=	Q_{max}=
4–12 yo female	$3.717 + 0.0463VV - 0.00003858VV^2$	$-23.6835(e^{-0.00576VV}) + 31.4008$
4–12 yo male	$3.03 + 0.0576VV - 0.0000757VV^2$	$-21.2405(e^{-0.010104VV}) + 26.0677$
>12 yo females	$4.10134 + 0.0605VV - 0.000079VV^2$	$9.589 + 0.089VV - 0.00008657VV^2$
>12 yo males	$7.27494 + 0.04633VV - 0.000027VV^2$	$8.79194 + 0.0878VV - 0.000078VV^2$
Total bladder capacity (VV + PVR)		
4–12 yo female	$3.37 + 0.048TBC - 0.0000354TBC^2$	$10.723 + 0.073TBC - 0.000042TBC^2$
4–12 yo male	$3.412 + 0.052TBC - 0.000061TBC^2$	$11.26 + 0.071TBC - 0.000051TBC^2$
>12 yo females	$3.987 + 0.055TBC - 0.0000205TBC^2$	$9.98 + 0.087TBC - 0.000068TBC^2$
>12 yo males	$7.16342 + 0.038TBC - 0.000021TBC^2$	$8.73647 + 0.082TBC - 0.000061TBC^2$
Males all ages	$TTQ_{max} = 52.8(e^{0.003267TBC}) - 50.497$	
Females all ages	$TTQ_{max} = -25.033(e^{-0.000789TBC}) + 26.792$	

Source: Based on FRANCO et al. [2]

Voiding Efficiency

Another potentially valuable job for uroflowmetry is that it can be an arbiter of voiding efficiency. Efficiency is the measure of the ability to empty the bladder fully and effectively as defined by the physics of voiding. There are numerous means of determining voiding efficiency some calculated using urodynamics but this is invasive. More simplistic forms rely on the PVR as a percentage of the initial pre-micturition volume [12] (%pvr), and another form is defined as the ability to empty effectively (VV/VV + PVR or 1–%PVR) [13].

A better way to look at efficiency is that it is a ratio of the useful work performed or the total energy used in the process of micturition. This was described by Griffiths et al. [8] in the form of an index with the actual flow rate/$vv^{0.66}$. They derived their formula from the continuity equation $Q = C\ Vol^{0.667} V_c$ where C is a constant and V_c is the contraction velocity. They describe this formula as a measure of voiding efficiency, but it is also identical to the concept of the flow index.

Since flow index = $Q_{max\ actual}/Q_{max\ estimated}$, we could then see that the FI can be seen as a surrogate for the efficiency of voiding and that it is capable of defining hyperefficient and hypoefficient voiding. If we rely on %PVR or 1−%PVR, we cannot capture the hypervoiders that are commonly seen with flow rates that exceed normal and potentially can even miss hypovoiders as well.

Efficiency can be defined as the ratio of $\frac{\text{actual work}}{\text{optimal work}}$. Since work is equal to the force times the volume of urine being moved, we can then work our way to the final equation:

$$\frac{Q_{\text{actual}}}{Q_{\text{optimal}}} = \text{efficiency} = \text{FI} \tag{6.4}$$

An important factor is that since these formulas relate to work, they are a viable proxy for the more accurate measure of efficiency defined by urodynamic means. The other difference with the Griffith formula is that this equation does not account for the total volume in the bladder which can include the PVR and throw off the efficiency significantly as we have seen from our bias and error analysis [4]. Our formula takes the PVR into account, and as seen by the work of Agarwal et al. [10], this method gives better results when total bladder volume is utilized.

Flow Shapes

The concept of flow shapes as something immutable has been propagated in the literature, but in reality, there is little more than conceptual drawings of idealized flow patterns. There are no actual parameters to help identify curves as one or the other except for staccato curves, but even these parameters are quite vague. In our paper [14] "Can a Quantitative Means Be Used to Predict Flow Shapes," we show that flow indexes are clearly capable of defining towers and plateaus. Interrupted and staccato shapes have too much variability to be capable of being predicted. The concept to view flow shapes as fractionated and smooth adds another dimension to the interpretation of flow shapes that strengthens its ability to make it reproducible. Using the flow index as a measure of voiding efficiency, we can describe flows as hyper- or hypoefficient voids. Combining the two measures has resulted in better inter-rater reliability [15] than using the standard five shapes system. Even utilizing this system produces less than auspicious reliability numbers. What can be relied on is that the FI is volume agnostic and can be used to compare disparate volume voids with good reproducibility.

How to Utilize the Flow Index and Modified Shape Methodology

We will present several examples of flows and demonstrate the benefits of using a more quantitative method to analyze the flows.

Example 6.1

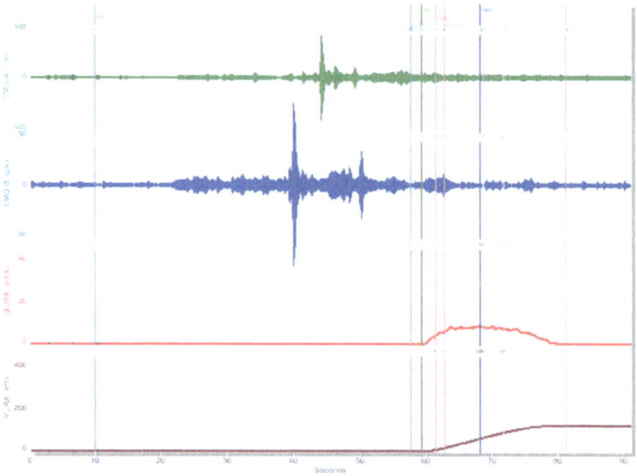

Study Results

Time to Max Flow	: 8.8 *s*	Void Time	: 21.8 *s*
Max Flow Rate	: 8.6 *ml/s*	Flow Time	: 20.0 *s*
Average Flow Rate	: 5.9 *ml/s*	Delay Time	: 49.3 *s*
Voided Volume	: 119.4 *ml*	Post Void	: 3 *ml*
EMG Lag Time	: 1.7 *s*	QMax FI	: 0.5

This is a 9-year-old male with chronic dysuria and some episodes of terminal dysuria along with nocturnal enuresis, with known autism and developmental delays. In this study, we see that there is a dual EMG study with pelvic floor activity in the uppermost line and abdominal EMG in the blue second line. There is some evidence of abdominal wall straining noted in this study in the early voiding phase. It is difficult to ascertain where the lag time would be measured in this case.

A prompt look at the numbers reveals that the Q_{max} flow index is 0.5 and the Q_{avg} flow index is 0.6. Both numbers are below the one standard deviation of 0.7 which would imply that this is out of the normal range and in the plateau curve range. The image is consistent with a plateau shape, but if the graph was drawn differently, it may have easily appeared like a bell. The curve is smooth, and the pelvic EMG does not appear to be active. This combined with low flow indexes would indicate that there may a persistent obstruction, i.e., bladder neck dysfunction, commonly seen in children with autism or a stricture which can develop from dysfunctional voiding. Underactive bladder is another possibility and would be very difficult to prove but cannot be ruled out in this case.

Therefore, this would be described as smooth flow with Q_{avg} FI = 0.6 and Q_{max} FI = 0.5 with PVR of 3 ml.

Example 6.2

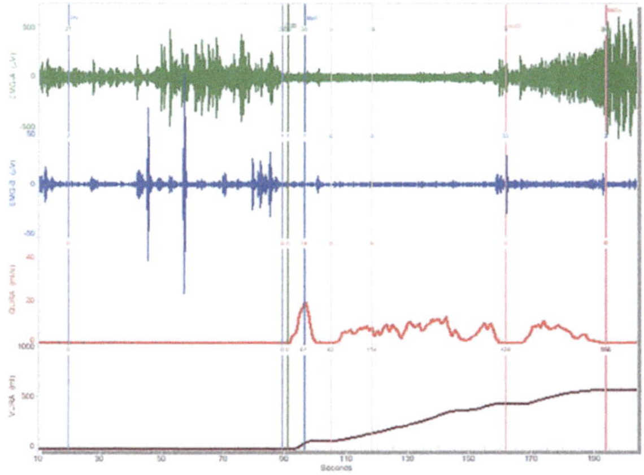

Study Results

Time to Max Flow	: 5.4 *s*	Void Time	: 102.8 *s*
Max Flow Rate	: 18.9 *ml/s*	Flow Time	: 88.2 *s*
Average Flow Rate	: 6.2 *ml/s*	Delay Time	: 71.1 *s*
Voided Volume	: 555.7 *ml*	Post Void	: 0 *ml*
EMG Lag Time	: 1.9 *s*	QMax FI	: 0.6

This is a 17-year-old female with history of segmentation anomalies in thoracic vertebra, left-sided reflux, and elongated bladder with open bladder neck and a normal filum with cord terminating at L2. She has a history of UTIs, incomplete bladder emptying, and nocturnal enuresis. In this study, we see a fractionated flow (elements of interrupted and staccato pattern), while the Q_{max} would be considered normal by most urologist based on standard nomograms and literature. In a quantitative methodology, this is an abnormal uroflow with Q_{max} FI = 0.6 and Q_{avg} FI = 0.5. The pattern is fractionated which typically goes along with some degree of abnormal voiding. The expected average flow rate for this flow is 12.4 ml/s for this patient while the expected Q_{max} is 31.5 ml/s. Examination of the EMG activity for both pelvic and abdominal shows that it is quiet till the last quarter of the study. Then there is abdominal straining and concomitant increase in pelvic floor activity. These findings bode more for a diagnosis of underactive bladder.

Example 6.3

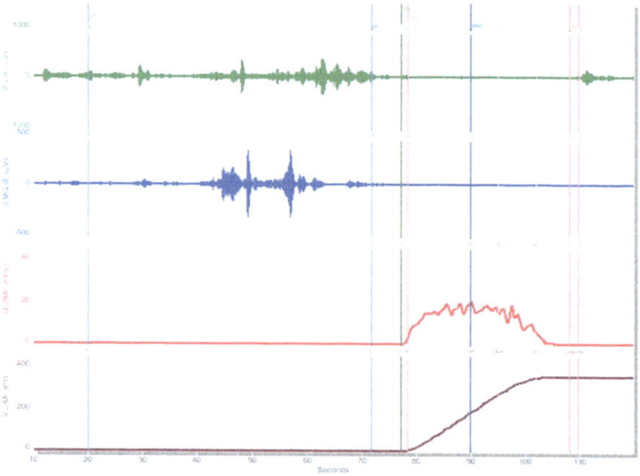

Study Results

Time to Max Flow	: 12.7 *s*	Void Time	: 32.5 *s*
Max Flow Rate	: 20.2 *ml/s*	Flow Time	: 27.8 *s*
Average Flow Rate	: 12.5 *ml/s*	Delay Time	: 57.1 *s*
Voided Volume	: 348.4 *ml*	Post Void	: 12 *ml*
EMG Lag Time	: 5.5 *s*	QMax FI	: 0.6

The patient is a 12-year-old female with a history of nocturnal enuresis and a mass noted by the bladder neck on ultrasound. This study represents a case of what appears to be a smooth bell curve with diminished peak flow rate in a 12-year-old female. We know that this is a smooth curve and the perturbations in the curve are due to how the urine hits the receptacle and is registered and not due to pelvic floor or abdominal activity because the EMG is quite during the curve production and the classic termination spike is evident at the end of voiding in the green uppermost curve. This helps verify that the EMG is still active and working properly.

This curve is not an ideal bell in effect since there is a diminished Q_{max} FI =0.6 which can be indicative of a potential bladder neck dysfunction or in this case an abnormal fold of tissue that was confirmed on cystoscopy. Q_{max} FI is diminished but we have achieved a Q_{avg} FI = 0.8 which is in the normal range. A closer look at the lag time indicates that it is almost 6 secs which is the cutoff for bladder neck dysfunction as outlined by Glassberg and Combs [16].

Example 6.4

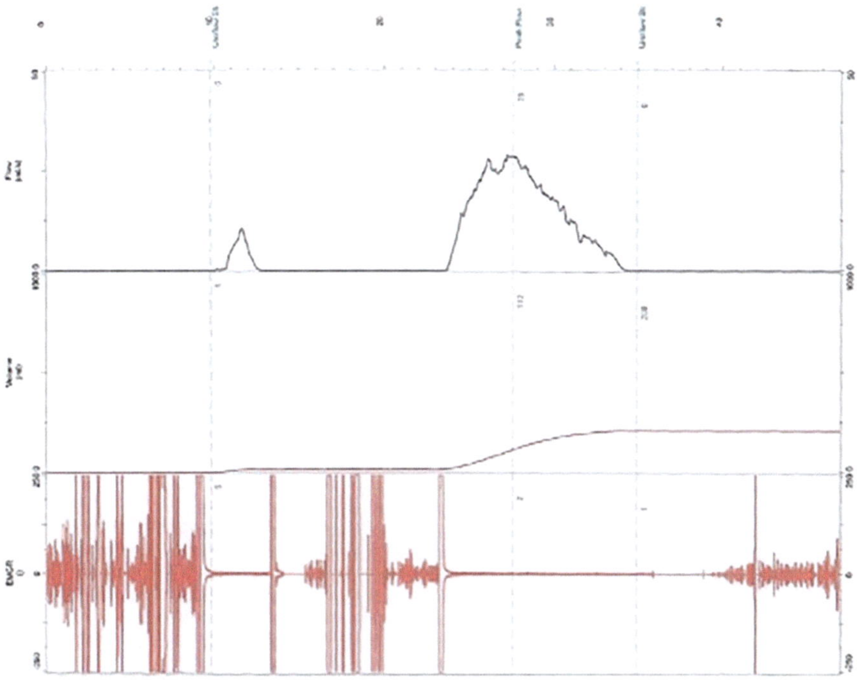

In this scenario, we have a 5-year-old female with a voided volume of 207 cc and a post-void residual of 18 cc that has a void with two peaks. How do we describe this void? Is it interrupted or is it a tower void? Utilizing the quantitative method, we can describe this as a fractionated void which when we look at the Q_{max} FI = 1.16 and Q_{avg} FI = 1.23 would qualify it as a bell curve based on the criteria that have been set of 0.7–1.3 as the bell interval. In reality, it does not matter. What we know is that this child regardless of the interruption in her flow has voided faster than expected for the volume in her bladder. Unfortunately, she has not emptied all the way which is likely due to the fact that she seems to have a very short lag time indicative of what we see with children with urgency. The initial delay in voiding where energy builds up and is dissipated can contribute to elevated residuals in these cases.

Example 6.5

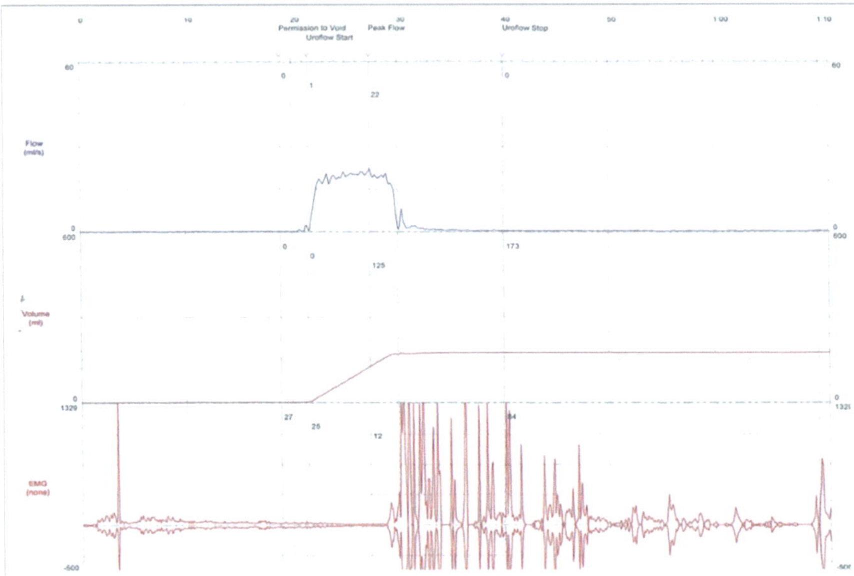

What type of curve is this? Doesn't look like a bell based on the ICCS and ICS curve descriptions. The VV = 173 and the PVR = 25 in this 7-year-old female patient. What we can safely say is that the curve is smooth and that the Qmax FI = 0.94 and Qavg FI = 1.07 which would safely fall in the bell curve category, but a closer look at the EMG reveals that there is a very prolonged lag time and the curve indicates that there is a very sudden rise with a delay in achieving peak velocity till late in the flow. Peak flow velocity is expected to be achieved within the first 50 mls of flow based on work by Rollema and Griffiths [17], and in this case, Qmax is not achieved till about ¾ through the flow. Again, the high flow velocities are indicative of a good contraction with some component of obstruction which in this case is likely the bladder neck due to lack of EMG activity during the void. The shape itself does not fall into any category, and describing this shape as a bell would be an injustice since this would lead people to assume that this is a normal void, which clearly it is not.

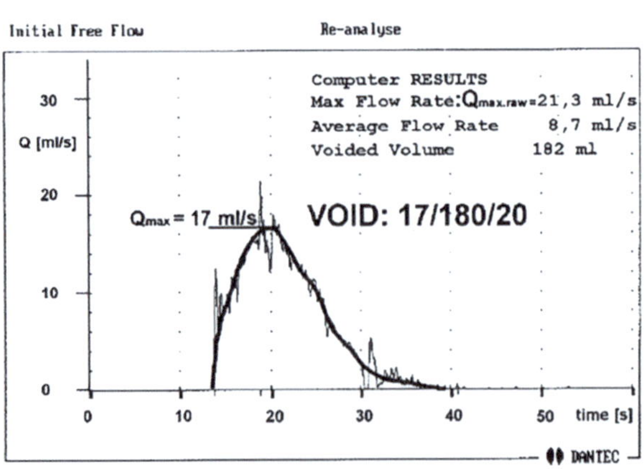

What we can safely say is that the curve is smooth and that the Q_{max} FI = 0.94 and Q_{avg} FI = 1.07 which would safely fall in the bell curve category, but a closer look at the EMG reveals that there is a very prolonged lag time and the curve indicates that there is a very sudden rise with a delay in achieving peak velocity till late in the flow. Peak flow velocity is expected to be achieved within the first 50 mls of flow based on work by Rollema and Griffiths [17], and in this case, Q_{max} is not achieved till about ¾ through the flow. Again, the high flow velocities are indicative of a good contraction with some component of obstruction which in this case is likely the bladder neck due to lack of EMG activity during the void. The shape itself does not fall into any category, and describing this shape as a bell would be an injustice since this would lead people to assume that this is a normal void, which clearly it is not.

Example 6.6

The Danger of Not Obtaining a PVR

A 14-year-old female with recurrent UTIs and the following uroflow parameters: VV = 671 cc, PVR = 250 cc, Q_{avg} = 23.9, expected Q_{avg} = 31.88, Q_{avg} FI = 0.74

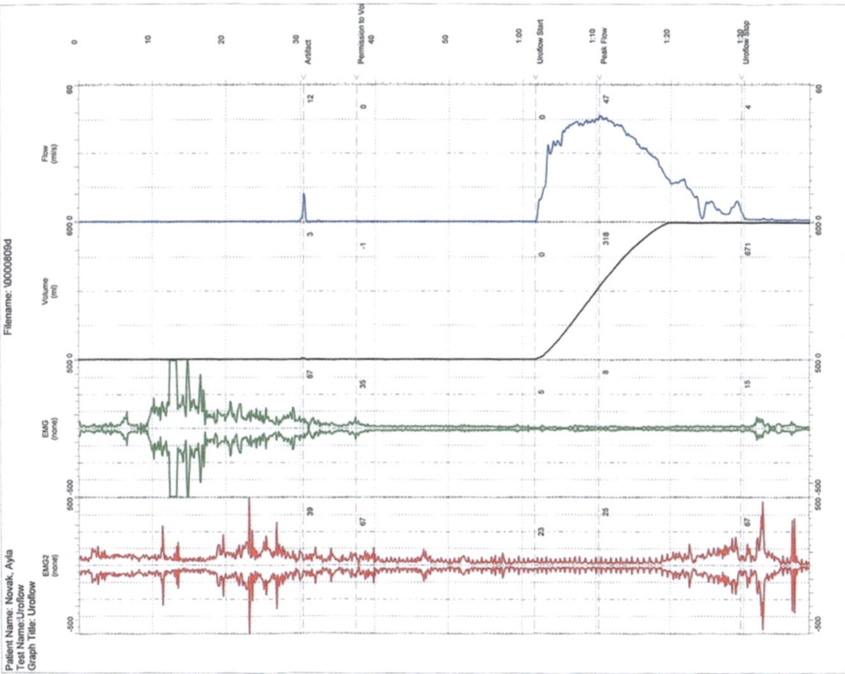

Q_{max} = 47, expected Q_{max} = 42.34, and Q_{max} FI = 1.11 with a smooth curve. Unfortunately, there is a PVR = 250 cc in this case and which indicates that this is a very abnormal void for this patient. A cursory look at the flow curve would have led anyone to believe this was a normal void. If she would not have had a PVR = 250 cc, the expected Q_{max} = 40.66 for a VV = 671 would lead to a Q_{max} FI = 1.15. This underscores the effect of overdistention on the bladder which leads to reductions in flow velocity as seen here.

Examination of the distance between the green line reveals that the lag time in this case approaches 20 secs which was confirmed on the voiding cystourethrogram that there is significant bladder neck dysfunction and high-grade reflux. The small blip in the blue line 30 secs before the large bladder contraction is motion artefact.

A quantitative approach in this case tells us that there is a discrepancy between the Q_{max} FI and the Q_{avg} FI which should alert us to the idea that something is abnormal.

By having all the tools available to us, we can clearly put together a diagnosis of underactive bladder and bladder neck dysfunction in this scenario. The bladder neck dysfunction if it persists through voiding generally leads to a plateau curve pattern as well as Q_{avg} FI below 0.7, which we are approaching. We do not see this; in this case, we see a contraction that naturally decays which is indicative of early fatigue seen in underactive bladders.

Example 6.7

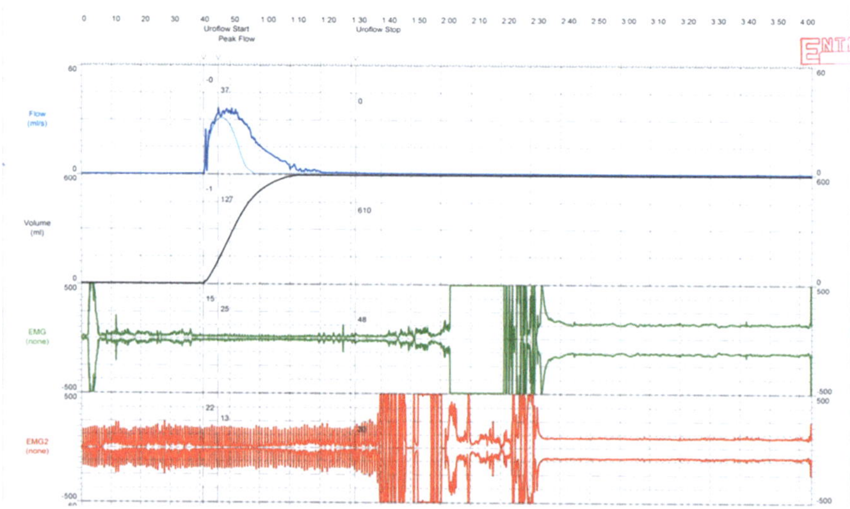

The patient is a 7-year-old male with urge incontinence, VV = 611, PVR = 26, Q_{max} = 36.6, Q_{avg} = 13.1, estimated Q_{max} = 35.79, estimated Q_{avg} = 11.78, Q_{max} FI = 1.02, and Q_{avg} FI = 1.11. The findings if looked at by standard means would indicate that this is an abnormal void based on the very high Q_{max}. In reality, both the Q_{max} and Q_{avg} are in the normal range for a bell curve and there is no increased EMG activity. This is a normal void except that it is a large-volume void.

Example 6.8

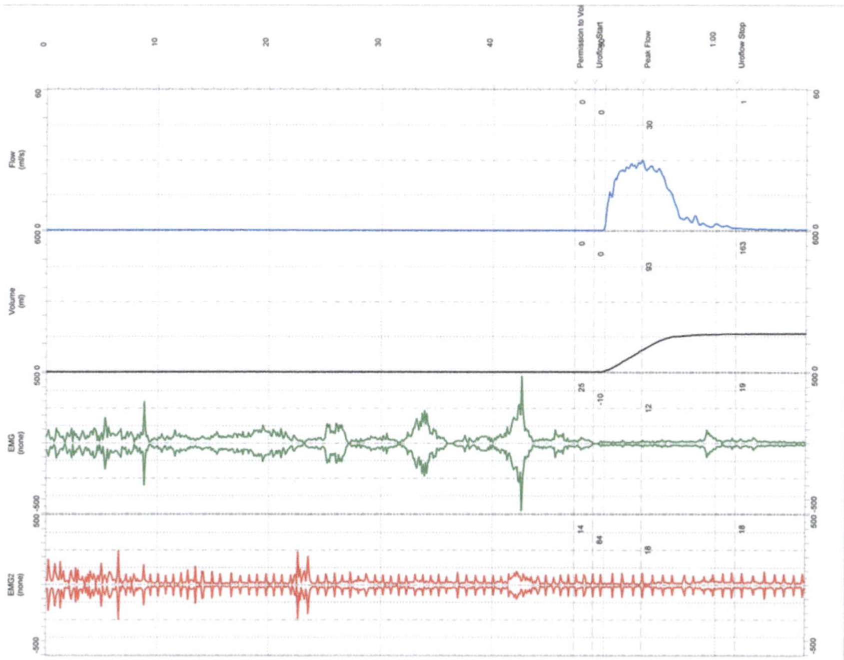

The patient is a 13-year-old male with urge incontinence, VV = 163, PVR = 13, Q_{max} = 30.2, Q_{avg} = 13.6, estimated Q_{max} = 22.11, estimated Q_{avg} = 13.21, Q_{max} FI = 1.02, ad Q_{avg} FI = 1.36.

The patient has a short lag time and the Q_{max} FI is 1.36 which is consistent with a tower void even though the curve appears to be in the shape of a bell.

In the quantitative method, this would be described as a smooth curve with a Q_{max} FI = 1.36 and Q_{avg} FI = 1.02. We would know that the patient voided with a smooth curve with some increased efficiency in achieving the *Qmax* indicating that the void is occurring faster than the normal patient. This finding is consistent with a child with urgency.

Example 6.9

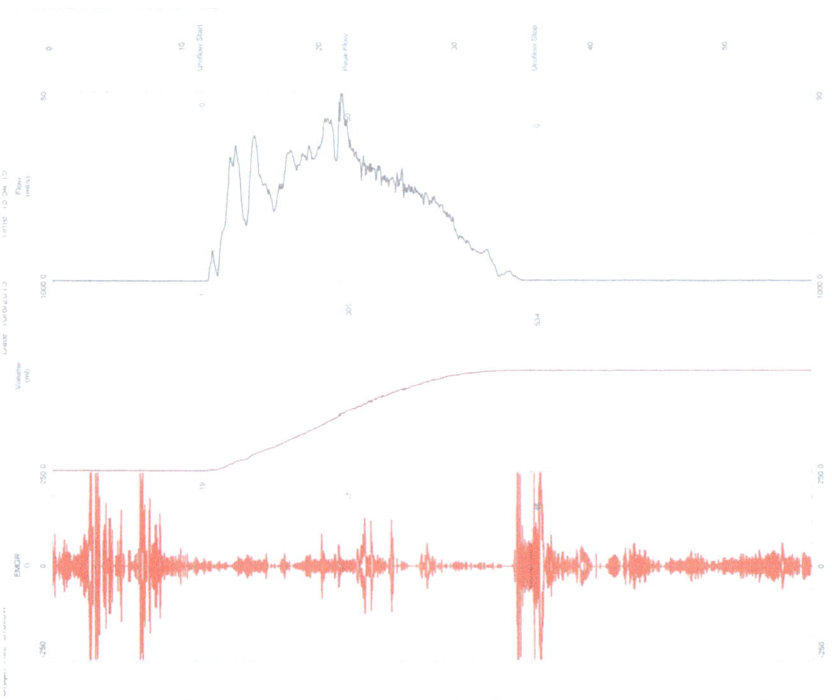

Patient is a 12-year-old male with VV = 533, PVR = 28, Q_{max} = 50.0, and Q_{avg} = 22.3. The question here is that this curve again does not fit in well in the standard ICCS paradigm. Is it a tower void or a staccato void? What really matters is that the flow appears to be fractionated and the EMG supports that with increased activity during the flow time, there are drops and spikes in the curve.

To assess whether this is a hypervoider or not, we need to know what the expected flow indexes are for this patient. Estimated Q_{max} = 35.54 yielding a Q_{max} FI = 1.4 and estimated Q_{avg} = 13.38 which yields a Q_{avg} FI = 1.6. The data is consistent with a hypervoider with a fractionated void. Using the ICCS nomenclature would not allow us to adequately describe this curve. Using the quantitative method, we can immediately properly visualize this void in our head without seeing it.

Conclusion

Understanding the basic laws of fluid dynamics allows the reader to have a better understanding of the processes involved in quantification of uroflowmetry. With a better understanding of what is being measured, we can then come to think about some of the problems we encounter in the field and begin to explain them in terms of the pathophysiology which makes greater sense. Not knowing and understanding the mechanics makes interpretation of the results like obtaining results from a black box, where we are disconnected from process and lack an understanding of what really is going on.

Declarations

Competing Interests The author(s) has no competing interests to declare that are relevant to the content of this manuscript.

Ethics Approval The author(s) declares that this manuscript does not include primary research with human participants.

The author(s) declares that this manuscript does not include primary studies involving animals.

References

1. Drake WM Jr. The uroflowmeter; an aid to the study of the lower urinary tract. J Urol. 1948;59(4):650–8.
2. Franco I, Shei-Dei Yang S, Chang SJ, Nussenblatt B, Franco JA. A quantitative approach to the interpretation of uroflowmetry in children. Neurourol Urodyn. 2016;35(7):836–46.
3. Netto JMB, Hittelman A, Lambert S, Murphy K, Collette-Gardere T, Franco I. Interpretation of uroflow curves: a global survey measuring inter and intra rater reliability. Neurourol Urodyn. 2020;39(2):826–32.
4. Franco I, Franco JA, Nussenblatt B. Can the idealized voider derived flow indexes be a measure of voiding efficiency and how accurate are they? Neurourol Urodyn. 2018;37(6):1913–24.
5. Bottacini M, Gleason D. Clinical neuro-urology. 1st ed. Boston: Little, Brown; 1979. p. xvi. 309 p.
6. Bottaccini MR, Gleason DM. Fluid mechanics of micturition. In: Krane RJ, Siroky MB, editors. Clinical neuro-urology. Boston: Little, Brown and Company; 1991. p. 93–108.
7. Von Garrelts B. Micturition in the normal male. Acta Chir Scand. 1958;114(3):197–210.
8. Griffiths DJ, Constantinou CE, van Mastrigt R. Urinary bladder function and its control in healthy females. Am J Phys. 1986;251(2 Pt 2):R225–30.
9. Mattsson S, Spangberg A. Flow rate nomograms in 7- to 16-year-old healthy children. Neurourol Urodyn. 1994;13(3):267–80.
10. Agarwal MM, Patil S, Roy K, Bandawar M, Choudhury S, Mavuduru R, et al. Rationalization of interpretation of uroflowmetry for a non-caucasian (Indian) population: conceptual development and validation of volume-normalized flow rate index. Neurourol Urodyn. 2014;33(1):135–41.
11. Yang SS, Chiang IN, Hsieh CH, Chang SJ. The Tzu Chi nomograms for maximum urinary flow rate (Qmax) in children: comparison with Miskolc nomogram. BJU Int. 2014;113(3):492–7.
12. Bosch JL, Kranse R, van Mastrigt R, Schroder FH. Dependence of male voiding efficiency on age, bladder contractility and urethral resistance: development of a voiding efficiency nomogram. J Urol. 1995;154(1):190–4.
13. Pulvino JQ, Duecy EE, Buchsbaum GM, Flynn MK. Comparison of 2 techniques to predict voiding efficiency after inpatient urogynecologic surgery. J Urol. 2010;184(4):1408–12.
14. Franco I, Franco J, Lee YS, Choi EK, Han SW. Can a quantitative means be used to predict flow patterns: agreement between visual inspection vs. flow index derived flow patterns. J Pediatr Urol. 2016;12(4):218e1–8.

15. Van Batavia JP, Pohl HG, Farhat WA, Chiang G, BaniHani A, Collett-Gardere T, et al. Is it time to reconsider how we document pediatric uroflow studies?: a study from the SPU voiding dysfunction task force. J Pediatr Urol. 2023;19(5):546–54.
16. Combs AJ, Grafstein N, Horowitz M, Glassberg KI. Primary bladder neck dysfunction in children and adolescents I: pelvic floor electromyography lag time--a new noninvasive method to screen for and monitor therapeutic response. J Urol. 2005;173(1):207–10; discussion 10–1.
17. Rollema HJ, Griffiths DJ, van Duyl WA, van den Berg J, de Haan R. Flow rate versus bladder volume. An alternative way of presenting some features of the micturition of healthy males. Urol Int. 1977;32(5):401–12.

Electromyography

7

Anne Wright and Poonam Guha Vaze

The combined action, the detrusor contraction, which pushes out the urine vis-a-vis state of relaxation of bladder neck and striated muscles of external sphincter and pelvic floor dictates the urinary flow. The activity of the last group of muscles is evaluated by the electromyography (EMG). It is the study of the electrical potentials generated by the depolarization of the perineal muscles.

When the bladder is filling up, the tone of the pelvic muscles/external sphincter gradually increases which reflects as increase in EMG activity. Sphincteric relaxation occurs as the first step of micturition which is followed by bladder neck relaxation, initiation of detrusor contraction and appearance of flow. Sphincteric relaxation is documented as EMG silencing which is seen immediately prior to voiding.

Practical Points

Surface Versus Needle

There are two types of electrodes—needle and surface. For all practical purposes, pediatric uroflowmetry always is done using surface electrodes.

A. Wright
The Children's Bladder Clinic, Evelina London Children's Hospital, London, UK
e-mail: Anne.Wright@gstt.nhs.uk

P. G. Vaze (✉)
Neotia Bhagirathi Woman and Child Care Centre, Newtown, Kolkata, India

Department of Pediatric Surgery, Nilratan Sircar Medical College and Hospital, Kolkata, India

S. Saha, P. Guha Vaze (eds.), *Comprehensive Atlas of Practical Pediatric Urodynamics*, https://doi.org/10.1007/978-981-95-2709-0_7

Types of Surface EMG Electrodes

Two types of electrodes are available—'snap on' and 'wired' (Fig. 7.1a, b). 'Snap-on' electrodes are more cost-effective in the long run as simple pediatric-sized ECG electrodes can be used which are rather cheap and universally available. EMG can be used for all patients irrespective of indication in the learning phase. Some machines work with wired electrodes, for example, wired neonatal 'dot' ECG electrodes. Fresh set of the electrodes along with the wire will be used for every patient. The running cost may be higher than snap-on electrodes.

Application

They are applied to the perineum, just anterior to the anus, at position eleven and one o' clock. It is important that the electrodes do not touch each other as this creates artefact. A grounding/reference electrode is applied 20 cm away from the primary electrodes—over a bony prominence (with no underlying muscle) such as the sacrum or iliac crest. The area of application should be absolutely dry, else the electrode will not stick; it should ideally be cleaned with alcohol gel, be dry and hairless. When using EMG during UDS, it may be preferable to apply the EMG electrode before inserting the rectal catheter as jelly used for rectal catheter insertion makes application of EMG electrode difficult.

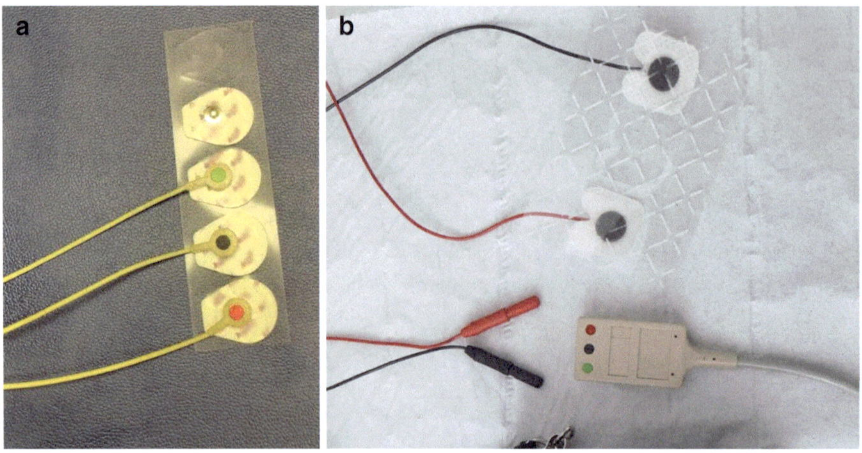

Fig. 7.1 Different types of surface EMG electrodes—'snap on' (**a**) and 'wired' (**b**). (Image courtesy (**a**): Dr. Jyoti Sharma, Consultant Pediatric Nephrologist, KEM Hospital, Mumbai)

Wetting Artefact

If urine falls on the electrode, it creates noise in the EMG reading as it is electrolyte-rich solution (Fig. 7.2a, b). So we routinely apply an adhesive barrier dressing on it to prevent wetting especially in girls and in boys who void in sitting position (Fig. 7.3).

Checking Working of the Electrodes

During coughing, there is reflex sphincteric contraction. So patient is asked to cough which causes an increase in EMG activity, thus confirming that the electrodes are working (Fig. 7.4).

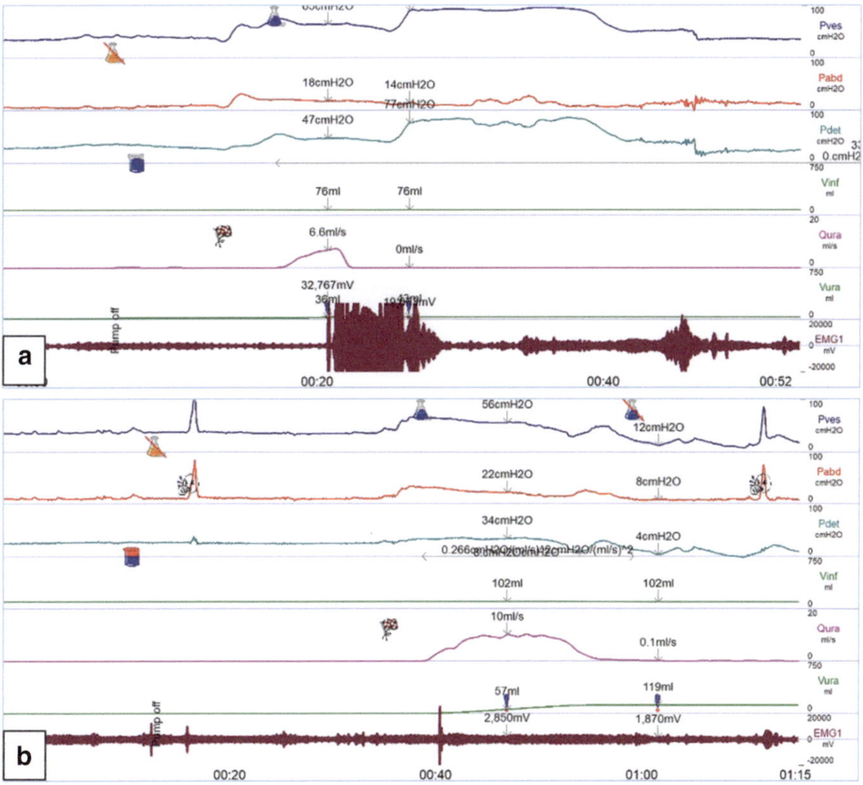

Fig. 7.2 EMG during *i*-UDS showing wetting artefact during the first void (**a**), whereas the second void (**b**) shows the actual EMG tracing when a barrier dressing is applied over it

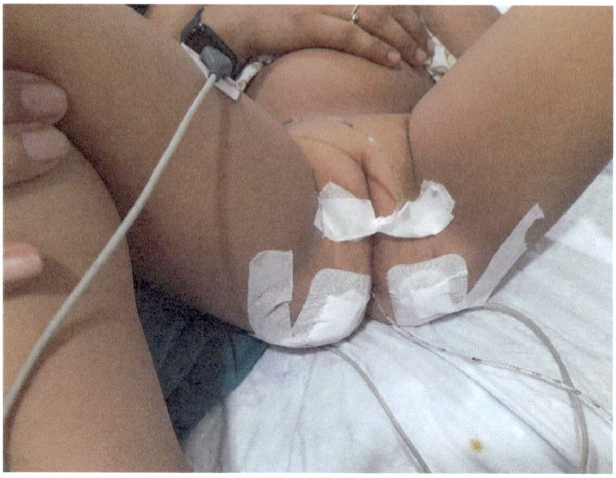

Fig. 7.3 Waterproof barrier dressing applied over the perineal EMG electrodes prevents wetting of the electrodes

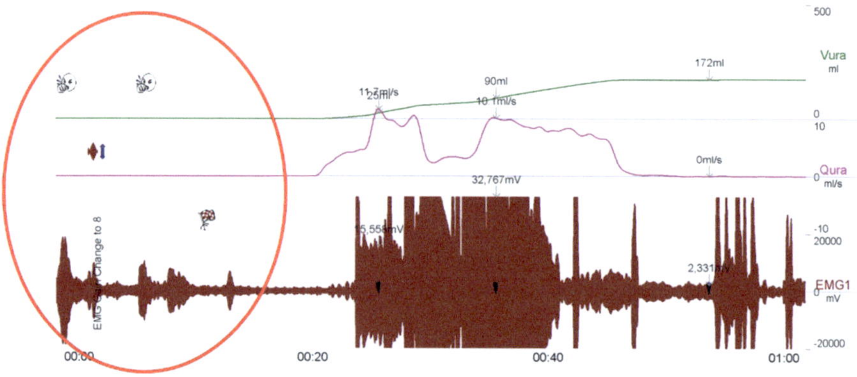

Fig. 7.4 EMG deflections checked when patient is asked to cough to (red circled portion of the tracing) confirm that the electrodes are working

Normal and Abnormal EMG Activity

Normally, the EMG activity is supposed to be absolutely silent throughout the void. Any abnormal EMG activity during voiding, which is substantiated by repeated assessments, and corroborates with the clinical scenario, suggests dysfunctional voiding (non-neurogenic)/detrusor sphincter dyssynergia (neurogenic dysfunction). Different patterns of abnormal EMG activity have been documented (Figs. 7.5, 7.6, 7.7, 7.8 and 7.9).

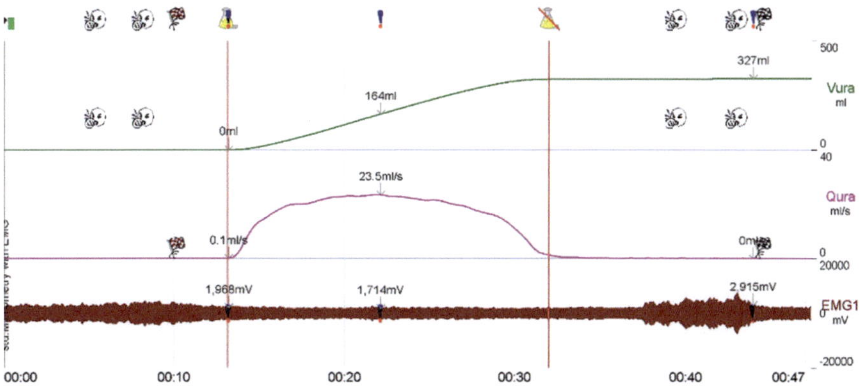

Fig. 7.5 Bell-shaped uroflowmetry curve with adequate EMG silencing during void

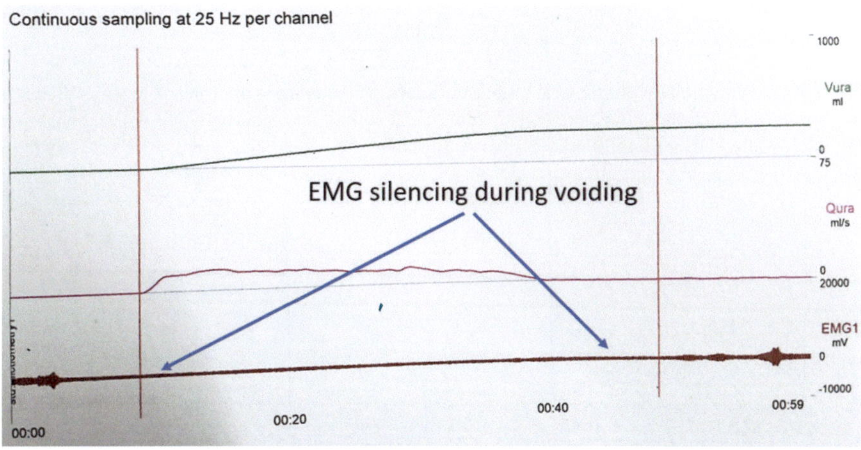

Fig. 7.6 Plateau-shaped uroflowmetry curve with normal EMG silencing during voiding

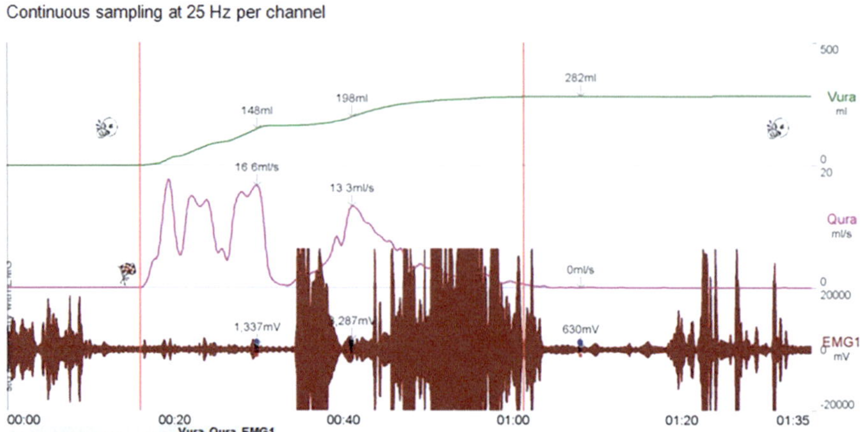

No	Icon	Description	Time	Vura ml	Qura ml/s	EMG1 mV
1		Cough	00:12			
2		Start void	00:14	0	0	1,074
4	!	Value Highlight	00:30	148	17	1,337
5	!	Value Highlight	00:41	198	13	3,287
7	!	Value Highlight	01:08	282	0	630
8		Cough	01:31			

Fig. 7.7 Dysfunctional voiding with a staccato/interrupted stream in an 8-year-old girl with bladder-bowel dysfunction with severe constipation, fecal soiling and recurrent UTI with USG showing thick-walled UB with mild bilateral pelvic fullness

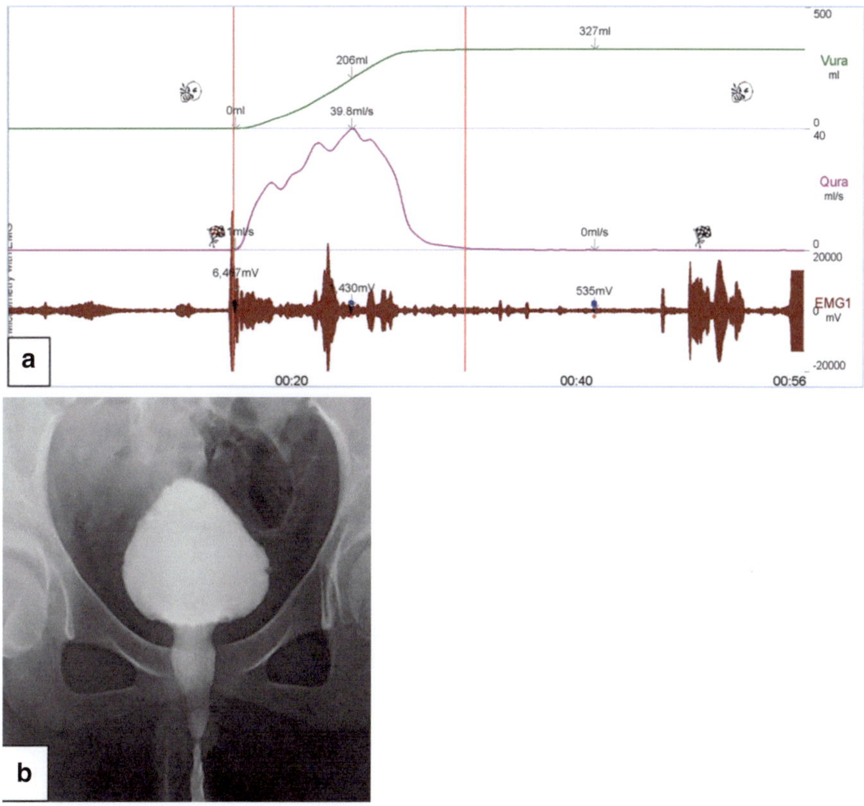

Fig. 7.8 (**a**, **b**) Dysfunctional voiding in a 10-year-old girl with bladder-bowel dysfunction with urgency incontinence/repeated UTI. Note that dysfunctional voiding may be seen with seemingly normal-appearing bell-shaped curves also

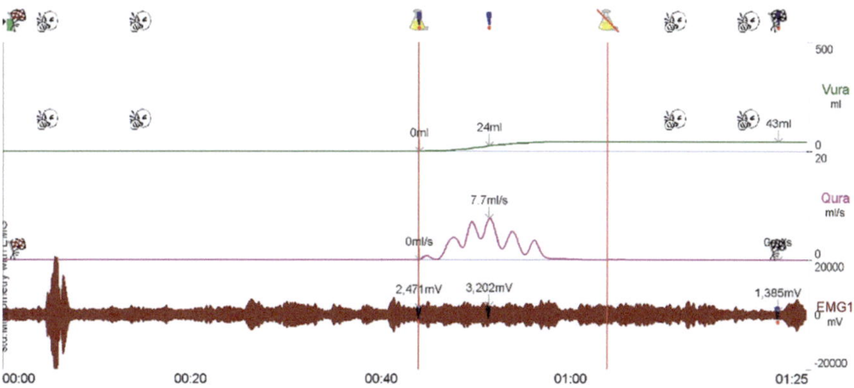

Fig. 7.9 Staccato curve with increased EMG activity throughout voiding. A 12-year-old girl, h/o transverse myelitis 5 months ago; having recurrent UTI with urgency, urge incontinence and significant PVR on USG—neurogenic DSD

EMG Activity During Invasive UDS

Abnormal EMG activity can also be noted while performing *i*-UDS during the filling and/or voiding phase (Figs. 7.10 and 7.11). Finding of increased EMG activity during voiding in the presence of catheter may be unreliable in non-neurogenic setting, as presence of catheter may cause some sphincteric irritation and resultant increase in EMG activity—it should be corroborated with EMG activity during free flow uroflowmetry.

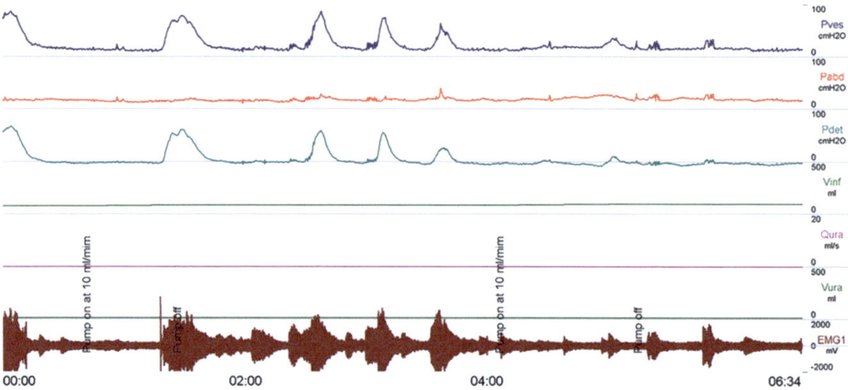

Fig. 7.10 An 8-year-old male child, known case of prematurity/perinatal hypoxic insult and cerebral palsy. He had history of recurrent episodes of UTI with bilateral gross VUR—underwent right-sided ureterostomy 2 years ago since when he has been stable. This is a segment of UDS tracing showing detrusor overactivity and increased EMG activity noted during all the episodes of detrusor overactivity

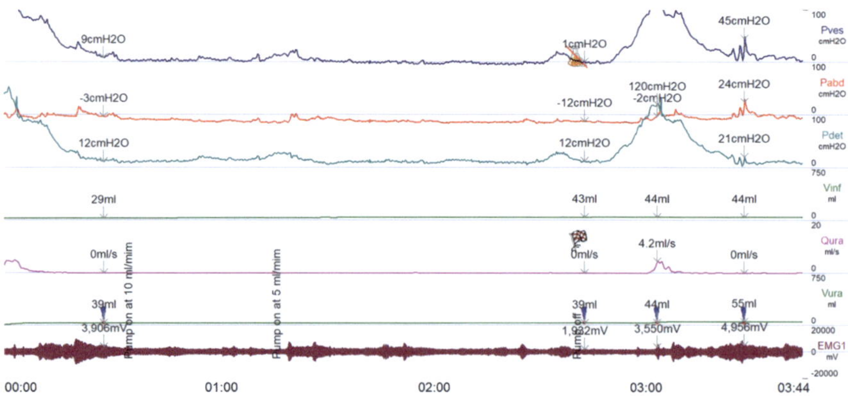

Fig. 7.11 A 12-year-old male child, known case of cerebral palsy. He had increased urinary frequency with poor urinary stream and episodes of UTI. Invasive UDS showed small-capacity bladder with detrusor overactivity. The figure shows a segment of UDS tracing showing a voiding contraction with high pressure void, poor flow rates and increased EMG activity during voiding, more in later half of the contraction. In children with spastic cerebral palsy, pseudo-DSD can be noted because of perineal muscle spasm

EMG Lag Time

It is the delay between silencing of EMG activity and appearance of flow on uroflowmetry curve. Normal EMG lag time is 2–6 sec. A short lag time of <2 sec signifies detrusor overactivity. A prolonged lag time of >6 sec and a depressed, often right-shifted, uroflow curve with quiet pelvic floor during voiding with LUTS, particularly hesitancy, suggests primary bladder neck dysfunction (Figs. 7.12, 7.13 and 7.14).

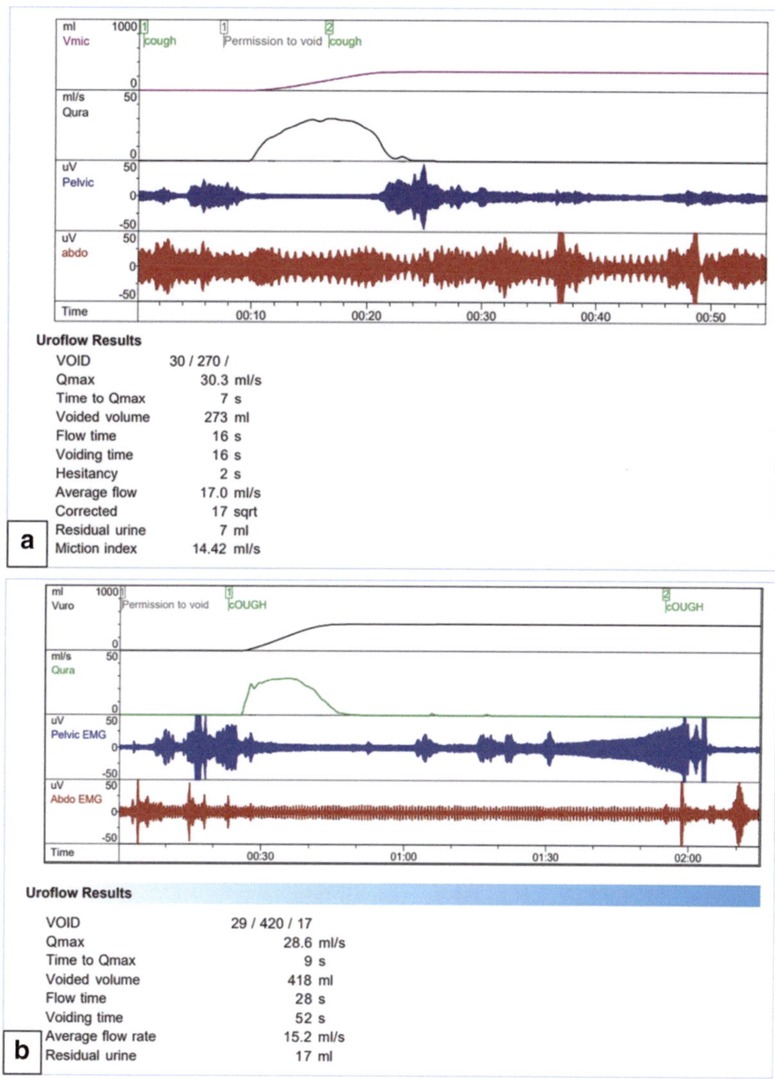

Fig. 7.12 An 11-year-old boy with day- and night-time wetting. Note that the scale in these flows is altered so that the y axis is reduced compared to the standard uroflowmetry ratio, and the bell shape is actually probably more like a tower. First uroflowmetry (**a**) was recorded at baseline. EMG lag time is reduced along with tower-shaped curve suggesting detrusor overactivity. (**b**) Same boy on treatment with trospium with better symptom control but ongoing evidence of urgency

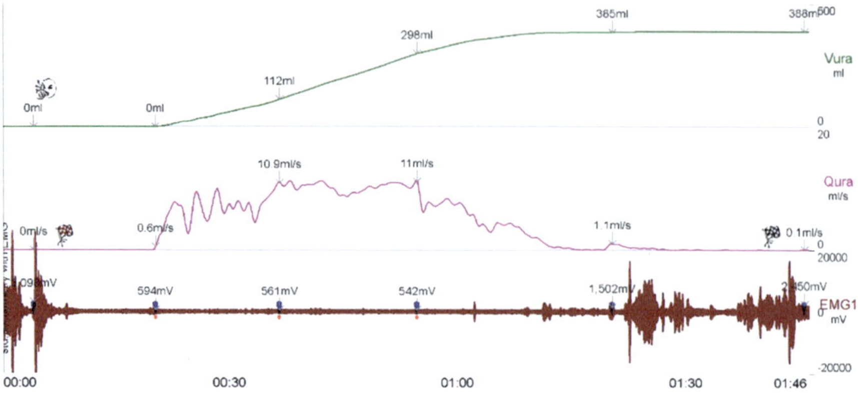

Fig. 7.13 EMG lag time of around 12 sec. EMG activity was seen to reduce immediately after command to void. Flow was recorded around 12 sec later suggesting a prolonged lag time (> 6 sec)

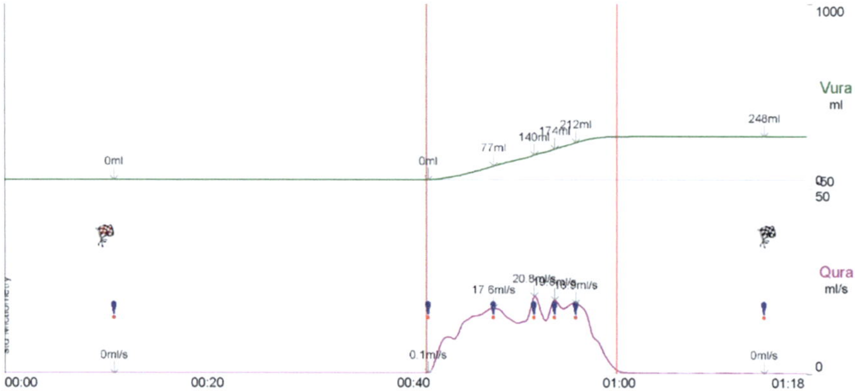

Fig. 7.14 Indirect evidence of increased lag time—delay of around 30 sec between command to void and beginning of flow. A 12-year-old child with history of hesitancy. The investigator was present during the study to observe the patient

Role of Dual-Channel EMG

If a patient strains while passing urine, there will be increase in EMG activity of the perineal muscles as well as the abdominal muscles, and perineal muscles contract as a capsule. Thus, it may give a false impression of dysfunctional voiding. For assessing contraction of the abdominal muscles simultaneously, a second set of electrodes is applied on the lower abdominal wall (Fig. 7.15) which can differentiate between true dysfunctional voiding and Valsalva voiding. In invasive urodynamics, the rectal catheter cancels the abdominal contractions, but in non-invasive uroflowmetry, the abdominal EMG becomes helpful.

In certain cases, dual EMG can differentiate between differing underlying causes of abnormal voiding (Figs. 7.16, 7.17 and 7.18). In an obstructed void, the lack of

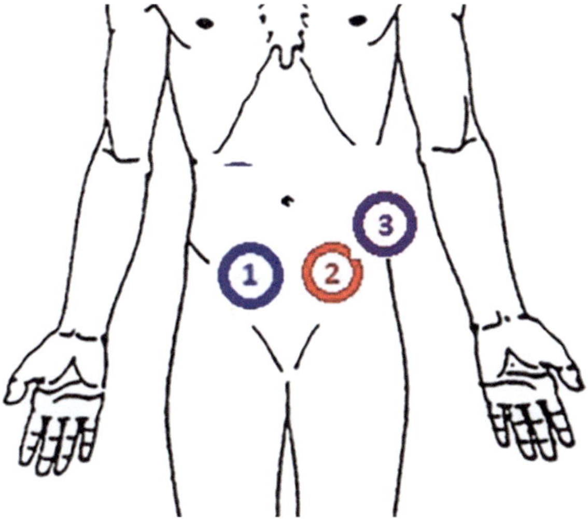

Fig. 7.15 Placement of EMG electrodes on abdominal wall

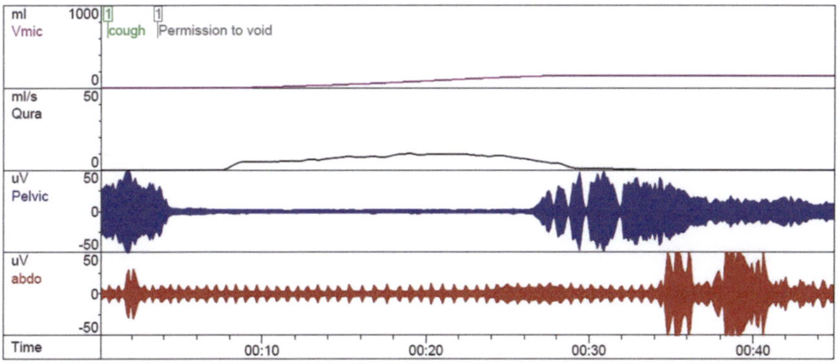

Uroflow Results

VOID	10 / 150 /
Qmax	10.0 ml/s
Time to Qmax	11 s
Voided volume	153 ml
Flow time	25 s
Voiding time	25 s
Hesitancy	4 s
Average flow	6.0 ml/s
Corrected	12 sqrt
Residual urine	6 ml
Miction index	3.67 ml/s

Fig. 7.16 A 12-year-old boy with treatment-resistant nocturnal enuresis with small-capacity bladder on diary and normal KUB ultrasound. OAB assumed to be underlying cause but uroflowmetry reveals obstructed flows with no evidence of dysfunctional voiding or abdominal straining pointing to anatomical obstruction; cystoscopy reveals late diagnosis PUV

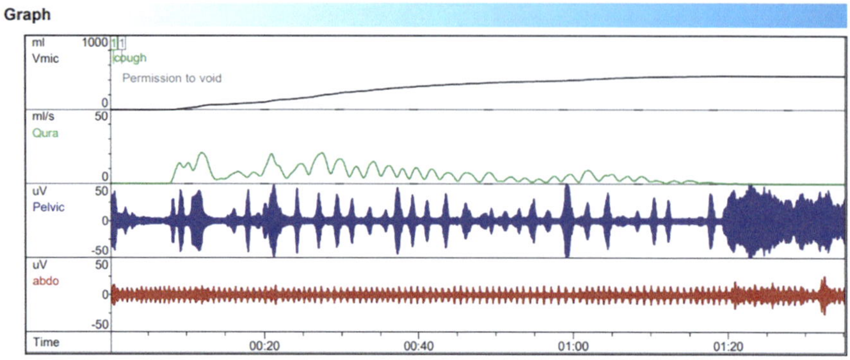

Uroflow Results

VOID	21 / 460 / 5
Qmax	20.8 ml/s
Time to Qmax	4 s
Voided volume	461 ml
Flow time	74 s
Voiding time	75 s
Average flow rate	6.3 ml/s
Residual urine	5 ml

Fig. 7.17 A 16-year-old girl with voiding postponement due to dislike of public toilets. She had history of infrequent voiding, poor flow and some difficulties with initiation and recent episode of urinary retention. Based on the history, she was believed to have underactive detrusor. Uroflow reveals dysfunctional voiding with no abdominal straining and complete emptying. Biofeedback therapy was successful

abdominal/pelvic floor activity points to an anatomical obstruction versus a functional obstruction. In the case of a staccato or interrupted flow, it can help with distinguishing between dysfunctional voiding and an underactive detrusor.

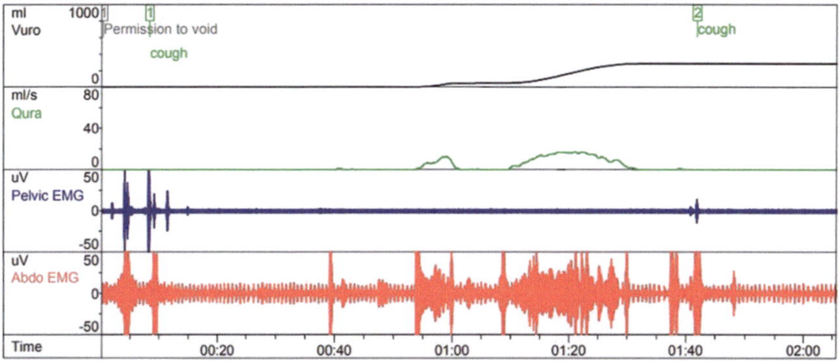

Uroflow Results

Qmax	16.7 ml/s
Time to Qmax	38 s
Voided volume	285 ml
Flow time	35 s
Voiding time	60 s
Average flow	8.1 ml/s
Residual urine	3 ml

Fig. 7.18 A 10-year-old girl with episodes of day- and night-time urinary incontinence and dislike of school toilets. Increasing difficulty with initiating voiding. MRI spine normal. Probable diagnoses were voiding postponer or dysfunctional voider. Uroflow/EMG shows poor flow pattern with abdominal contraction and no perineal EMG activity, thus suggesting underactive detrusor contraction with Valsalva voiding. This was further confirmed on urodynamics and she was started on CIC

Declarations

Competing Interests The author(s) has no competing interests to declare that are relevant to the content of this manuscript.

Ethics Approval The author(s) declares that this manuscript does not include primary research with human participants.

The author(s) declares that this manuscript does not include primary studies involving animals.

Suggested Reading

1. Babu R, Gopinath V. Role of uroflowmetry with electromyography in the evaluation of children with lower urinary tract dysfunction. Indian J Urol. 2015;31(4):354–7. https://doi.org/10.4103/0970-1591.166469. PMID: 26604449; PMCID: PMC4626922.
2. Bercovich S, Morag R, Sivan B, et al. A comparative study between EMG uroflowmetry with and without a catheter in children. BMC Urol. 2024;24:196. https://doi.org/10.1186/s12894-024-01575-9.
3. Clothier JC, Wright AJ. Dysfunctional voiding: the importance of non-invasive urodynamics in diagnosis and treatment. Pediatr Nephrol. 2018;33:381–94. https://doi.org/10.1007/s00467-017-3679-3.

4. Combs AJ, Van Batavia JP, Horowitz M, Glassberg KI. Short pelvic floor electromyographic lag time: a novel noninvasive approach to document detrusor overactivity in children with lower urinary tract symptoms. J Urol. 2013;189(6):2282–6. https://doi.org/10.1016/j.juro.2013.01.011. Epub 2013 Jan 9.
5. Samijn B, Van Laecke E, Vande Walle J, Pascal A, Deschepper E, Renson C, Van den Broeck C. Uroflow measurement combined with electromyography testing of the pelvic floor in healthy children. Neurourol Urodyn. 2019;38(1):231–8. https://doi.org/10.1002/nau.23836. Epub 2018 Oct 12.
6. Van Batavia JP, Combs AJ, Fast AM, Glassberg KI. Use of non-invasive uroflowmetry with simultaneous electromyography to monitor patient response to treatment for lower urinary tract conditions. J Pediatr Urol. 2014;10(3):532–7. https://doi.org/10.1016/j.jpurol.2013.11.015. Epub 2013 Dec 17.

8 When Do We Need Invasive UDS? The "UDS Question"

Poonam Guha Vaze and Jyoti Sharma

i-UDS gives us a wealth of information about the functioning of the urinary bladder, but being invasive, its indications are restricted.

The data obtained from the study may:

- Provide insight into the diagnosis—where the diagnosis is not clear
- Direct treatment approach—in cases which do not show response to conventional treatment
- Give us a baseline information about bladder function so that any change or worsening in the future can be compared with

i-UDS has a concrete role in management of patients with known neurogenic etiology and in certain follow-up cases of PUV; its role in management of patients of non-neurogenic/functional bladder dysfunction is controversial.

Irrespective of the indication of the study, it is important to analyze why do we need the study. The "UDS question(s)"—in other words, the points in the diagnosis or treatment planning that are missing from the available investigation results which we want to be answered by the *i*-UDS—needs to be framed before performing or ordering an *i*-UDS (Fig. 8.1). These questions help us to perform/plan the test in a way so that all the questions are answered appropriately—how to go about the study, how many cycles, what provocations to ask for, any special maneuvers needed, when to ask patient to void, and so on. This makes the results of the study valuable in treatment planning.

P. G. Vaze (✉)
Neotia Bhagirathi Woman and Child Care Centre, Newtown, Kolkata, India

Department of Pediatric Surgery, Nilratan Sircar Medical College and Hospital, Kolkata, India

J. Sharma
Pediatric Nephrologist, KEM Hospital, Pune, India

S. Saha, P. Guha Vaze (eds.), *Comprehensive Atlas of Practical Pediatric Urodynamics*, https://doi.org/10.1007/978-981-95-2709-0_8

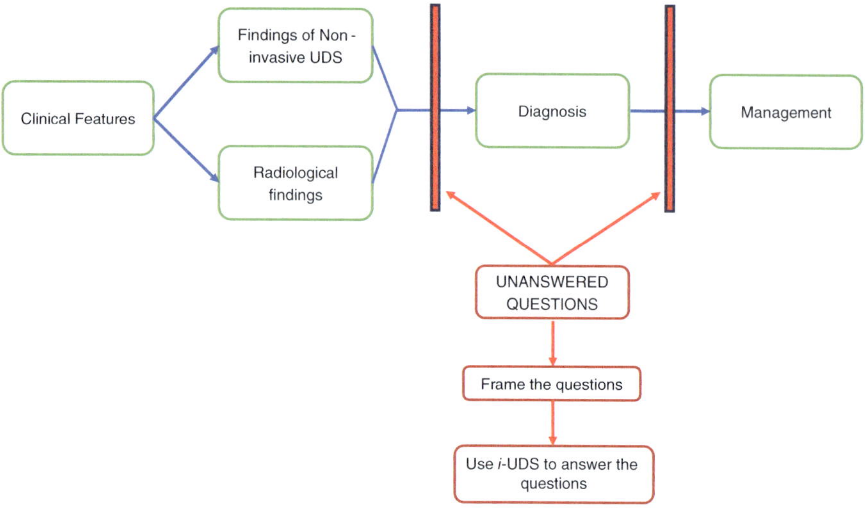

Fig. 8.1 The "UDS question"—the unanswered questions

A few examples to illustrate the thought process underlying a UDS question are as follow:

- If a patient of neurogenic bladder has weak bladder outlet and is being planned for bladder neck procedure, our question will be to assess the filling phase parameters. So during the study, we would need to perform one study wherein we fill the bladder without occluding the urethra and document the leak point pressures. Then we perform the second fill when we keep the urethra occluded preventing the leak and assess compliance/overactivity as the bladder fills up.
- In a child with VUR and recurrent UTI, *i*-UDS will be needed to determine whether the VUR is primary or secondary. We would need to check whether there is any evidence of significant overactivity or poor compliance which would point toward secondary nature of VUR and would mandate stabilization of the bladder before correction of VUR. If MCU shows VUR to be present only during voiding, voiding pressures also need to be assessed to check for any high-pressure voiding.
- In a child who presents with features of urgency and urinary incontinence, *i*-UDS shows overactivity and the child is often seen to leak/void during an episode of strong overactive contraction. Before starting anticholinergics, we need to document that child has the ability to void on her own voluntarily and can empty her bladder. So we have to perform a second fill on her and ask her to void at a point when she is not having overactivity. We check whether she can void voluntarily and whether the bladder empties completely. If she is able to void voluntarily, then anticholinergics can be safely added, whereas if she is not able to do so, she may actually land up in retention with anticholinergics and may need CIC.

- If a follow-up patient of PUV is stable on anticholinergics and we want to assess whether the medications can be stopped, we can perform the UDS after stopping the anticholinergics for a week and assess how the bladder behaves without the medication. On the other hand, if the child has urinary incontinence in spite of the present doses of anticholinergics, we can perform the study when the medications are on to check whether the current doses are sufficient.
- A patient who has history of leaking urine when laughing (giggle incontinence) has to be made to laugh out loud during the test to manifest leak. Also, an effort should be made to check whether there is any overactivity/leak at other times, that is, by performing other provocative maneuvers like coughing/Valsalva which would be unlikely in true "giggle" incontinence.

We have tried to formulate the UDS questions in the common scenarios of neurogenic bladder, PUV, and non-neurogenic/functional bladder as an illustration to identify the patients who can benefit from *i*-UDS and to frame UDS questions (Figs. 8.2, 8.3 and 8.4).

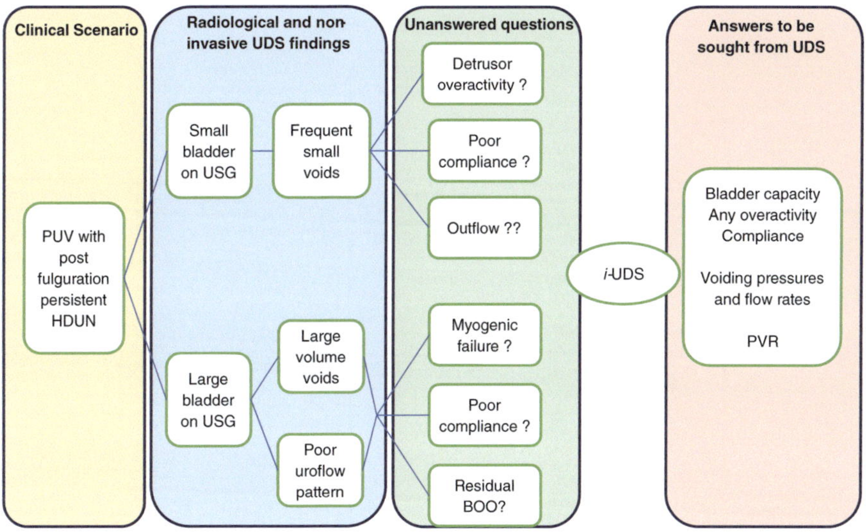

Fig. 8.2 UDS question in setting of PUV

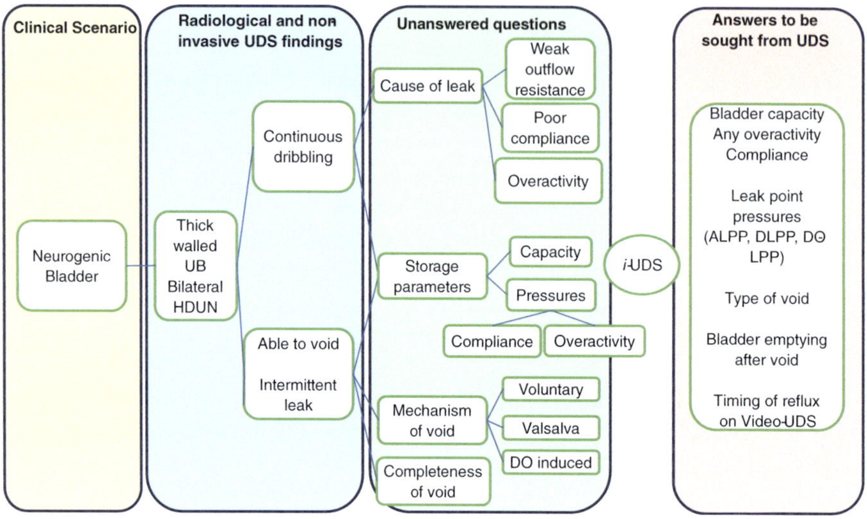

Fig. 8.3 UDS question in setting of neurogenic bladder

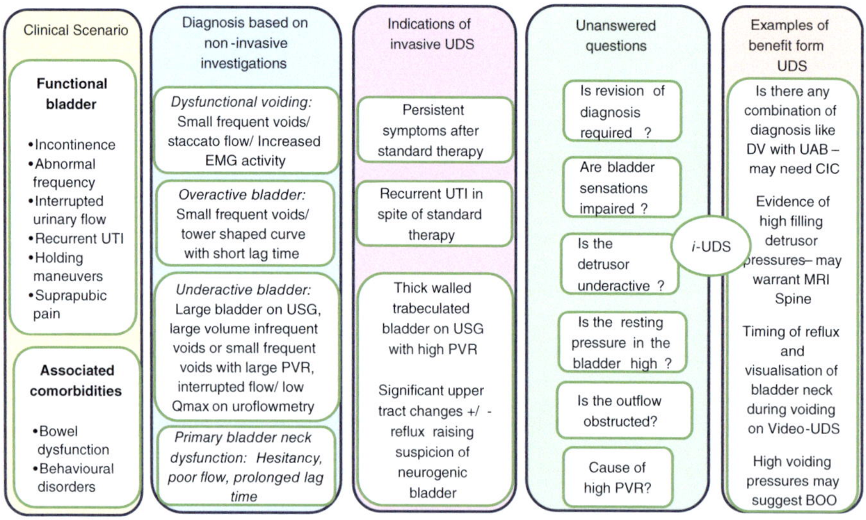

Fig. 8.4 UDS question in setting of functional bladder dysfunction

Declarations

Competing Interests The author(s) has no competing interests to declare that are relevant to the content of this manuscript.

Ethics Approval The author(s) declares that this manuscript does not include primary research with human participants.

The author(s) declares that this manuscript does not include primary studies involving animals.

Suggested Reading

1. Bauer SB, Nijman RJ, Drzewiecki BA, Sillen U, Hoebeke P. International Children's Continence Society Standardization Subcommittee. International Children's Continence Society standardization report on urodynamic studies of the lower urinary tract in children. Neurourol Urodyn. 2015;34(7):640–7. https://doi.org/10.1002/nau.22783. Epub 2015 May 21. PMID: 25998310.
2. Drzewiecki BA, Bauer SB. Urodynamic testing in children: indications, technique, interpretation and significance. J Urol. 2011;186(4):1190–7. https://doi.org/10.1016/j.juro.2011.02.2692. Epub 2011 Aug 16. PMID: 21849190.
3. Tekgul S, Stein R, Bogaert G, Undre S, Nijman RJM, Quaedackers J, 't Hoen L, Kocvara R, Silay MS, Radmayr C, Dogan HS. EAU-ESPU guidelines recommendations for daytime lower urinary tract conditions in children. Eur J Pediatr. 2020;179(7):1069–77. https://doi.org/10.1007/s00431-020-03681-w. PMID: 32472266.

How to Perform *i*-UDS

9

Poonam Guha Vaze

1. Patient preparation
   (a) Antibiotics
   (b) Rectal preparation
   (c) Sedation
   (d) Whether to stop or continue anticholinergics?
2. Position of the patient
3. Catheter insertion and fixation
   (a) Urethral
   (b) Rectal
4. Making the connections
5. Performing the study
   (a) Filling phase
   (b) Voiding phase
   (c) Ending the test
   (d) How many cycles?

Patient Preparation

Urine testing A routine urine test is recommended before the procedure to document absence of any ongoing infection. If there is any evidence of infection, appropriate antibiotic therapy should be instituted before the procedure.

P. G. Vaze (✉)
Neotia Bhagirathi Woman and Child Care Centre, Newtown, Kolkata, India

Department of Pediatric Surgery, Nilratan Sircar Medical College and Hospital, Kolkata, India

S. Saha, P. Guha Vaze (eds.), *Comprehensive Atlas of Practical Pediatric Urodynamics*, https://doi.org/10.1007/978-981-95-2709-0_9

Antibiotics There is divided opinion about use of pre-procedural antibiotics. We prefer to give a prophylactic dose of antibiotics usually cephalexin or co-amoxiclav started one day prior to and continued for one day after the test.

We have performed post-procedure urine routine tests in all our patients and have documented a UTI rate of around 1% (2 out of 250 patients). Both the patients were follow-up cases of PUV and had gross VUR. After these two cases, in patients with gross VUR, we have started retaining the urethral catheter in situ for 15–20 minutes after completion of the procedure to drain out the returning refluxed urine from the bladder so that we can further reduce any chances of UTI.

Sedation Catheterisation is an unpleasant part of the procedure, but rest of the procedure is painless. Many young children become anxious and apprehensive during the procedure—they become uncooperative and pose resistance while performing the test.

Studies have reported that use of sedation in the form of intravenous ketamine or midazolam (oral/nasal/rectal/IV) does not affect the filling phase urodynamic findings especially capacity and compliance.

We have observed that detrusor overactivity frequently manifests itself when child is active and may disappear if child is sleeping/calm (Fig. 9.1a, b). Findings in children with functional voiding disorders may get altered when child is sedated. Also, if the child is sedated, voiding may not be recorded altogether; only filling phase may be assessed. Thus, many crucial findings may be missed if the child is sedated.

We usually perform the procedure without any sedation and make use of other incentives like videos on mobile phones, sweetmeats, star-stickers, smiley stamps and presence of one or both parents to keep the children engaged and feel at ease (Fig. 9.2).

Rectal preparation Most of the children who are advised urodynamics for assessment of detrusor function also have some element of constipation as a comorbidity. If the rectum is loaded during the procedure, several problems may appear.

- Rectal catheter may fail to read abdominal pressures properly because of tamponade effect of stools and may give dampened readings.
- Significant rectal contractions may be recorded making evaluation of detrusor pressure tracing difficult (Fig. 9.3).
- The patient may feel desire to pass stools or even evacuate the rectum when the study is going on and continuing the study may become impossible.

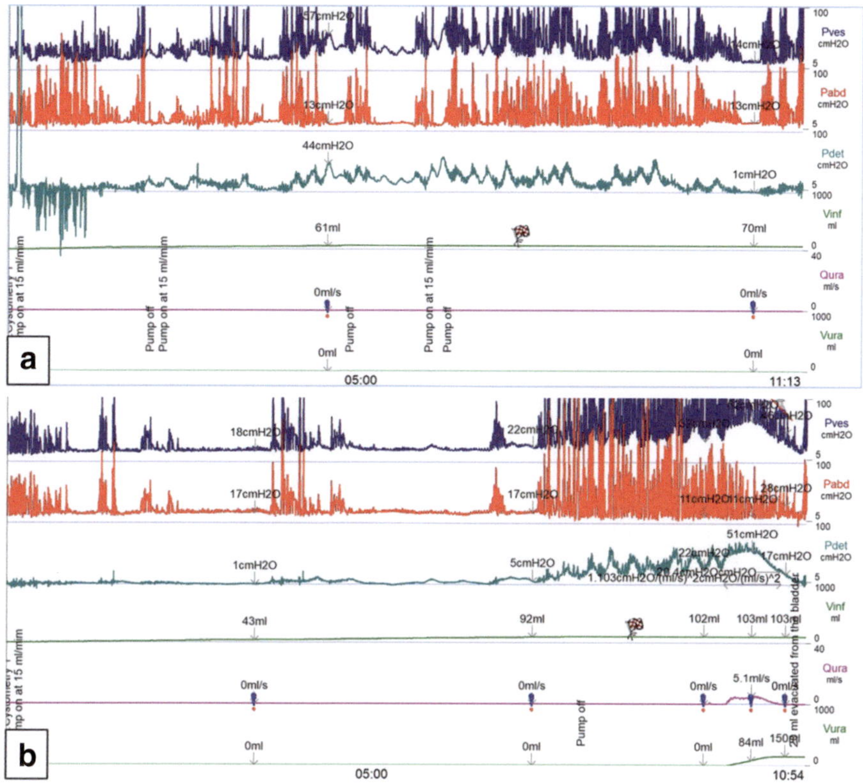

Fig. 9.1 A 3-year-old girl, follow-up case of anorectal malformation, having recurrent UTI and shows gross VUR on MCU. Child was irritable throughout the study during first cycle (**a**) when UDS tracing shows severe overactivity. During the second study (**b**), child was calm up to 90 ml fill when no overactivity was noted; overactivity as noted after 90 ml fill when child became irritable

Thus, we recommend to withhold oral laxatives a night before and introduce a per-rectal bisacodyl or glycerine suppository (depending on the age of the child) 12 hours before the procedure to ensure an empty rectum during the test.

Whether to Stop or Continue Anticholinergics?

It depends on the question that we want to answer through the urodynamic study and the clinical scenario.

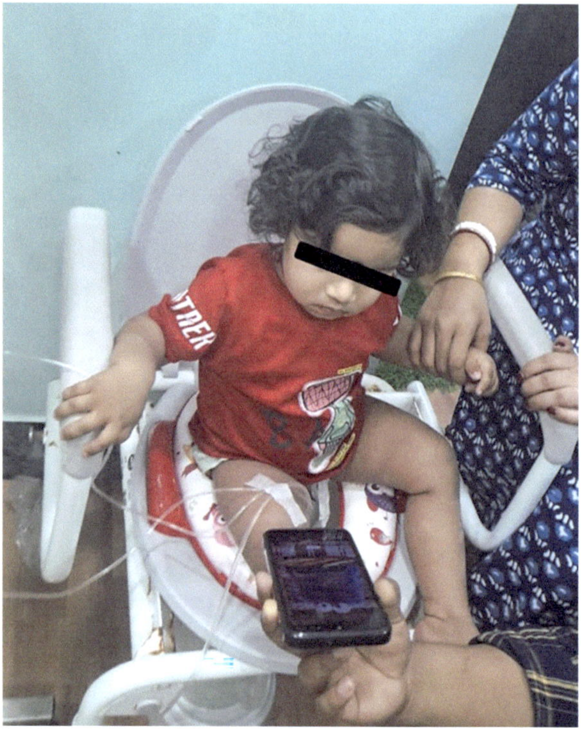

Fig. 9.2 A 1-year-old child watching video on mobile phone and allowing the test to be done in a peaceful manner

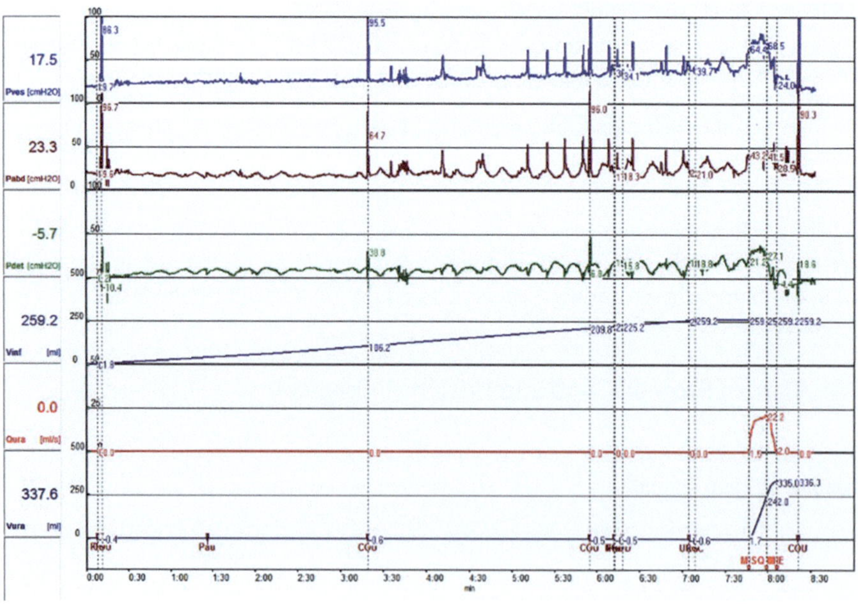

Fig. 9.3 UDS tracing showing continuous deflections in the abdominal tracing due to loaded rectum. These deflections cause artefacts (negative deflections) to appear in the detrusor tracing which may be mis-interpreted as detrusor overactivity. The vesical tracing on the other hand shows only a gradual upward slope suggesting reduced compliance and no overactivity at all

We stop the anticholinergics if:

(a) First urodynamic evaluation—If a child is undergoing a urodynamic investigation for the first time, we would like to stop the medications and then perform the test to assess the baseline bladder function.
(b) UDS being performed to check whether anticholinergics can be stopped—If the child has documented evidence of overactivity and has been stable on anticholinergics, voiding diary shows normal voided volumes and we are planning to stop the medications, we may stop the medication before repeating the UDS to check whether the bladder is stable without the anticholinergics.
(c) To ascertain the cause of persistent HDUN in otherwise stable post-PUV child—If a follow-up case of PUV is otherwise stable, has good voided volumes and flow, but has persistent HDUN, we need to differentiate whether the HDUN is because of subclinical bladder dysfunction or prolonged use of anticholinergics. It is preferable to stop the medications and reassess the USG/voiding diary and perform the UDS.
(d) Voiding parameters need to be studied—Anticholinergics reduce detrusor pressures as a whole - both during filling and voiding. So voiding detrusor pressures may not rise even if there is outflow tract obstruction. So, we stop the medications if we want to assess the voiding pressures.

We continue anticholinergics if the child is a follow-up patient of neurogenic bladder/PUV with a *bad* bladder and is on anticholinergics. We would like to continue the medications while doing the UDS to check whether there is any residual overactivity or reduced compliance even while being on the drugs; if so, then doses of the medications may have to be increased; or if we find the bladder to be absolutely stable, the doses may be reduced.

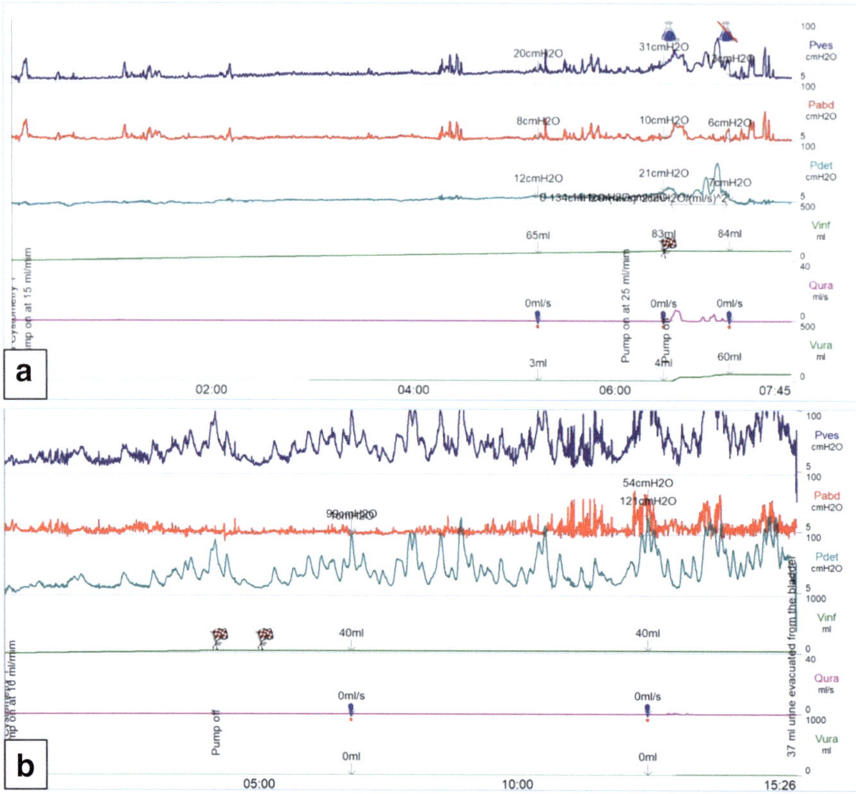

Fig. 9.4 A 3-year-old male child, follow-up case of PUV, was doing well on anticholinergics (oxybutynin 2.5 mg BD). First study (**a**) done while he was on medications showed a good capacity stable bladder with no overactivity. But he showed increased PVR on USG. So he was planned for stopping anticholinergics. Second study (**b**) was performed 6 months later after stopping anticholinergics for 1 week which reveals severe overactivity. Parents also complained that as soon as anticholinergics were stopped, he started having wetness of pants. Thus, in this patient, anticholinergics need to be continued

In any case where we want to stop the medications before the test, we stop anticholinergics as well as beta-3 agonists 1 week before the procedure (Fig. 9.4).

Position of the Patient

Whenever feasible, the child should be allowed to void in the posture he/she is comfortable in. To study the filling and voiding phase, the child has to be positioned so that the urine falls into the funnel overlying the uroflowmetry jar.

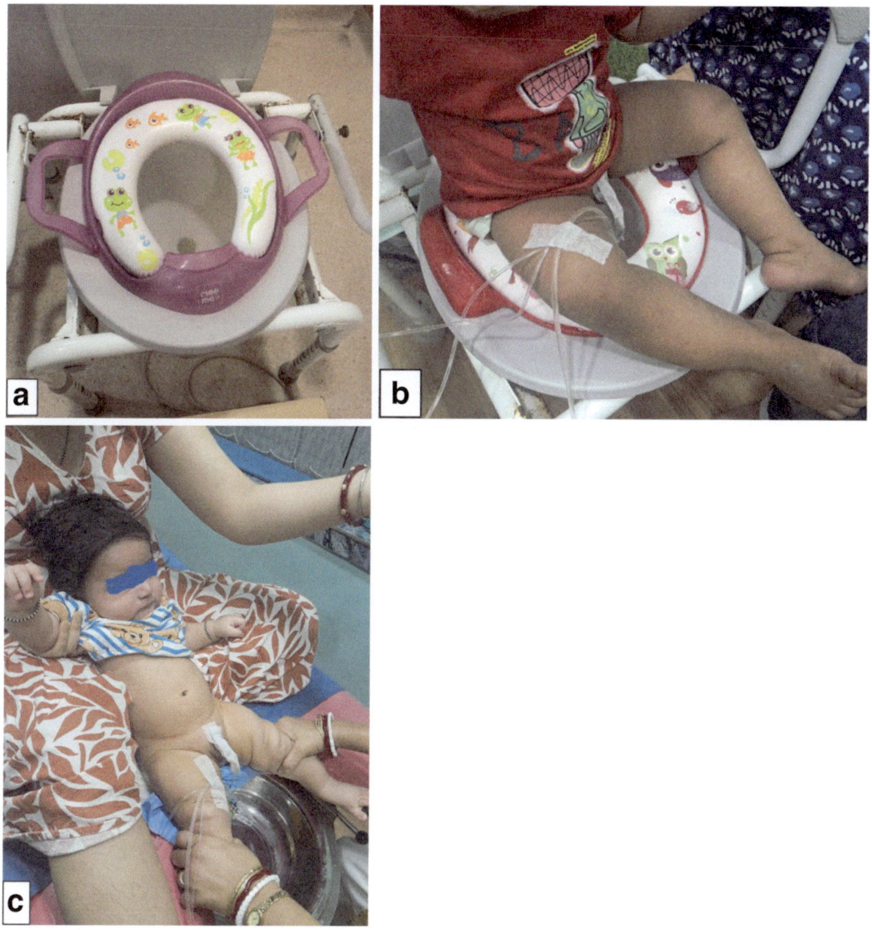

Fig. 9.5 (**a**–**c**) Seating options in young children.

We perform most of the studies in sitting position with the child seated comfortably over the commode chair. Young children need a commode seat reducer over the conventional commode seat (Fig. 9.5a, b).

For young babies/infants, the baby is positioned at the edge of the table reclining on the mother's lap so that the voided urine falls on the uroflowmetry funnel (Fig. 9.5c).

For children whom we do not expect to void or those who are extremely irritable and pull off the catheters, we perform the study in supine position and study only the filling phase.

For boys who are uncomfortable in voiding in sitting position, we allow them to stand during voiding.

Catheter Insertion and Fixation

Choosing the right size The smallest size catheter should be introduced for the test as size of the catheter can influence the voiding pressures and flow rates. We use 6 Fr double-lumen catheter for all children and adolescents till the age of 18 years.

Catheterisation Before catheterisation, patency of both the ports should be checked. Catheterisation should be performed after proper lubrication to minimise urethral irritation. Else, child will withhold micturition. In children with PUV, if the bladder neck is very prominent, the stiff double-lumen catheter may not negotiate across the shelf created by the bladder neck, and placing a finger per rectally may be helpful.

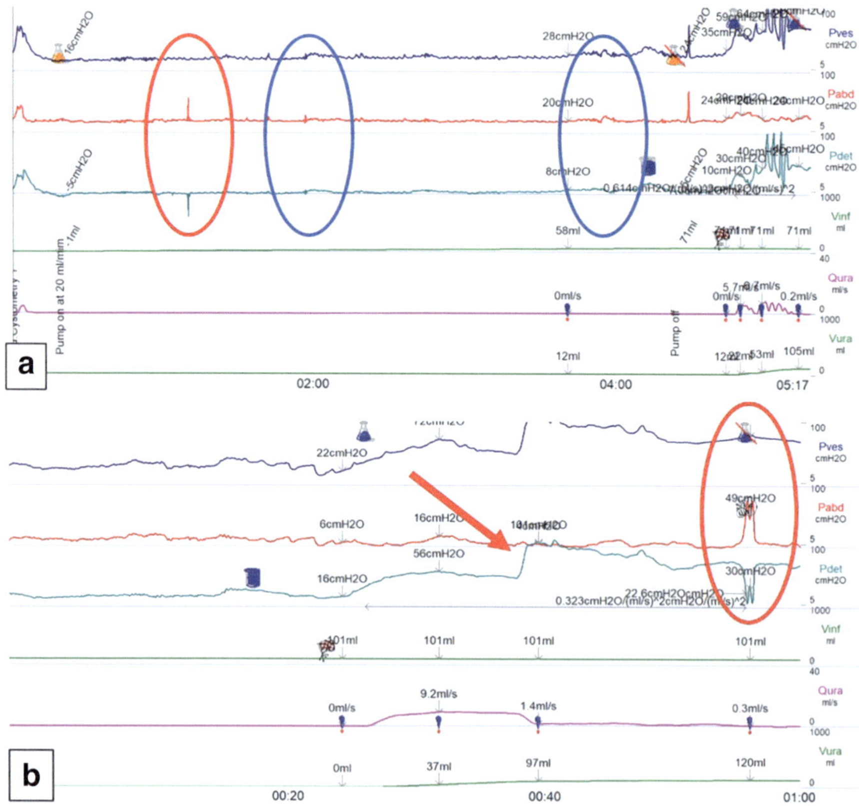

Fig. 9.6 (**a**) UDS tracing showing no deflection in vesical tracing while checking cough impulse in early part of the curve (red oval), whereas normal activity is seen in the later part of the tracing (blue oval). Vesical catheter starts reading when the bladder fills up and kink in the catheter gets corrected. (**b**) Voiding phase of a UDS curve shows sudden and sustained rise of detrusor pressure at the end of the void (red arrow) and absence of cough deflection thereafter (red oval). This is caused by kinking of the catheter as the bladder empties

Length of catheter to be inserted The length of catheter that is introduced in the bladder is of paramount importance. If a longer length of catheter is in the bladder, it tends to get kinked when the bladder is empty/collapsed and fails to read. It starts reading when the catheter gets space to straighten itself out, that is, there is some volume of urine in the bladder. Thus, the catheter fails to read in early part of filling and during later half of voiding (Fig. 9.6a, b).

We introduce the catheter in the bladder for a length of 12 cm in infants and children up to 7 years, 15 cm for elder boys and 20 cm for post-pubertal boys. Whereas in girls, we introduce it for 5–7 cm in girls younger than 4 years and for a length of 10 cm in elder girls.

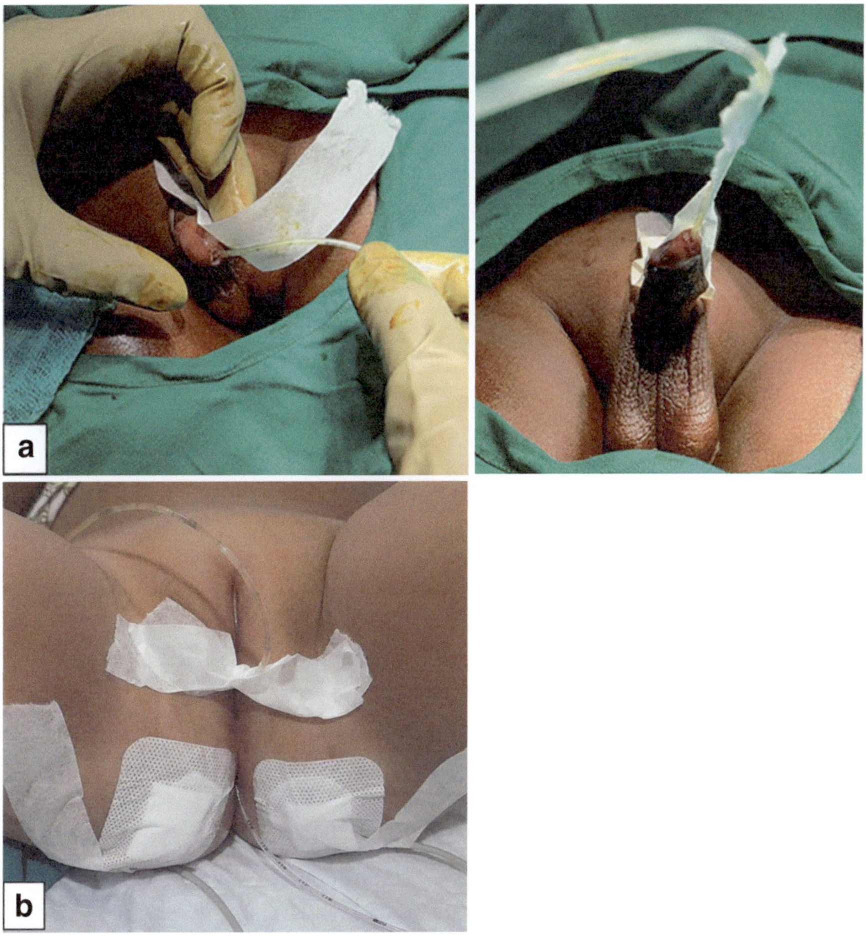

Fig. 9.7 Fixation of urethral catheter in boys (**a**) and girls (**b**)

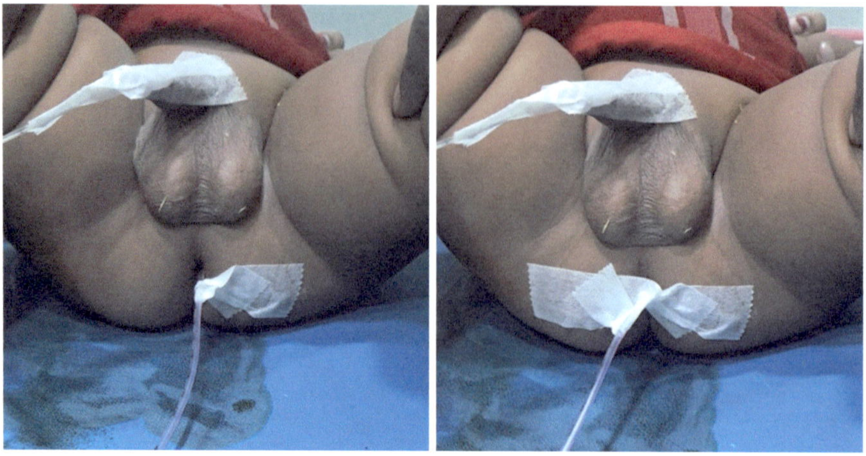

Fig. 9.8 Fixation of rectal catheter

Fixation of Catheter Fixation of the catheter should be such that it should allow urine to flow out unimpeded by the side of the catheter, but the catheter should not slip out due to force of urine flowing out during voiding. Occlusion of the urethral/preputial orifice may lead to false finding of outflow tract obstruction. We use 1 inch micropores applied in a particular fashion to achieve these goals (Fig. 9.7a, b). These have been adopted after several combinations and permutations. This technique has given us good results in the last 450 cases.

Fixation of rectal catheter is also important because children tend to push out the rectal catheter if they strain to pass urine. Technique of fixation of rectal catheter is shown in Fig. 9.8.

EMG Electrodes Electrodes are applied after wiping the area dry. The active electrodes are applied on either side of the anus, and the reference electrode is applied on the thigh/abdomen. We usually apply a waterproof dressing like G-Dress/Tegaderm over the electrodes to prevent wetting by urine (Fig. 9.7b).

Special Situations

Absent or Lax Anus

In patients with anorectal malformation or neurogenic bladder, anus may be either absent or may be very lax. In such cases, rectal catheter cannot be introduced or, if introduced, do not read properly as the abdominal pressure leaks out through the lax anus. In such cases, a nasogastric tube (NGT) can be introduced and used for

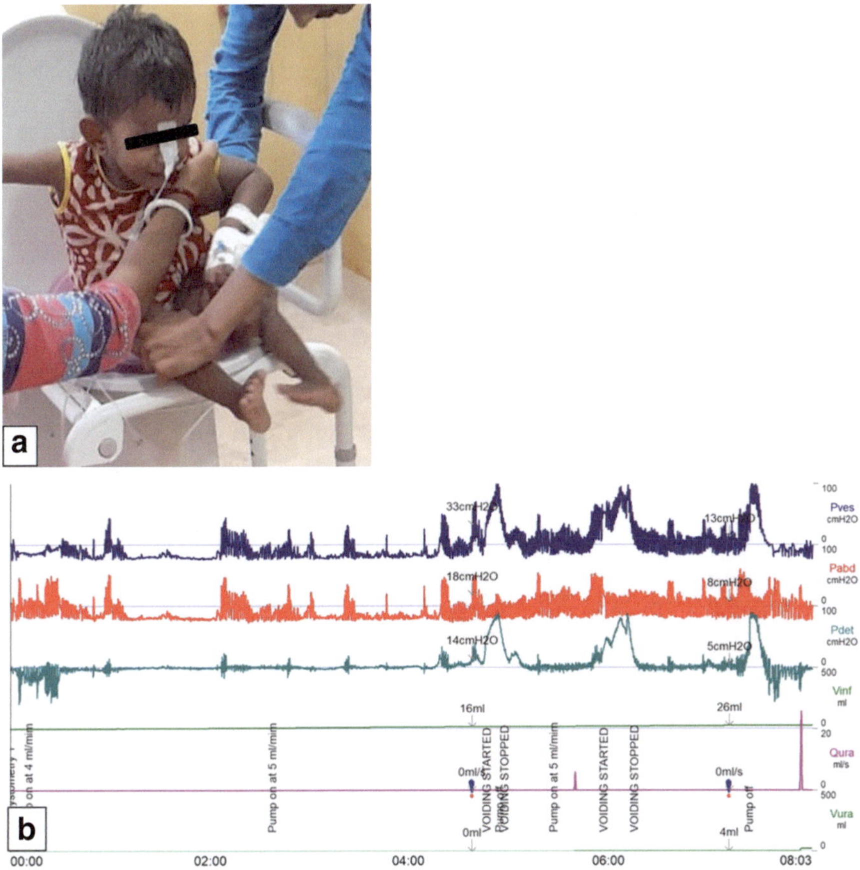

Fig. 9.9 (**a**) A 2-year-old child with neurogenic bladder/bowel with lax anus having an NGT in situ for measuring Pabd. (**b**) UDS tracing of a 2-month-old male child with an intermediate type of anorectal malformation, partial sacral agenesis and recurrent UTI. NGT was used for monitoring Pabd due to absent anus

measuring the abdominal pressure (Fig. 9.9a). The results are equivalent to or better than using a rectal catheter (Fig. 9.9b). Although it is uncomfortable for the patient, it is a useful bail-out technique in select cases.

Vesicostomy

Children with vesicostomy pose two problems—leak of infused fluid through the vesicostomy and small bladder volume. In children with vesicostomy, we keep the vesicostomy occluded by digital compression or by a Foley's balloon, introduce the catheter per urethrally and perform the study with a very slow filling rate. Catheter

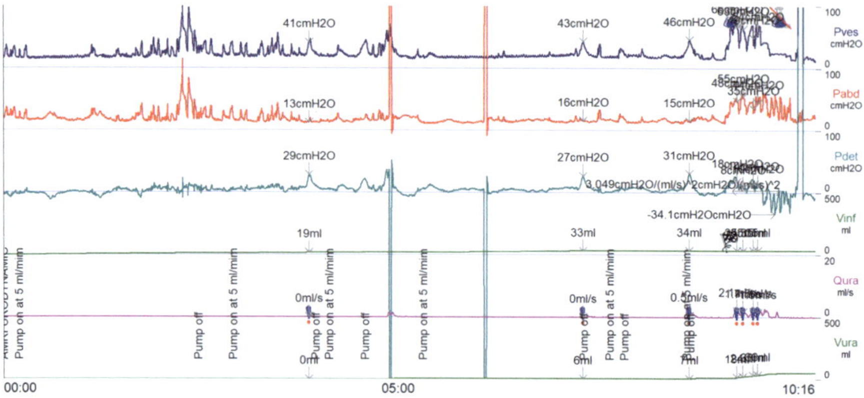

Fig. 9.10 A 4-year-old male child, follow-up case of PUV, with vesicostomy in situ—UDS performed by blocking the vesicostomy with a Foley through the vesicostomy and inflating it with 1 ml. Filling has been performed at 5 ml/min

can also be introduced through the stoma, but occluding the stoma with the catheter passing through it becomes difficult (Fig. 9.10).

In children with SPC, we remove the SPC catherter and introduce the catheter through the SPC opening. After the test is over, the SPC can be reintroduced.

Ureterostomy

Stoma in a non-refluxing ureter does not make a difference in the performance of *i*-UDS. Refluxing ureterostomy can cause loss of infused fluid through the stoma. We observe the child to note if there is any leak through the stoma due to reflux and note the point on the tracing (Fig. 9.11a, b). During rest of the study, we keep the

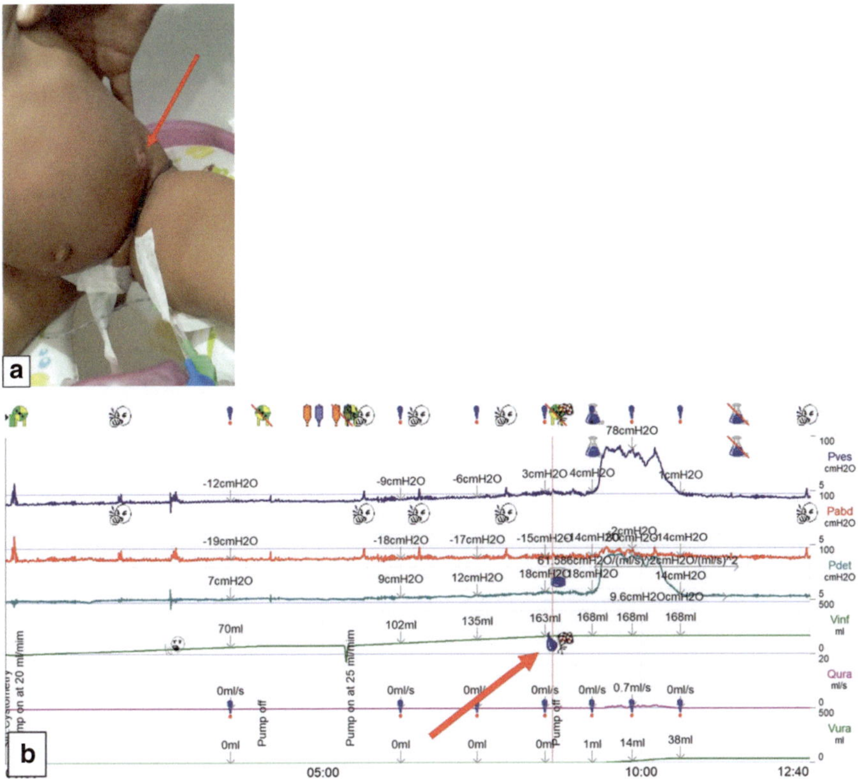

Fig. 9.11 (**a**) *i*-UDS being performed in a child with ureterostomy in situ. (**b**) UDS tracing of a 6-year-old girl with NNNB with right refluxing ureterostomy in situ. She passes urine mostly through the stoma and occasionally per urethrally. UDS shows point of reflux through ureterostomy as 'leak' sign (marked by red arrow) after which it was kept occluded during voiding. It shows that reflux appears at 160 ml volume at Pdet of 16 cm H2O

stoma occluded by digital compression and finish the study as usual. This gives an idea about the bladder capacity or pressures at which reflux appears.

We have also used the ureterostomy for catheterisation instead of per-urethral catheterisation as it allows unimpeded voiding to be observed.

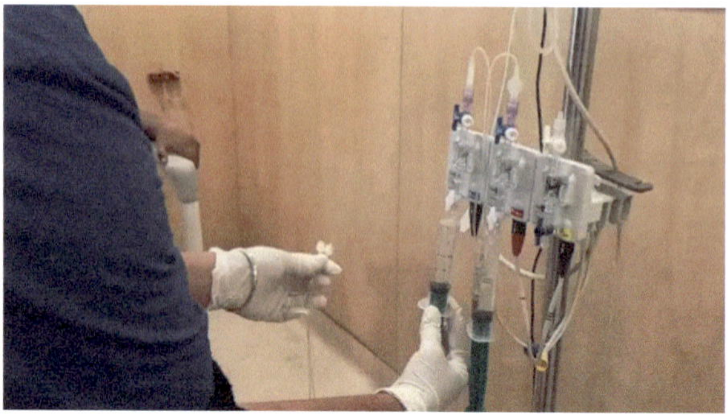

Fig. 9.12 Flushing the catheter before connecting them

Connecting Catheters to the Machine

Flushing

Importance of flushing the catheters during a urodynamics test cannot be overstated. In the water-charged systems, the pressure transducer reads the pressure across a continuous column of fluid from the bladder/rectum till the transducer sensor. Presence of tiny air bubbles can break the continuity of this column and dampen the pressure readings. Flushing removes any micro-bubbles which may be present in the tubings and allows the pressure reading to be recorded appropriately (Fig. 9.12).

The sequence that needs to be followed religiously is

$$\text{Flush} \rightarrow \text{Zero} \rightarrow \text{Connect} \rightarrow \text{Flush} \rightarrow \text{Cough impulse} \rightarrow \text{Start}$$

Flushing has to be repeated each time if any of the tubing connections are disconnected/ reconnected as these actions introduce air bubbles into the system.

Zeroing

Once the pressure monitoring lines are flushed, their open end is held at the level of pubic symphysis and the bed height/transducer height is adjusted so that they come to lie at the same level and the Pves/Pabd are at zero level; at this point, the 'zero' icon on the software is clicked.

We use a simpler technique which has worked well with us. We do not adjust the heights of the transducer/bed. After flushing the catheters, we hold the open end of the catheters at the level of pubic symphysis of the patient and press the 'zero' icon. When we start the study, instead of starting at 'zero', the Pves and Pabd start at some value depending on height of the transducer relative to the bed, but the Pdet starts at 'zero'. We interpret the changes to values of Pves/Pabd with reference to their values at initiation of the study, whereas the interpretation of values of Pdet remains unchanged. For example, if the value of Pabd at the beginning of the study is recorded as 12 cm H2O and Abdominal Leak-Point Pressure (ALPP) is documented at 75 cm H2O, the actual ALPP would be 63 cm H2O (75–12)

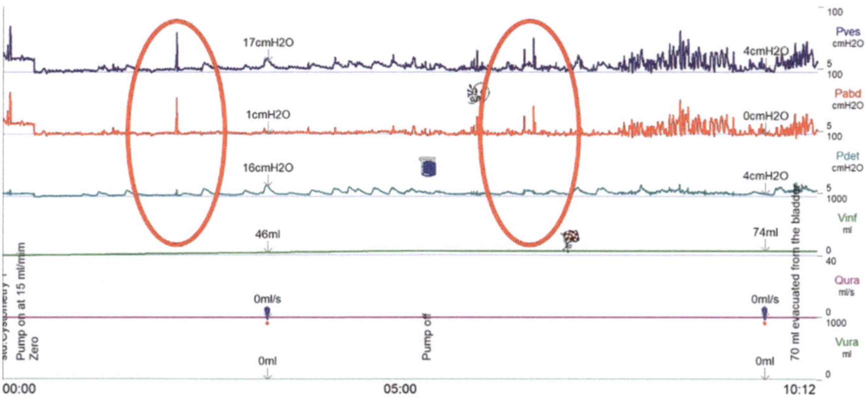

Fig. 9.13 UDS tracing showing cough impulses (red ovals)

Making the Connections

The tubes need to be oriented properly and connected to their respective counterparts. The common colour coding followed by most urodynamics systems are:

- Green port of the double-lumen urethral catheter → pump tubing
- Blue port of the double-lumen urethral catheter → vesical pressure monitoring line (*B*LUE for *B*ladder)
- Rectal catheter → rectal pressure monitoring line (*R*ED for *R*ectum)

Cough Impulse

After the connections are established and catheters are flushed, we need to confirm whether both the catheters are reading well. It is done by asking the patient to cough. It results in sudden sharp deflections in both the rectal and vesical tracings. Under ideal circumstances, both the deflections should be of same magnitude and cancel each other out so that there is no deflection in the detrusor tracing when the patient coughs (Fig. 9.13).

Checking for cough impulse should be done at the beginning of procedure and periodically thereafter to check if both the catheters are reading well. If the deflection in one of the catheters is dampened, the catheter needs to be flushed.

If the catheter is inserted too far inside the bladder, it fails to read in early part of fill when the bladder is empty and starts reading when the bladder is filled up with 10–20 ml saline. Thus, cough impulse may be unbalanced in early part and autocorrects itself after 10–20 ml fill.

In a young child, who will not cough on command, simple suprapubic compression will give adequate deflection in both the catheters.

Performing the Study

Bladder behaviour needs to be assessed during the filling and voiding phases.

Filling Phase

Rate of fill The recommended rate of fill is usually 10% of expected bladder capacity. To calculate the rate of fill, whenever feasible, it is better to have a voiding diary before performing the invasive urodynamic study, as the rate of fill should be adjusted to 10% of functional bladder capacity. For example, a 9-year-old child, who is a follow-up case of PUV, would have an expected bladder capacity of 270 ml whereas the voiding diary may show his functional capacity to be around 100–120 ml. In this child, the fill should be done at 10–15 ml/min rather than 25–30 ml/min. If the detrusor is found to be stable with no overactivity, fill rate may be temporarily increased to 2–3 times the original rate to unmask any underlying overactivity as a provocative maneouvre.

Capacity Filling is stopped when the child complains of significant urge to void or suprapubic pain, a young child becomes irritable and EBC or functional capacity is reached, > 150% capacity is reached or detrusor pressures are persistently around or above 40 cm H2O or there is significant spontaneous leak/ dribble of urine.

Total capacity is recorded as the voided volume + PVR at the end of the study. This may not always match the filled volume. Children with high pressure (poorly compliant/overactive) bladders tend to have some diuresis during the study and the voided volume + PVR may be surprisingly high compared to the filled volumes. On the contrary, in children with gross VUR, the bladder may empty itself completely with most of the urine getting refluxed into the upper tracts. The voided volumes may be smaller compared to the filled volumes with no PVR being documented immediately after the void.

Compliance Normally during filling, detrusor pressures should remain near 'zero'. Sustained rise of pressure above baseline which does not return to the baseline is called reduced compliance.

Assessment of compliance may become tricky in the presence of prolonged tonic overactivity or in patients with severe repeated waves of overactivity (especially if the child is irritable). Tonic overactivity usually subsides on stopping the flow for a few minutes and the detrusor pressure reduces. Repeating the study in case of an irritable child makes assessment of compliance easier as children tend to be less irritable during the second study and overactivity improves to some extent (Fig. 9.14a, b).

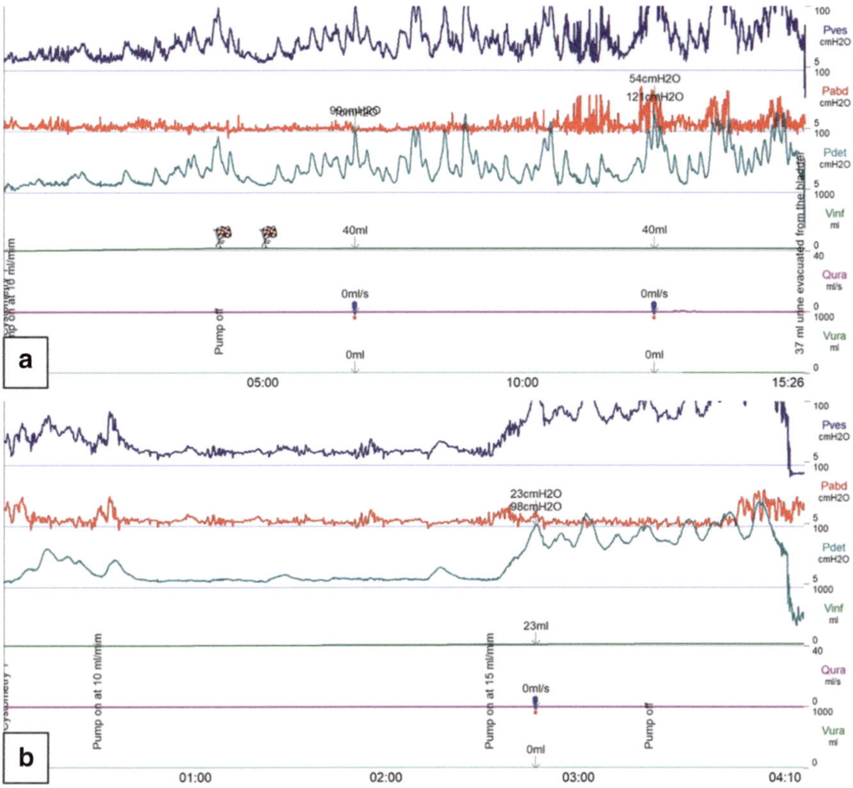

Fig. 9.14 UDS tracings of a 3-year-old child, follow-up case of PUV (both the studies were performed in the same sitting). First study (**a**) shows severe detrusor overactivity—assessment of compliance is difficult. Second study (**b**) shows relatively less overactivity in the intervening part when it is apparent that the compliance is normal for the assessed volume

Overactivity Any transient rise of detrusor pressure which comes down to the baseline is called overactivity or involuntary detrusor contraction. If there are no spontaneous waves of overactivity, provocative maneuvers are performed—like coughing/Valsalva/change of posture or rapid filling to unmask any latent overactivity.

Leak The timing and approximate volume of leak should be documented. If there is a ureterostomy, it should be documented at which point does urine start refluxing out through the ureterostomy after which it should be kept occluded by digital compression.

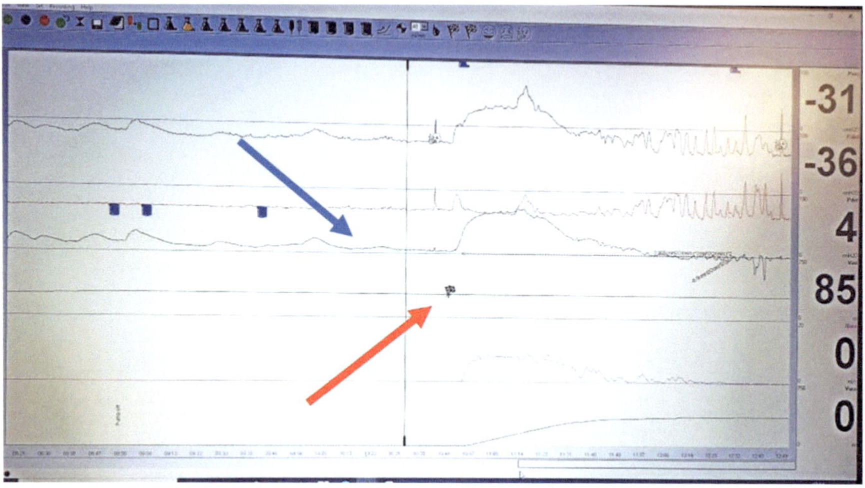

Fig. 9.15 Voiding command (red flag, marked by red arrow) should be preferably given once overactivity has abated (blue arrow). Voiding command is followed by voiding detrusor contraction

Sensation It is difficult to ascertain bladder sensations in young children. Young children usually start crying when the bladder is full. In older children, sensations such as first sensation, first urge, severe urge, pain and suprapubic discomfort can be marked.

Voiding Phase

Young children (< 1 ½ years) void spontaneously; children between 1 ½ and 5 years usually withhold voluntary micturition; elder ones void on request.

Wherever feasible, voiding command should be given once wave of detrusor overactivity has ended. Else, voiding parameters may be altered (Fig. 9.15).

In young children, it is difficult to differentiate between involuntary leak due to terminal overactivity and a voluntary void. This can be differentiated only when the child is old enough to verbalise. Slowing the rate of infusion may delay void due to terminal overactivity, and few smaller waves of overactivity may be noted before the terminal void in case of overactivity-associated void.

If a young child is not voiding spontaneously, after 150% of EBC is reached, the child should be given cues to void and the point should be recorded on the graph.

Volume and flow rate can be recorded only if the study is done in sitting/standing position.

Pdet during void—Pdetmax, Pdet @ Qmax, after-contraction are noted

Residual volume—Post-void residue should be documented before removal of the catheter. Both the lumens of the catheter should be aspirated. Although PVR may be ascertained by handheld bladder scanners, emptying the bladder at the end of the procedure reduces the chances of post-procedure UTI in hostile bladders.

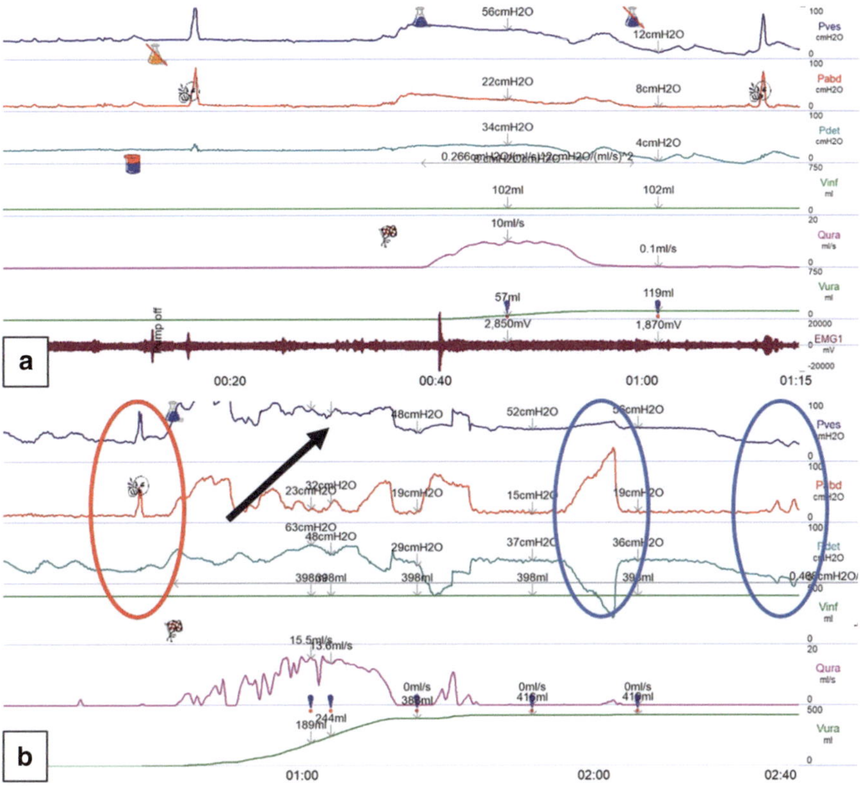

Fig. 9.16 (**a**) Voiding phase of a UDS study showing cough impulses before and after voiding. (**b**) Voiding phase of a UDS study showing cough impulse before void (red oval) but no deflection in vesical tracing after the void (blue ovals). Black arrow denotes the point where vesical catheter got kinked and malfunctioned

Ending the Study

Cough impulse should be documented at the end of the fill to document that both the catheters are working till end of the procedure (Fig. 9.16a). Often during voiding, the catheter may get kinked within the bladder and stop reading. Interpretation of the voiding pressures should be done only till the point when the catheter was reading (Fig. 9.16b).

The study should be stopped and saved on the software.

Number of Studies to Be Performed

We usually perform two studies for most of the patients.

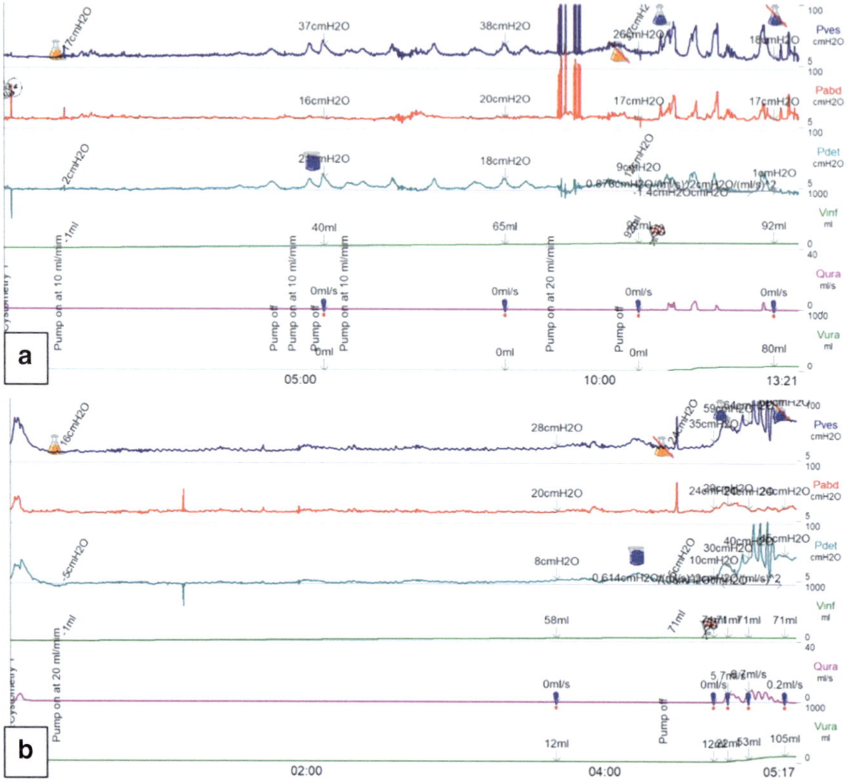

Fig. 9.17 First study (**a**) and second study (**b**) of a 3-year-old child, follow-up case of PUV, (performed in the same sitting) showing significant overactivity during the first study but none during the second study. He had history of increased voiding frequency and intermittent dribbling, so the findings of the first study are accepted

For studying voiding parameters, usually the second void is more reliable as the child is more apprehensive during the first void.

The observations may be different during both the studies. Most commonly, one of the studies may show overactivity whereas the other does not. Few children show overactivity only in either supine or sitting position and not in the other. Also, children are usually more apprehensive during the first study when overactivity gets manifested. During the second study, when child is calmer, overactivity disappears or appears later during filling (Fig. 9.17a, b) If findings during the two studies are different, the usual voiding behaviour/voiding diary is taken into account to decide which finding to consider.

In a case of neurogenic bladder, if the first study shows all the required parameters like compliance, overactivity, leak point pressure, etc., then the second study may not be required.

Declarations

Competing Interests The author(s) has no competing interests to declare that are relevant to the content of this manuscript.

Ethics Approval The author(s) declares that this manuscript does not include primary research with human participants.

The author(s) declares that this manuscript does not include primary studies involving animals.

References/Suggested Reading

1. Bauer SB, Nijman RJ, Drzewiecki BA, Sillen U, Hoebeke P, International Children's Continence Society Standardization Subcommittee. International Children's Continence Society standardization report on urodynamic studies of the lower urinary tract in children. Neurourol Urodyn. 2015;34(7):640–7. https://doi.org/10.1002/nau.22783. Epub 2015 May 21. PMID: 25998310.
2. Cheriyan A, George AJP, Devasia A, Chandrasingh J. Can rectal catheters be avoided during paediatric urodynamic studies? Arab J Urol. 2019;18(1):41–6. https://doi.org/10.1080/2090598X.2019.1668176.
3. Drzewiecki BA, Bauer SB. Urodynamic testing in children: indications, technique, interpretation and significance. J Urol. 2011;186(4):1190–7. https://doi.org/10.1016/j.juro.2011.02.2692. Epub 2011 Aug 16. PMID: 21849190.
4. Özmert S, Sever F, Tiryaki HT. Evaluation of the effects of sedation administered via three different routes on the procedure, child and parent satisfaction during cystometry. Springerplus. 2016;5(1):1496. https://doi.org/10.1186/s40064-016-3164-7. PMID: 27652069; PMCID: PMC5013006.
5. Sözübir S, Celik A, Emir N, Avanoglu A, Ulman I. Consistency of urodynamic parameters in children with detrusor instability: how many times should the bladder be filled? Urol Int. 2005;75(2):129–32. https://doi.org/10.1159/000087166.
6. Sweeney H, Marai S, Kim C, Ferrer F. Creating a sedation service for pediatric urodynamics: our experience. Urol Nurs. 2008;28(4)
7. Thevaraja AK, Batra YK, Rakesh SV, Panda NB, Rao KLN, Chhabra M, Aggarwal M. Comparison of low-dose ketamine to midazolam for sedation during pediatric urodynamic study. Paediatr Anaesth. 2013;23:415–21. https://doi.org/10.1111/pan.12046.
8. Wen JG, Djurhuus JC, Rosier PF, Bauer SB. ICS educational module: cystometry in children. Neurourol Urodynamics. 2018;37:2306–10. https://doi.org/10.1002/nau.23729.

Basics of Curve Interpretation

10

Poonam Guha Vaze and Sirish Yande

Lines in a Standard Curve

Any particular invasive urodynamics tracing depicts the following lines in variable order and color coding (Fig. 10.1):

1. Pves
2. Pabd

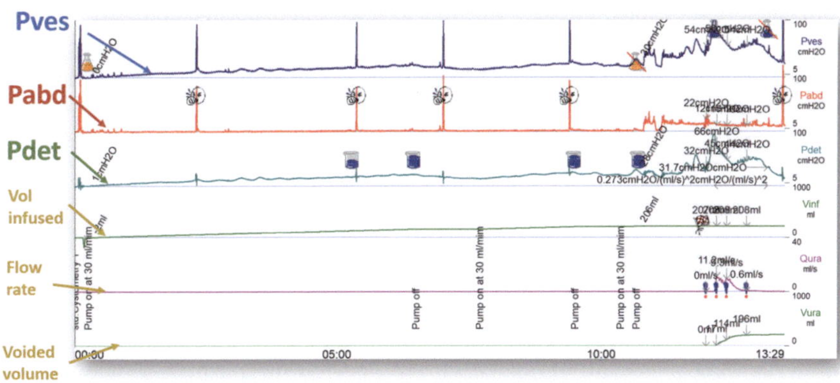

Fig. 10.1 Standard urodynamic curve

P. G. Vaze (✉)
Neotia Bhagirathi Woman and Child Care Centre, Newtown, Kolkata, India

Department of Pediatric Surgery, Nilratan Sircar Medical College and Hospital, Kolkata, India

S. Yande
Crystal Centre, MMF- Ratna Memorial Hospital, Pune, India

S. Saha, P. Guha Vaze (eds.), *Comprehensive Atlas of Practical Pediatric Urodynamics*, https://doi.org/10.1007/978-981-95-2709-0_10

3. Pdet
4. Volume infused
5. Flow rate
6. Voided volume

The last two parameters (Flow Rate and Voided Volume) are similar to the parameters of uroflowmetry. Deflection in these parameters is seen the following situations:

1. Significant leakage of fluid (if any) during the storage phase
2. Flow rate during the voiding phase

The limits of each of these parameters depicted on the graph can be changed depending on the clinical situation. For example, upper limit of pressures (Pdet/Pves and Pabd) is usually set at 100 cm H2O. If we see that the pressures are going up to 150 cm H2O, i.e., outside the range of 100 cm H2O, we can increase the limit to 150 or 200 cm H2O. Similarly, we can set the volume-infused limit till 200 ml for small children or 1000 ml in older children.

Different Symbols Used in a Curve

Different symbols can be used in the curve to demonstrate special events occurring during the test, for example, sensations like first sensation, normal urge, strong urge, urgency, and pain; maneuvers like cough/Valsalva; change of posture; leak; crying; command to void; and starting and stopping of micturition (Fig. 10.2). These are inserted by the examiner at relevant points so that any person other than the investigator looking at the curve can interpret the events that occurred during the test. For example, we should be able to differentiate a significant leak due to involuntary detrusor contraction from a detrusor contraction during a voluntary void by the markers that have been placed by the investigator (Fig. 10.3a, b).

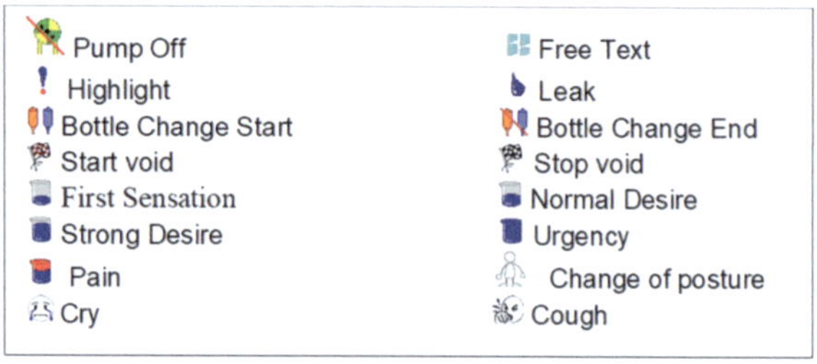

Fig. 10.2 The common symbols that can be inserted in the urodynamics system by Albynn

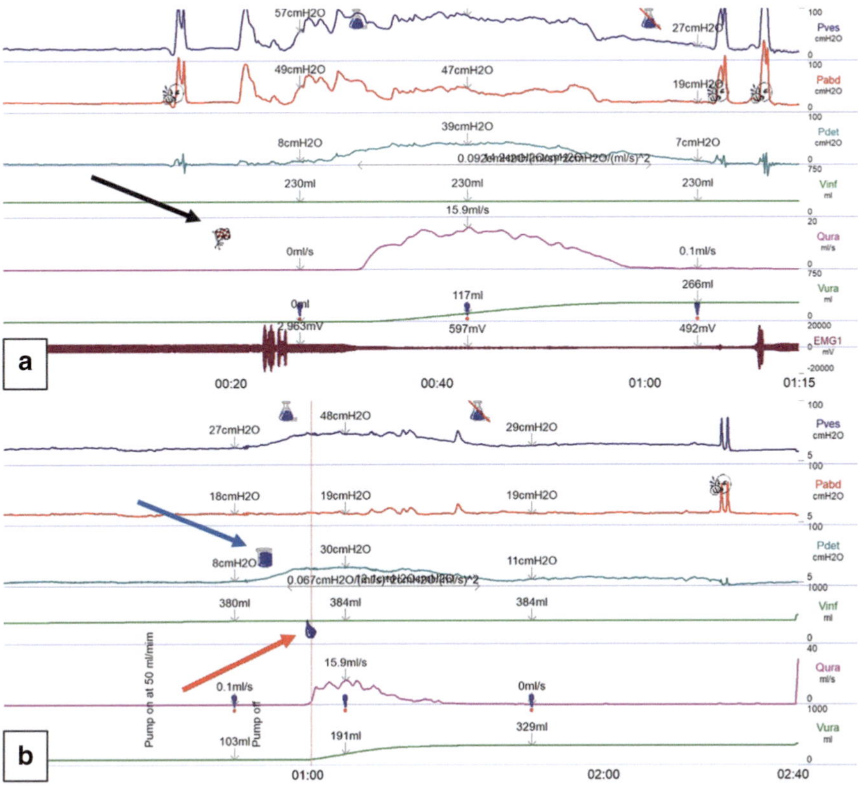

Fig. 10.3 (**a**) Voiding phase of a UDS curve showing voiding command (black arrow) followed by appearance of detrusor contraction and flow. Thus, this shows voluntary void. (**b**) shows another voiding phase where detrusor contraction starts involuntarily and patient complains of urge to pass urine (blue arrow) followed by urine leak (red arrow) and involuntary complete void. Thus, this shows terminal overactivity with leak

What Does Each Pressure Tracing Indicate

- *Pves* = *vesical catheter reading* = abdominal pressure + detrusor pressure
- *Pabd* = *rectal catheter reading* = abdominal pressure (+ rectal pressure)
- *Pdet* = *Pves—Pabd*

The software measures Pves and Pabd and calculates Pdet.

Depending on which traces are showing deflections, we can determine which pressure changes are responsible for deflections (Table 10.1), (Figs. 10.4, 10.5, 10.6 and 10.7).

Table 10.1 Deflections in the curves and their inferences

	Pves	Pabd	Pdet
Straining/coughing/crying (Figs. 10.4 and 10.5)	✓ (Positive)	✓ (Positive)	✗
Rectal contraction (Fig. 10.6)	✗	✓ (Positive)	✓ (Negative)
Detrusor contraction (Fig. 10.6)	✓ (Positive)	✗	✓ (Positive)

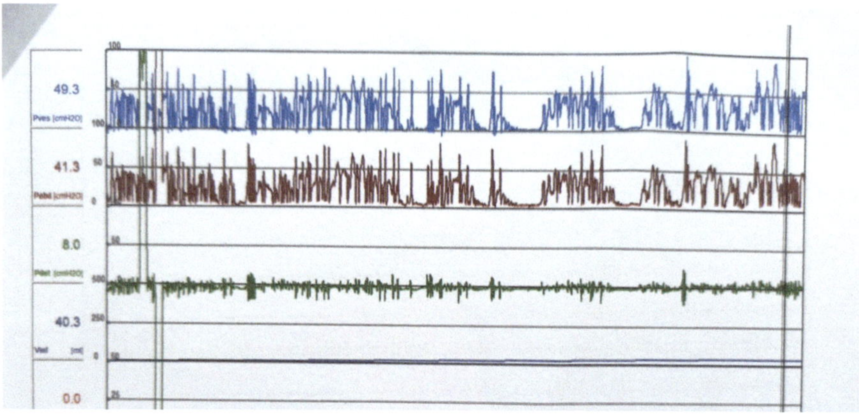

Fig. 10.4 Continuous deflections in both rectal and vesical tracing are caused by continuous crying of the child. The Pdet tracing is stable indicating a stable bladder

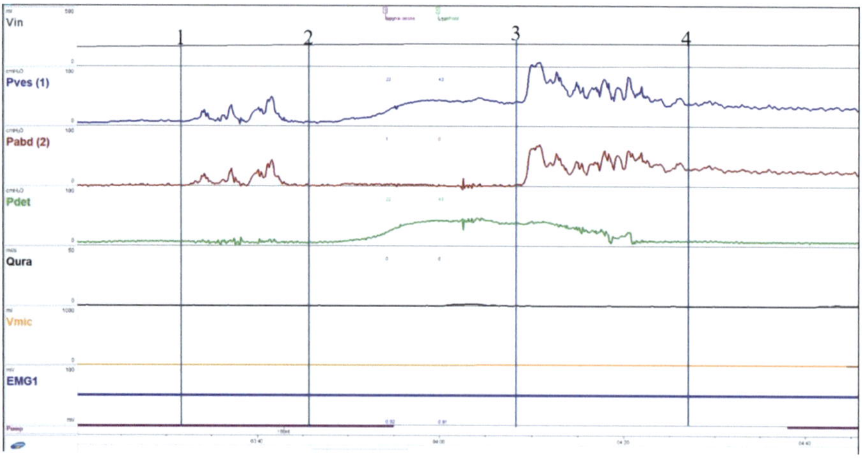

Fig. 10.5 Interplay of pressure measurements in an 8-year-old boy (BLUE = Pves, RED = Pabd, and GREEN = Pdet). Interval between points 1 and 2 denote coughing impulses (change in abdominal pressures only). Interval between points 2 and 3 denotes a detrusor contraction. (Note there is no change in rectal pressure trace.) Interval between 3 and 4 shows a combination of detrusor contraction and abdominal straining (note pressure subtractions are perfect)

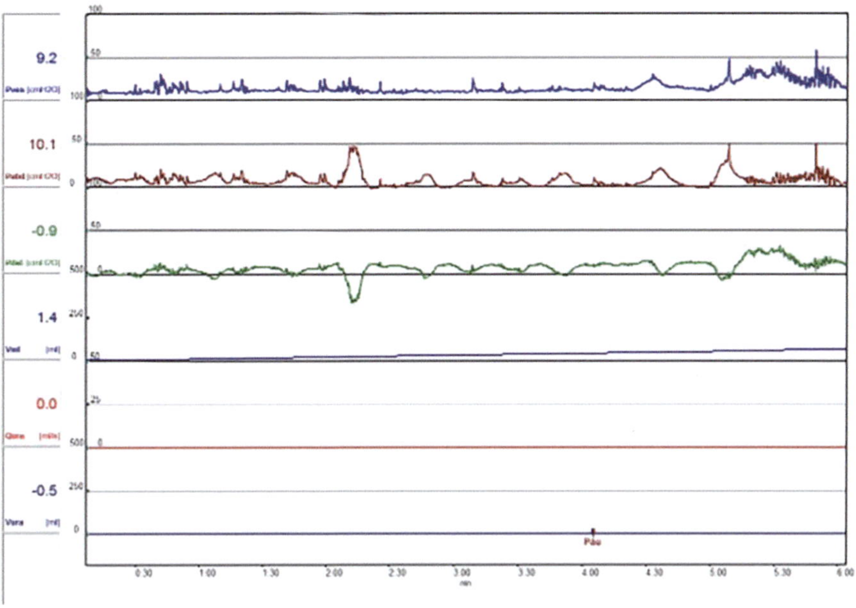

Fig. 10.6 Positive deflections in rectal tracing only, causing artifactual negative deflections in Pdet tracing. (This is not an instrument artefact. Contractions from rectal origin shows a true positive deflection. Since the software is programmed to SUBTRACT the Pabd from Pves, the detrusor pressure line will show a corresponding negative deflection.) Such waves in rectal catheter are usually caused due to intermittent rectal contractions in neurogenic dysfunction and in a constipated child

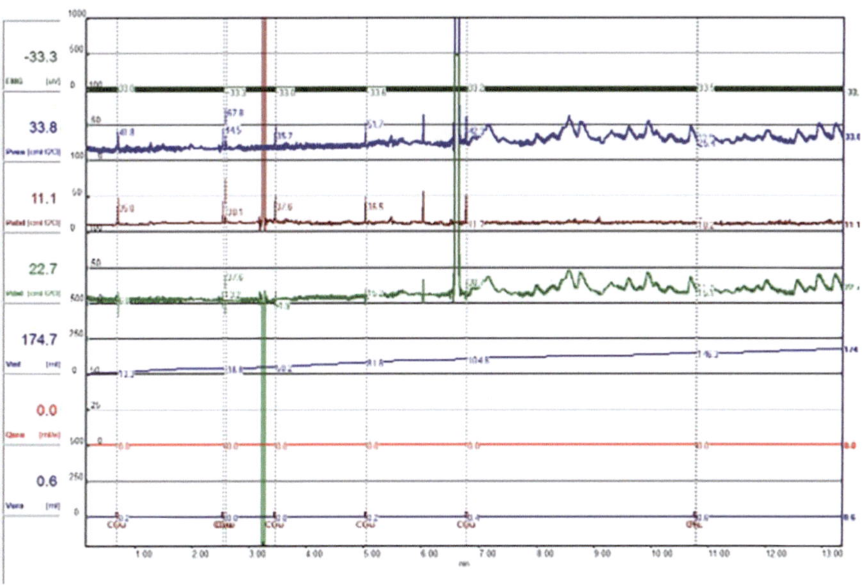

Fig. 10.7 Deflections in the vesical tracing only, resulting in positive deflections in the Pdet tracing, suggest detrusor contractions implying detrusor overactivity

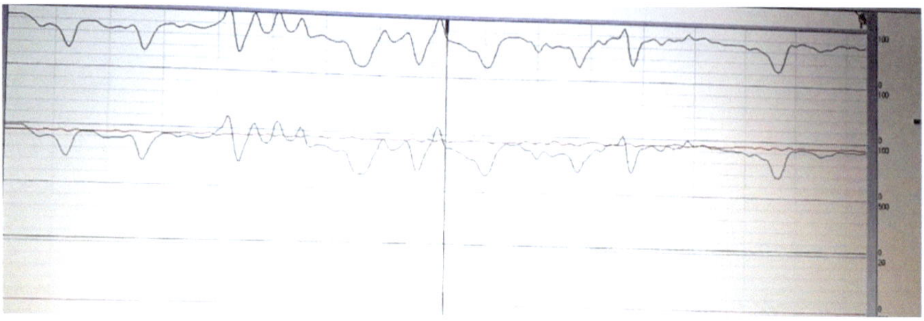

Fig. 10.8 No rectal catheter tracing is seen. Only vesical catheter tracing is seen with continuous deflections in either direction. It is impossible to ascertain the cause of such deflections as detrusor contraction/straining by the child

Is Rectal Pressure Measurement Essential?

Several centers in India and elsewhere perform urodynamics routinely without a rectal catheter. On the other hand, we use rectal/abdominal pressure monitoring catheter in *all* patients.

If we have to assess only the filling phase in an absolutely calm and obedient child, insertion of a rectal catheter may be omitted.

In the absence of rectal catheter reading, it is difficult to differentiate whether vesical catheter deflections are caused by straining or due to detrusor contractions, especially if the child is irritable/crying (Fig. 10.8). Also, if midway during the study the vesical catheter reading gets dampened, it is difficult to assess as there is no other catheter for comparison. In the absence of rectal catheter, it is impossible to assess the voiding detrusor pressures as the component caused by straining cannot be subtracted.

Problems with Rectal Pressure Measurement?

There is a downside to using rectal catheter as well. An abnormal activity in the rectal catheter can lead to false interpretation of detrusor hypocompliance/overactivity if the observer is not vigilant enough (Figs. 10.9 and 10.10). Thus, we have to assess deflection in all the three traces to come to a conclusion about the detrusor behavior.

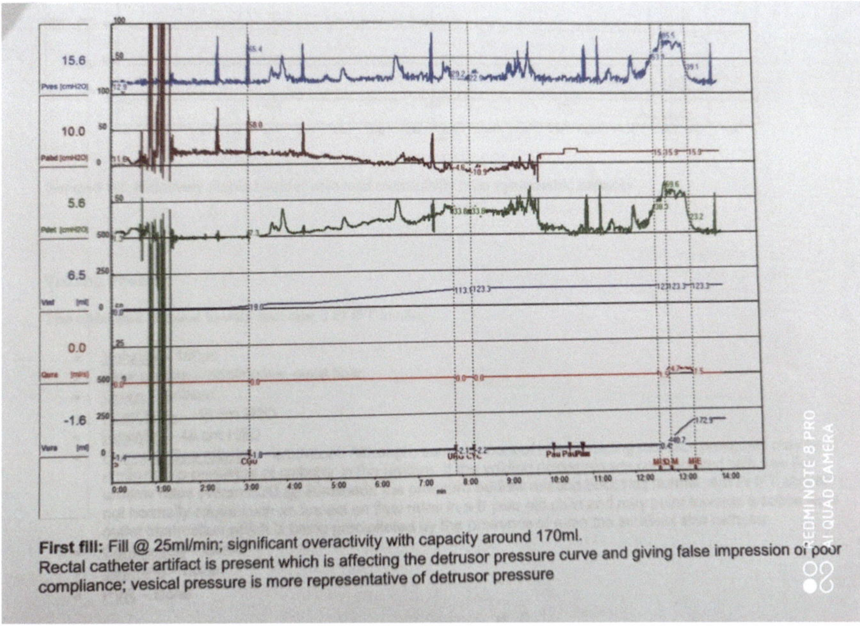

Fig. 10.9 The Pdet tracing shows an upward slope suggesting poor compliance and intermittent peaks denoting detrusor overactivity. The Pves tracing on the other hand shows the corresponding peaks of detrusor overactivity but does not show any deflection denoting poor compliance. The upward slope of Pdet tracing is caused by downward movement of the Pabd tracing and then it is seen to stop reading in the later one-third of the trace. The rectal catheter slipped out during the study which resulted in the deflection in the abdominal tracing which has caused an artifactual elevation of Pdet. In such situations, analysis of Pves is essential

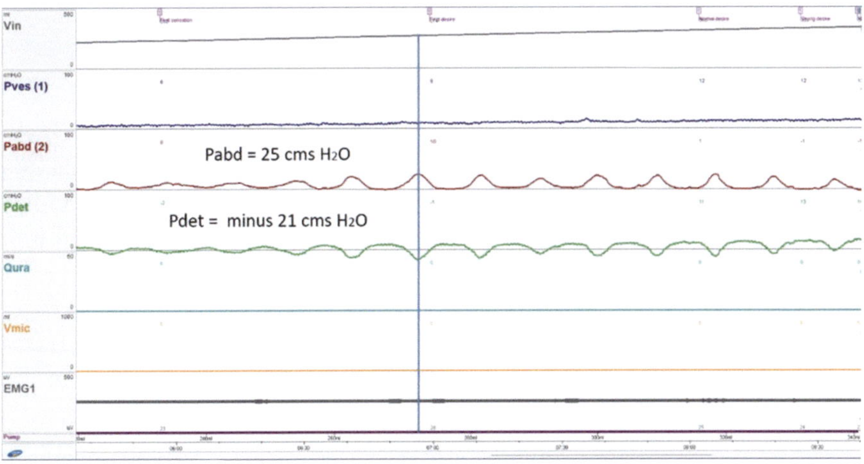

Fig. 10.10 Rectal contractions causing severe interference in the interpretation of detrusor pressure. Rectal waves are common in neuropathic affection of the lower urinary tracts. This is not an artefact but is a natural response. In this tracing, each rectal wave causes negative deflection in the detrusor pressure trace whereas the Pves tracing is showing a stable bladder

Fig. 10.11 Checklist for interpretation of UDS curves

Checklist for interpreting UDS curve

- Fill rate:
- All three tracings – Yes/ no
- Is cough response balancing OK – Yes/ no
- Is the rectal pressure tracing stable – Yes/ no
- Is voiding phase included – Yes/ no

Filling Phase

- Capacity
- Compliance
- Overactivity
- Leakage
- Sensation

Voiding phase

- Volume
- Qmax
- PdetQmax
- PVR

Checklist for Interpreting an *i*-UDS Tracing?

Figure 10.11 enumerates the points to be assessed whenever we try to read a UDS tracing.

Parameters to Be Assessed in Filling Phase

Capacity

Expected capacity of bladder is calculated according to age

- <2 years—wt in Kg × 7 = (mls)
- >2 years—(age + 1) × 30 = (mls)

Bladder capacity during the study is calculated as:

$$\text{Capacity} = \text{voided volume} + \text{PVR}$$

Many patients with high filling pressures/overactivity tend to have diuresis during the study. Thus, the "capacity" may be actually much higher than the infused/filled volume. For example, if we have filled a bladder with 200 ml, he voids 190 ml with a PVR of 60 ml. His total capacity would be 250 ml and not 200 ml.

Bladder capacity is reported as small capacity or large capacity if:

- <50% EBC—small capacity
- > 150%—large capacity

If there is a high-grade reflux with grossly dilated upper tracts, performing urodynamics blindly gives us a false impression of large capacity bladder. Performing Video-UDS in such a situation gives a better visualization of the size of the bladder (Fig. 10.12).

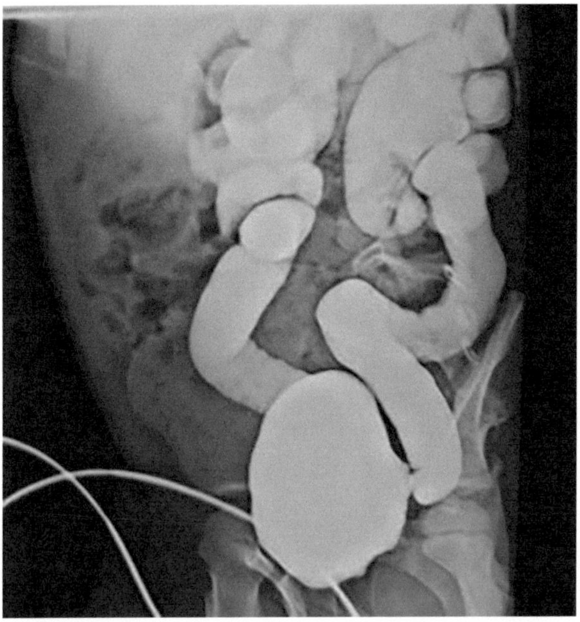

Fig. 10.12 Bilateral gross reflux with size of renal pelvis almost similar to that of bladder. UDS without video screening will give a false estimation of bladder capacity

Compliance

The detrusor pressures should be normally "zero" throughout the filing phase, i.e., the bladder should allow filling to occur with no rise of detrusor pressures. If the bladder loses its elasticity, the pressure rises when it fills up; thus, its compliance reduces.

Compliance is calculated as

$$\text{Compliance} = \frac{\Delta V}{\Delta P}$$

The higher the compliance is, the more stretchable is the bladder

Normal compliance > 30 ml/cm H2O

Normal "End Fill Pdet" should be < 10 cm H2O at capacity or 5% of child's normal capacity.

If the pressure starts rising during filling and does not come down to the baseline, the compliance is poor (Fig. 10.13). The slope of the curve gives us an idea about degree of loss of compliance—the steeper the slope, the poorer is the compliance.

Detrusor compliance is a pure function of the bladder volume and is defined as unit change in detrusor pressure per unit change in bladder volume. The rate of change therefore is expected to be a uniform straight line, as long as the rate of filling is constant. Also, if the rate of fill is very high, there may be reflex increase in bladder pressures which stabilizes or reduces once the flow is reduced (Figs. 10.14, 10.15 and 10.16)

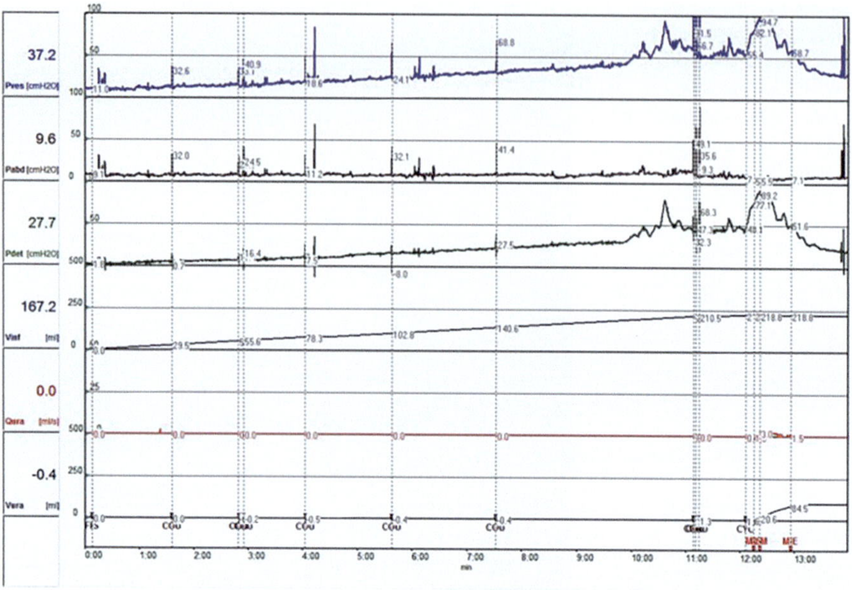

Fig. 10.13 Pdet is seen to rise continuously and not returning to baseline. Upgoing slope of the curve denotes poor compliance

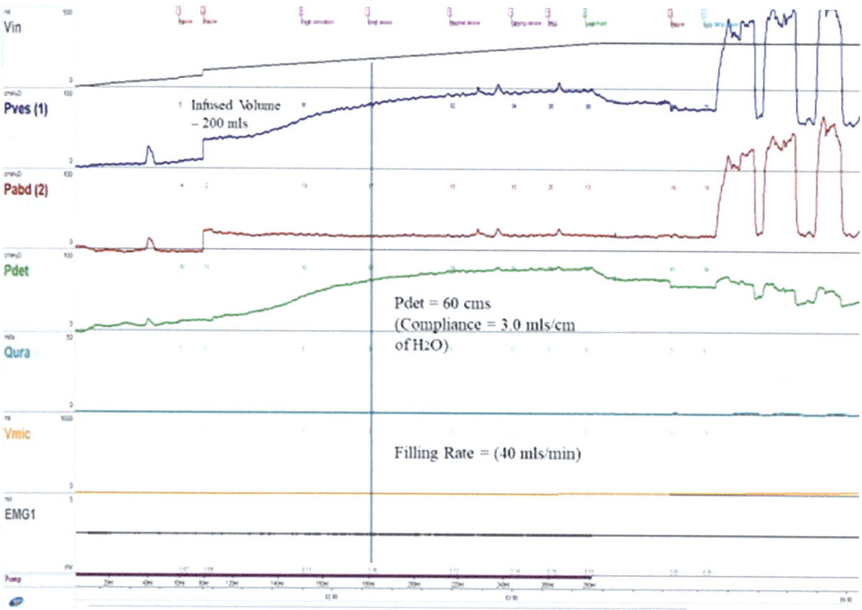

Fig. 10.14 Unrealistically high Pdet and low compliance being recorded at the filling rate of 40 mls/sec

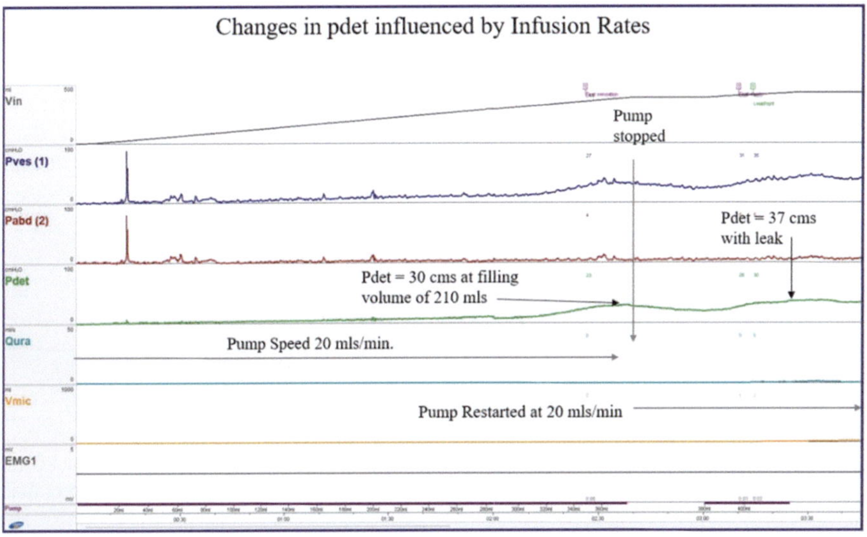

Fig. 10.15 Pdet is seen to rise exponentially at 210 ml volume to 30 cm H2O which plateaus off when the pump is stopped. It rises again after the pump is restarted and reaches 37 cm H2O when leak is documented

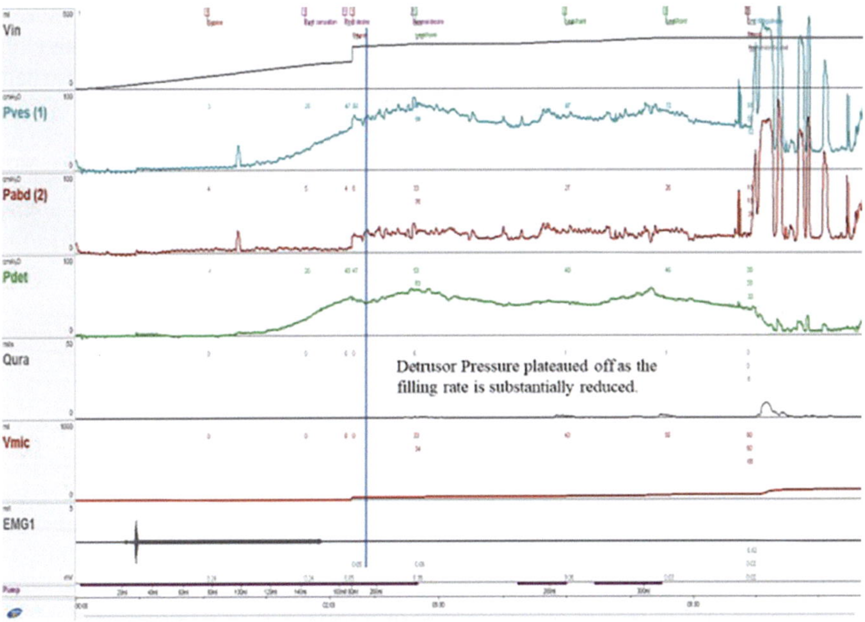

Fig. 10.16 Pdet rises with a steep curve. The curve plateaus and even reduced slightly when the fill rate is reduced. True detrusor compliance should therefore be measured at a point where the Pdet does not rise anymore during slow fill cycle

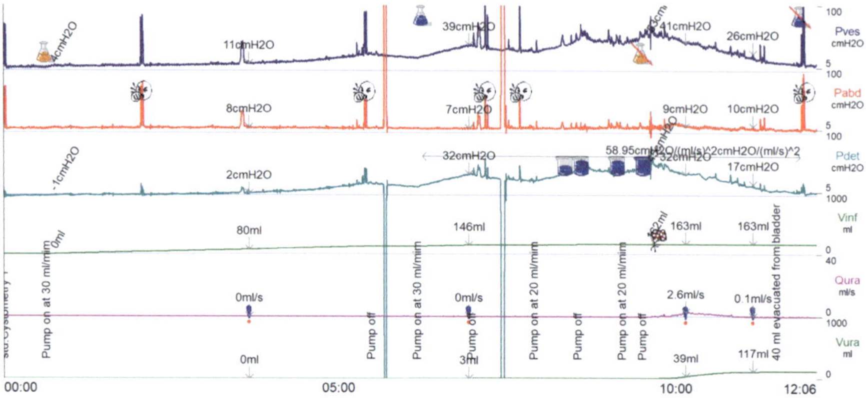

Fig. 10.17 Compliance was normal in first half of fill and reduced in second half of fill. Pdet reaches 95 cm H2O at 160 ml which reduces once patient voids. As the pressure rise starts at 80 ml, the compliance is to be calculated as 0.8 (80 ml/95 cm H2O) from 80 ml to 160 ml fill rather than 1.7 (160 ml/95 cm H2O) from 0 to 160 ml

The rise in detrusor pressures during filling may not be uniform throughout the fill despite uniform fill rates. It may remain stable for the initial part and then start rising after a particular volume (Fig. 10.17). In such cases, we should note the volumes after which the pressures start rising and the compliance should be measured for the volume when the pressure is rising. This has an important bearing with CIC volumes in bad bladders. If we can keep the CIC volumes below the threshold when the pressure starts rising, damage to upper tracts will be prevented.

Such variable rise of detrusor pressures can also be seen in cases of massive VUR or a bladder diverticulum (Fig. 10.18) wherein the detrusor pressures remain stable till the diverticulum or upper tracts fill up and then the reduced compliance manifests as rise in pressure. Such structural abnormalities can cause challenging problems in the estimation of true detrusor compliance.

Overactivity

If there are intermittent detrusor contractions during filling, the Pdet curve is seen to rise momentarily and comes down to baseline. This is known as detrusor overactivity (DO) (Fig. 10.19).

Overactivity can be normally seen in 10% of infants. Some overactivity may be seen near capacity and may be considered physiological. Overactivity seen in any other situation is pathological.

Overactivity may be due to neurogenic cause (neurogenic DO) or idiopathic.

It may be phasic or terminal. An involuntary detrusor contraction which is strong enough and culminates in complete voiding or leak of significant amounts of urine is known as terminal overactivity.

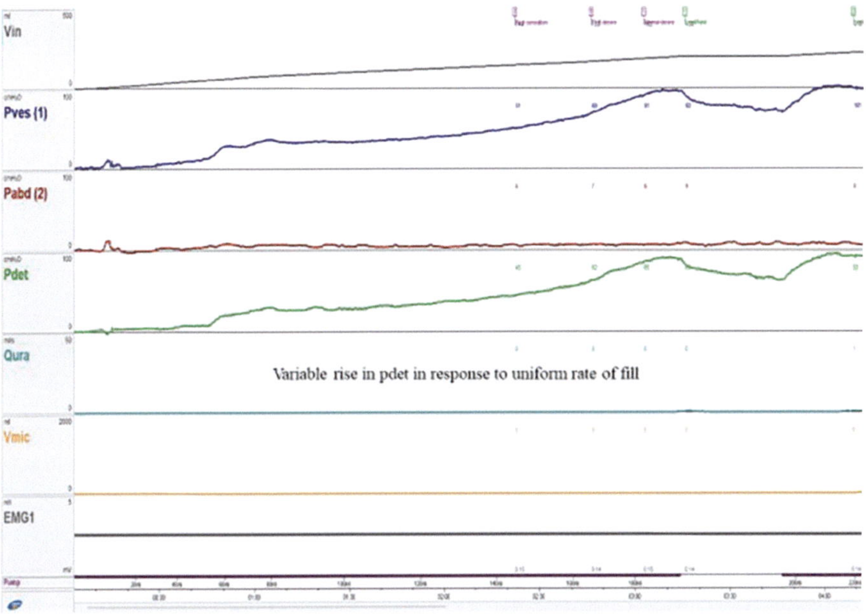

Fig. 10.18 Variable rise in Pdet in the presence of a large bladder diverticulum. Such structural abnormalities can cause challenging problems in the estimation of true detrusor compliance

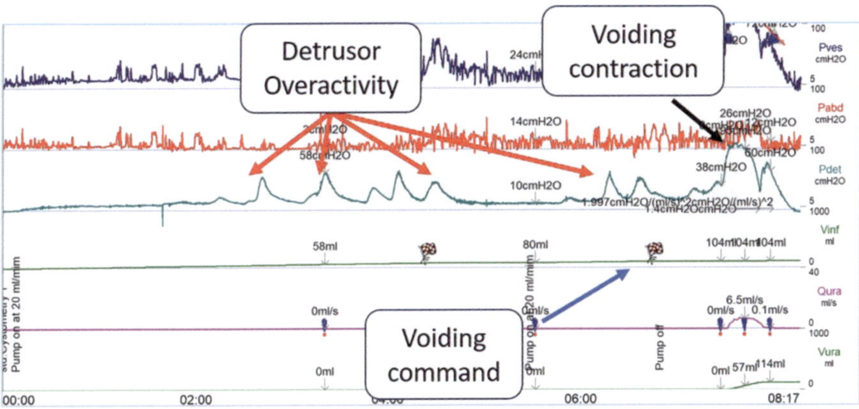

Fig. 10.19 Severe overactivity in a 4-year-old child with bladder outflow obstruction. Note that involuntary DO contraction should be differentiated from voiding detrusor contraction which the child initiates voluntarily to void (differentiation may be difficult in young children)

It may be spontaneous or provoked. In many children, DO may be manifested when the child is irritable/crying or performing some activity. Bladder may be absolutely stable when the child is calm (Fig. 10.20). This explains the absence of nocturnal symptoms when the child is sleeping in many children who have DO-associated

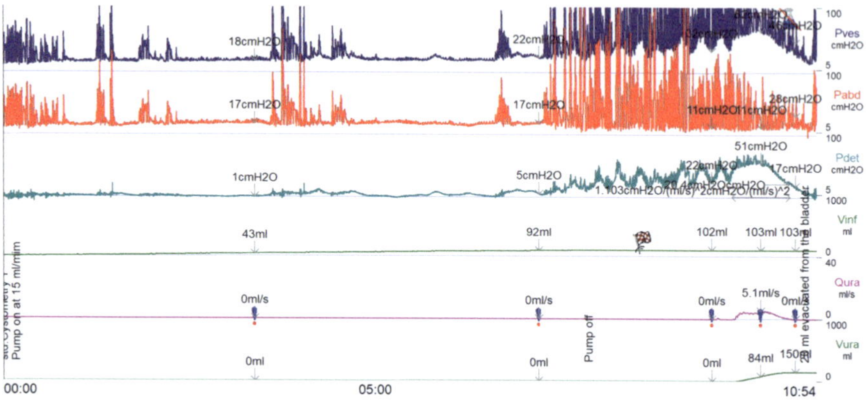

Fig. 10.20 No DO is seen in early part of fill when child is calm. Severe DO is seen after 90 ml fill when child gets irritable (irritability/ straining is evidenced by continuous deflections in both rectal and vesical tracing)

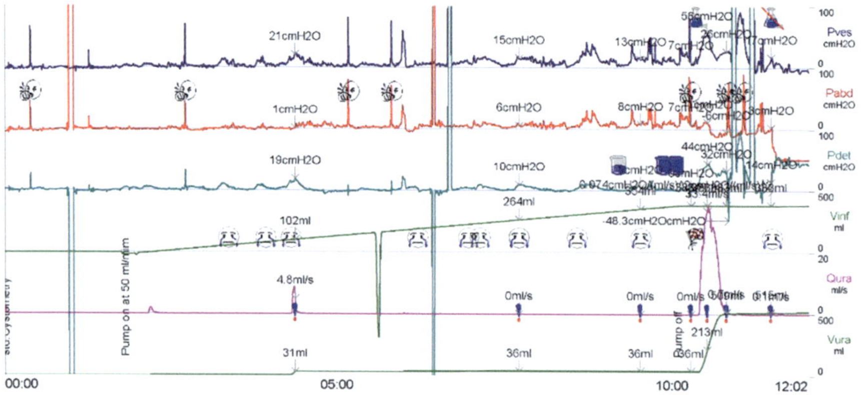

Fig. 10.21 UDS tracing of a 12-year-old girl with bladder bowel dysfunction complaining of significant suprapubic pain even after appropriate bowel clearance. Filling phase shows low-amplitude DO with pressures ranging from 5 to 10 cm H2O; on one occasion, the pressure was seen to reach 19 cm H2O, but the patient complained of pain during each of the episodes of DO (marked by "cry" symbol). So although the DO contractions are very weak, they are significant as they are causing symptoms

leak during the day. Thus, if we use sedation while performing the study, such findings may be masked.

There may or may not be symptoms of urgency or leak during the episodes.

Both the ICS and ICCS documents do not lay down any cutoff limit of pressure rise to define DO, but it is generally regarded at 15 cm H2O. We have had children complaining of urgency or suprapubic pain with detrusor contractions of even 5 cm H2O (Fig. 10.21). Hence, any phasic (demonstrable) rise in detrusor pressure during the filling phase should be regarded as "detrusor overactivity."

Sensations

ICS guidelines 2016 recommend the following bladder sensations to be recorded:

- *First sensation of filling* (FSF)—"Tell me the moment when you perceive that your bladder is not empty anymore."
- *First desire to void* (FDV)—"Tell me when you have the first sensation that normally tells you to go to the toilet, without any hurry, at the next convenient moment."
- *Normal desire to void* is marked when the patient reaches a bladder volume and feels the sensation that he/she "normally" would go to pass urine.
- *Strong desire to void* (SDV)—"The moment that you would definitely visit the nearest toilet to pass urine." There should be no pain or any fear of losing urine.

ICS (2016) recommends that incontinence, fear of leakage, pain, or other signs or symptoms during the test should be specifically marked on the urodynamic graph.

ICCS defines reduced bladder sensation as diminished awareness throughout bladder filling and absent bladder sensation as no bladder sensation whatsoever. Both can be observed in children with an underactive detrusor, a neuropathic bladder, or a comorbidity of diabetes mellitus (Fig. 10.22).

Younger children cannot inform any bladder sensations but indicate pain/sense of full bladder by behavior changes/changes in facial expression/crossing of legs/crying. If a child does not show any behavioral change even after filling up to 150% of EBC, we can presume reduced or absent sensation and stop the filling.

Elder children can report bladder sensations appropriately and they should be recorded whenever the child is verbal enough.

Children usually complain of urge to void/pain during periods of DO.

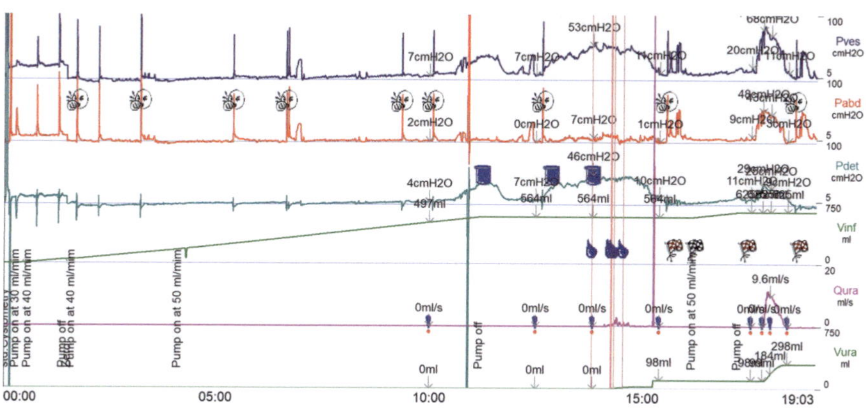

Fig. 10.22 A 14-year-old girl with type I DM and diabetic neuropathy. USG shows large bladder with thick walls, upper tract changes, and significant PVR. No bladder sensations were reported till 500 ml fill suggesting reduced bladder sensations. She reported urgency during episodes of DO which appeared at 500 ml fill

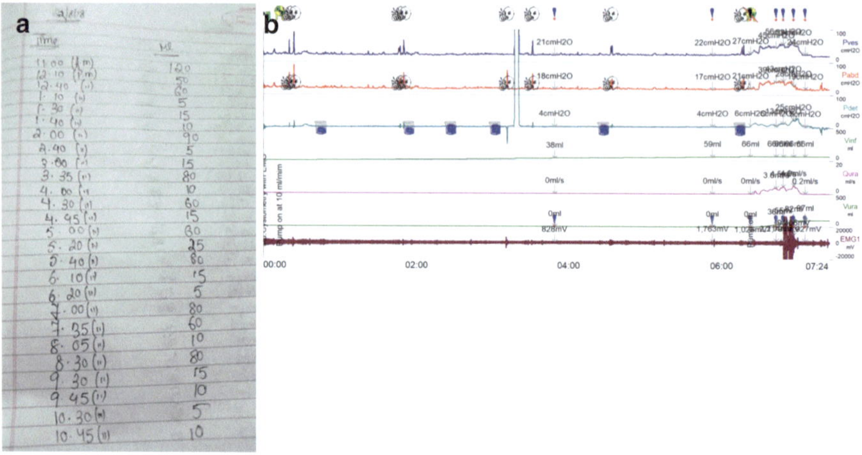

Fig. 10.23 (**a**) A 7-year-old boy with extraordinary high daytime-only urinary frequency. He is seen to have a small capacity bladder with urge to void from beginning of fill with no apparent rise in detrusor pressures—"SENSORY URGENCY" (**b**) A 24-hour voiding diary of the same child showing extraordinary high daytime-only frequency

We have seen a separate subset of patients who complain of urge to void from beginning of study even before the filling is started although there is no evidence of DO. They allow bladder filling to continue if they are distracted in conversations. We label them as "SENSORY URGENCY." We have seen this finding very commonly in children presenting with increased urinary frequency either due to extraordinary increased daytime-only frequency (Fig. 10.23a and b) or bladder bowel dysfunction. These children also typically have a low-pressure-low-flow pattern during voiding phase; thus, we do not use anticholinergics in them. These children usually respond to aggressive management of constipation over a period of 2–4 weeks.

Leakage

A normal bladder does not leak anytime during filling.

Leak may be seen if detrusor pressures are exceptionally high in spite of a competent outlet or if the outlet is incompetent to variable degrees.

An outlet which is very loose will allow urine to leak out as soon as the bladder starts filling up.

Detrusor Leak Point Pressure (DLPP) is defined as the lowest detrusor pressure at which urinary leakage occurs in the absence of a detrusor contraction or an increase in abdominal pressure (Fig. 10.24). Classically, end fill pressures of DLPP >40 cm H2O is considered as high risk for upper tract damage, but studies have shown that pressure of >20 cm H2O is a better predictor of upper tract changes.

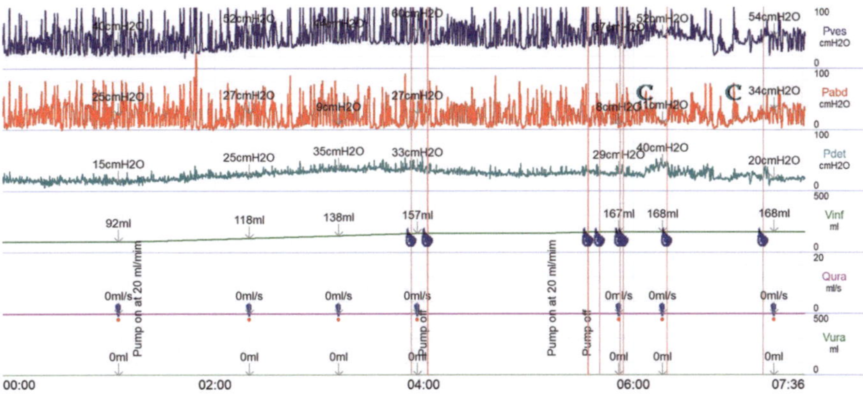

Fig. 10.24 A 3-year-old girl with neurogenic bladder showed gross bilateral HDUN and thick-walled UB on USG. UDS showed large capacity bladder (170 ml; EBC 120 ml) with leaks appearing at 160 ml at Pdet around 30–40 cm H2O in the absence of any DO or coughing—DLPP 30 cm H2O at 160 ml volume. The symbol "C" shows that Crede's maneuver was performed to assess leak

Also, animal studies have shown that ultrastructural changes begin appearing in the detrusor if the bladder is exposed to pressures as low as 10 cm H2O for 24 hours.

Detrusor Leak Point Pressure (DLPP) has a direct relevance to the safety of the upper urinary tracts in bladder dysfunction due to neurologic causes.

However, the exact magnitude of the resting bladder pressure required to produce upper tract dilatation remain a matter of controversy.

McGuire (1981) in his classic study of children with neurogenic bladder dysfunction had recommended a DLPP figure of 40 cms of H2O, beyond which upper tract are at risk of dilatation and renal dysfunctions. But many studies subsequently showed that DLPP figures of greater than 20 cms are capable of producing upper tract damage in this group of patients. By and large, it is seen that the higher the storage pressure, the higher are the chances of deterioration of the upper urinary tracts.

Besides DLPP, there are other factors such as neurogenic detrusor overactivity, VU reflux, reduced bladder capacity, detrusor hypocompliance, and episodes of urinary tract infection which may contribute to renal deterioration in the long term.

There are some clear technical issues about the standardization of measurement of DLPP:

- Abdominal pressure rise may interfere.
- Presence of gross UV reflux/diverticula may dissipate intravesical pressures and add errors.
- Size of catheter may influence the measurement.
- Theoretically, the dynamics of the urethra could be altered by the presence of urethral catheter in two ways.

In summary, the resting value of detrusor pressure relates to two important aspects of neurogenic bladder dysfunction.

- It is the pressure at which natural leakage would occur.
- The value of resting pressure is sustained in the bladder and theoretically impedes the antegrade flow of urine from kidneys to the bladder, thus culminating into dilatation of the upper tracts and renal deterioration.

Such a bladder needs emptying periodically to ensure low sustained detrusor pressures either by intermittent catheterization or a combination of CIC with oral medications, periodic intradetrusor injection of botulinum toxin or augmentation of the urinary bladder (augmentation cystoplasty).

Urodynamic evaluation of the storage function should mandate two important urodynamic parameters:

- Leak-specific bladder pressure
- Leak-specific bladder volume (Fig. 10.25)

Abdominal Leak Point Pressure (ALPP) is defined as the intravesical pressure at which urine leakage occurs because of increased abdominal pressure in the absence of a detrusor contraction. Leakage is caused by an increase in abdominal pressure when there is an incompetent urethra (Figs. 10.26 and 10.27).

Detrusor Overactivity Leak Point Pressure (DO-LPP) is the detrusor pressure during an episode of detrusor overactivity when leak is seen (Fig. 10.26).

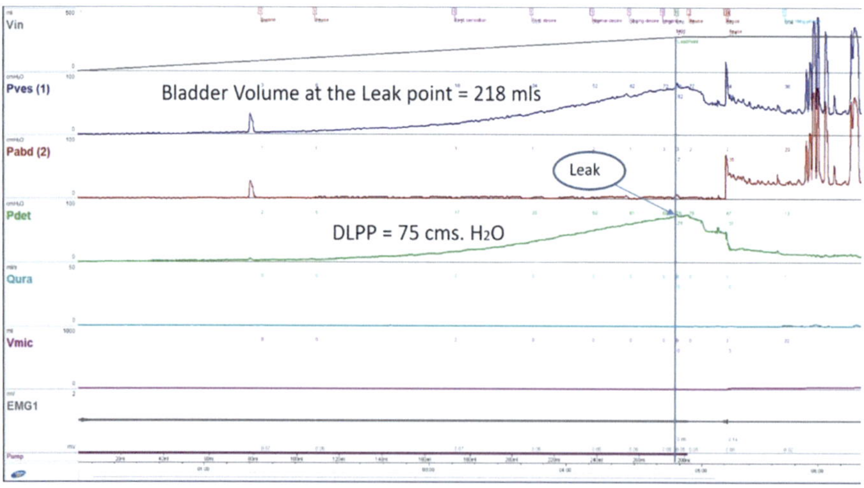

Fig. 10.25 Urodynamic tracing of an 11-year-old girl with meningomyelocele. She presented with continuous dribbling urinary incontinence with a moderate upper tract dilatation. Filling cystometry shows severely hypocompliant bladder with leakage at 75 cms of H2O and leak-specific bladder volume of 208 mls

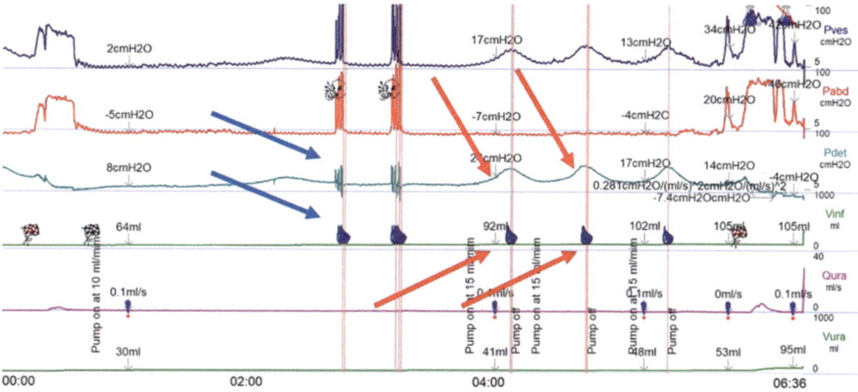

Fig. 10.26 A 7-year-old boy with neurogenic bladder, not on any management. USG shows normal upper tracts with thick-walled bladder. He showed leak during coughing in the absence of any DO (blue arrow) suggesting weak bladder outlet—ALPP 60 cm H2O. He also had severe detrusor overactivity. Red arrows show leak during episodes of DO—DO-LPP 50 cm H2O

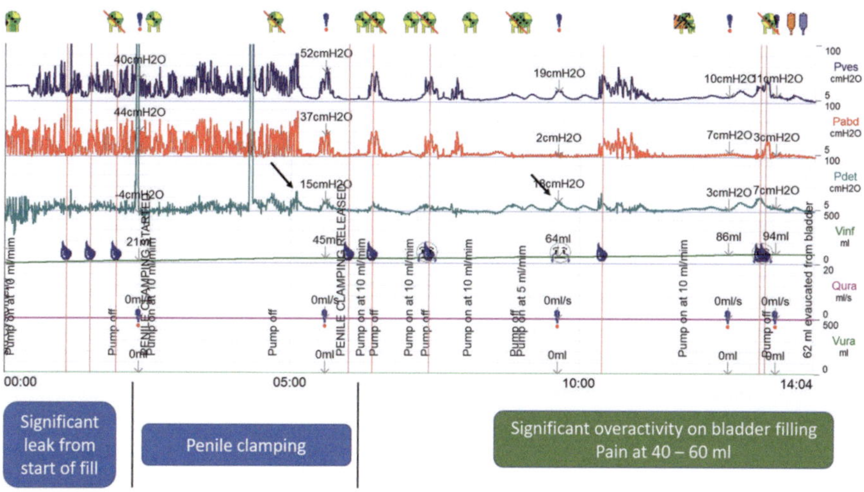

Fig. 10.27 A 4-year-old boy with neurogenic bladder, normal upper tracts and bladder on USG. Started leaking shortly after filling was started showing very weak bladder outlet. Penile clamping was done to allow bladder filling which manifested detrusor overactivity when the bladder was filled up

Terminal overactivity is usually a wave of strong involuntary detrusor contraction when patient leaks substantial amount or whole of the urine (Fig. 10.28). ICS recommends that command to void may be given during terminal overactivity when leak appears. In such cases, we usually repeat the study and give command to void at a volume which precedes the usual volume for occurrence of terminal

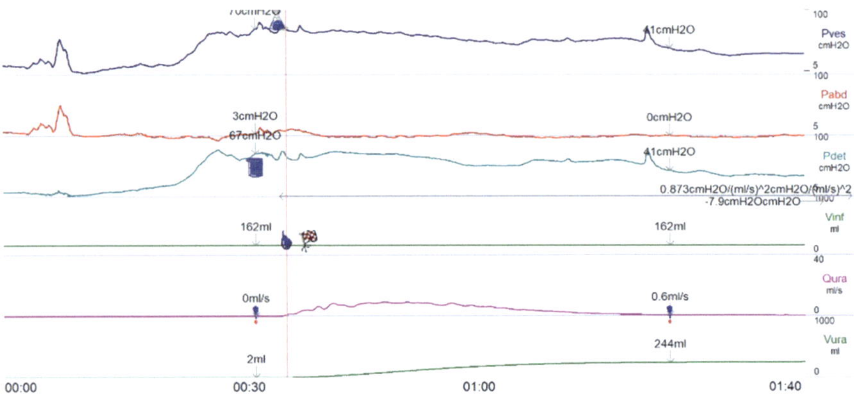

Fig. 10.28 A 15-year-old boy with overactive bladder. Terminal overactivity is seen at 160 ml fill (marked by sign for urgency) when patient starts to leak which is shown by "leak" sign. After the leak appears, he is given command to void and he finishes rest of the void. These annotations help us to understand the events which occurred during the study

overactivity and assess whether the patient can initiate voluntary void. Very often, in patients with neurogenic bladder, they have the ability to void only during periods of involuntary detrusor contraction but cannot initiate void on their own.

Parameters to be Assessed in Voiding Phase

Physics of Voiding

The detrusor contracts and provides the force to push the urine out. The outlet provides variable degrees of resistance to outflow by virtue of relaxation/contraction of bladder neck/sphincter or presence/absence of anatomical narrowing.

The work done by the detrusor manifests as flow rate and detrusor pressure. If outflow resistance is normal or low, detrusor pressure does not rise much and a good flow rate is achieved. If the outflow resistance is high, lower flow rate is achieved and detrusor pressures are high.

If the force generated by the detrusor is small, both the pressure and flow rates are low. If the force generated by detrusor is high, supranormal flow rates are achieved with pressures being normal (Fig. 10.29).

When pressure-flow dynamics is studied, we can study the Qmax as well as the detrusor pressure during different phases of flow. Qmax gives an indirect idea about detrusor contractility if Qmax is normal or supranormal. But if Qmax is low, to differentiate between detrusor underactivity and obstructed outflow, we need to know the Pdet during voiding.

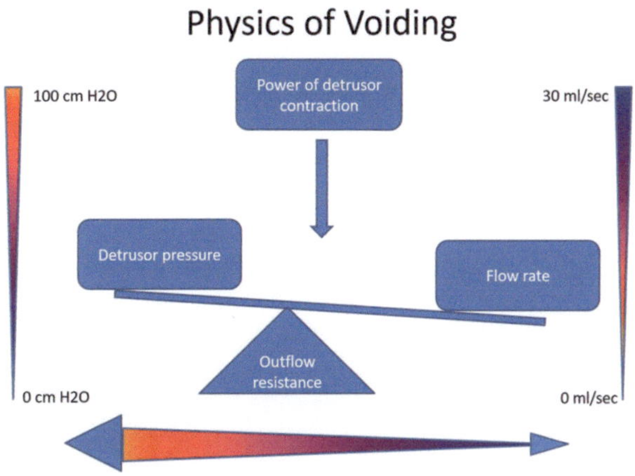

Fig. 10.29 Effect of interplay of outflow resistance and detrusor contraction on detrusor pressure and flow rates

Standard Pressure-Flow Parameters in Children

Inadequacies in Current Nomenclature

There are no normative values of pressure-flow parameters in children. Nomenclature used in literature for depicting pressure-flow parameters in children is varied and confusing and the reference standards are rather descriptive.

The usual voiding pressures in neurologically normal boys in standard fill cystometry is quoted as 127 cm H2O in the ICCS document.

Definition of bladder outflow obstruction (BOO):

(a) ICS—"A high voiding detrusor pressure (usually >74 cm H2O in boys) with a low urine flow indicates bladder outflow obstruction; low pressure with a low flow indicates underactive detrusor."
(b) ICCS—Anatomical obstruction results in a low and constant maximum flow, despite high detrusor pressure and complete relaxation of the external urethral sphincter.

Definition of underactive detrusor:

- ICCS—If a detrusor contraction is inadequate in magnitude and duration to effectively empty the bladder, it is referred to as detrusor underactivity during voiding.

Several parameters have been assessed in different studies and there is no uniformity in the literature. "Maximum voiding pressure" in infants has been variedly reported to be 100–200 cm H2O and older children as 70–100 cm H2O.

Pressure-Flow Indices: Deductions from Adult Data

We routinely perform pressure-flow studies in children. We found the existing literature very confusing and inadequate to be put to practical use. So we tried using the nomenclature proposed for adult studies instead. We have observed that the data obtained from properly conducted pressure-flow studies can provide essential information to guide treatment planning.

Various parameters have been used to objectively assess voiding in adults.

- Qmax—maximum flow rate during the void
- Pdet at Qmax—detrusor pressure recorded at maximum urine flow rate
- Pdetmax—maximum registered detrusor pressure during voiding
- PVR

It has been shown that Pdetmax and PdetQmax are discrete parameters and have different connotations. They can be easily recorded in most children (Fig. 10.30).

Several nomograms and indices have been developed to quantify detrusor contractility and outflow resistance in elderly men with prostatic hyperplasia which have also been extrapolated to men of all ages. Commonest of these is the relation between PdetQmax and Qmax in the form of BOOI and BCI.

$$\text{BOOI} — \text{bladder outlet obstruction index} — \text{Pdet at QMax} - 2 \times \text{Qmax}$$
$$\text{BCI} — \text{bladder contractility index} — \text{Pdet at Qmax} + 5 \times \text{Qmax}$$

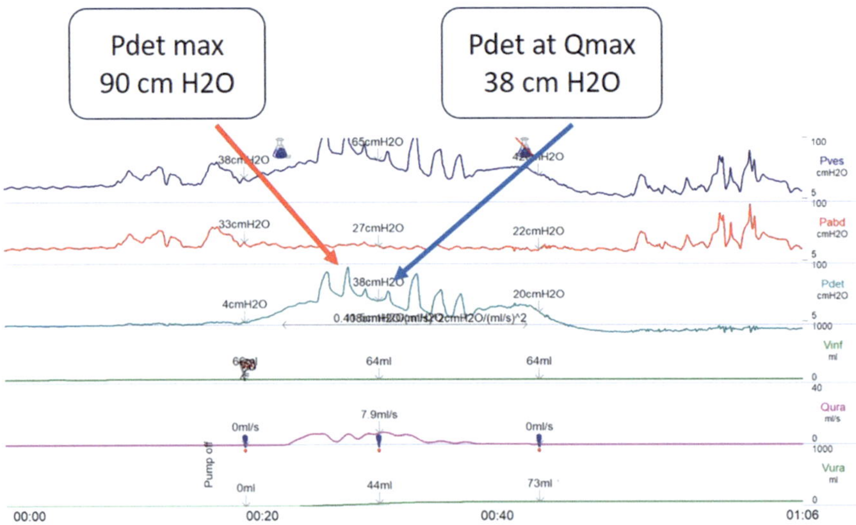

Fig. 10.30 Voiding phase of a UDS tracing showing Pdetmax and Pdet at Qmax

Based on these formulae, outflow tract in adults can be divided into obstructed, equivocal, and unobstructed according to their BOOI:

- BOOI >40 = obstructed
- BOOI 20–40 = equivocal
- BOOI <20 = unobstructed

Similarly, detrusor contractility in adults can be divided into strong, normal, and weak based on BCI:

- BCI > 150—strong contractility
- BCI 100–150—normal contractility
- BCI < 100—weak contractility

Our Observations About Reference Values in Boys

We have observed that the Qmax reduces in the presence of a 6 Fr catheter in all age groups. For *similar voided volumes*, UDSQmax and UFQmax correlated significantly but the value of UDSQmax is around 27% lower than the value of UF Qmax.

We have observed that the PdetQmax does not vary with age and is normally around 40 cm H2O. Pdetmax varies with age as younger children show more episodes of sphincteric contraction during voiding in the presence of catheter which raises the Pdetmax.

We have also observed that the range of BOOI in boys is similar to that in adults and BOOI >40 in follow-up children with PUV correlates with small for age capacity bladders. We found BCI to vary with age as a major part of BCI is contributed by Qmax which varies with age.

Pressure-Flow Parameters in Girls

Pressure-flow parameters in women have been found to be different from that of men. Women have shorter and wider urethra and thus reduced outflow resistance compared to men. Thus, voiding detrusor pressures are generally lower and flow rates are higher in women than in men. Hence, indices of BOOI and BCI are not applicable in women and separate sets of indices have been devised.

Blaivas and Groutz developed a nomogram based on Pdetmax and free uroflowmetry Qmax, defining four regions in the graph: no obstruction, mild, moderate, and severe obstruction (Fig. 10.31). They defined BOO as a free Qmax <12 mL/sec combined with a Pdet Qmax of >20 cm H2O in pressure-flow study, or obvious radiographic obstruction in the presence of a sustained detrusor contraction of >20 cm H2O, or urinary retention or the inability to void with a transurethral catheter in place despite a sustained detrusor contraction of >20 cm H2O.

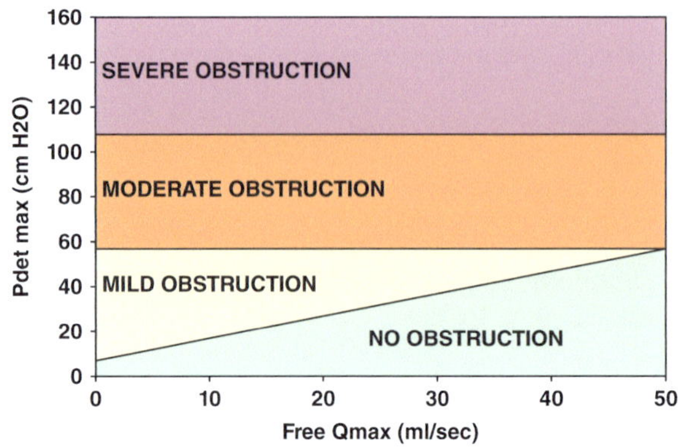

Fig. 10.31 Blaivas and Groutz nomogram for assessing BOO in women. (Adapted from: Blaivas and Groutz [5])

We have observed a similar trend of pressure-flow parameters in girls. In the absence of any outflow tract obstruction, the voiding detrusor pressures in girls are usually less than 40 cm H2O.

Different Voiding States

In general, pressure-flow studies will identify three fundamental voiding states:

1. Low detrusor pressure and high flow rate (unobstructed)
2. High detrusor pressure and low flow rate (obstructed)
3. Low detrusor pressure with low flow rate (poor detrusor contractility).

Although it is important to understand these three fundamental patterns, it is equally important to realize the limitations of such categorization. Unfortunately, pressure-flow studies do not always allow for an absolute classification into one distinct category. Borderline cases exist as well as cases in which there is a combination of impaired contractility and obstruction (Fig. 10.32). Figures 10.33, 10.34, 10.35, 10.36, 10.37, 10.38, 10.39 and 10.40 show different UDS traces with varying pressure-flow relations.

Pitfalls in the Interpretation of Pressure-Flow Findings in Children

While the storage parameters can be assessed with a reasonable accuracy in children (with due precautions), voiding parameters cannot be evaluated reliably in children. There are various reasons for this statement:

1. Presence of the cystometry catheter can cause a mechanical occlusion or obstruction in the urethra and can skew the flow rate.
2. For this reason, detrusor pressure measured during the voiding process may be recorded very high due to mechanical obstruction in the urethra.

		Qmax		
		High	Normal	Low
Pdet	High		Probable obstruction	Obstruction
	Normal	Probable overactivity	Normal	Probable obstruction + underactivity
	Low	Overactivity	Normal	Underactive detrusor

Fig. 10.32 Inference of different flow rates and corresponding detrusor pressures

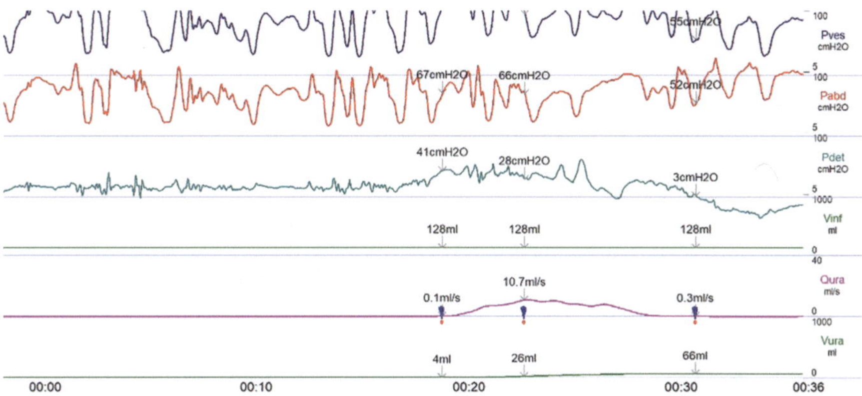

Fig. 10.33 Normal pressures and flow rates—*un*obstructed outflow—2.7-year-old boy, follow-up case of PUV with intermittent dribbling. Filling phase showed detrusor overactivity (not shown in the figure), but voiding parameters were normal

3. A relatively stiffer catheter in the urethra in children can variably alter the dynamics of the urethra during the voiding process.
4. Finally, presence of a gross VUR (or a large bladder diverticulum) can potentially dissipate the pressure inside the bladder and may give a much lower figure of the voiding detrusor pressure than the real pressure that the bladder has generated inside.

The observed voiding pattern during pressure-flow study should be corroborated with the pattern observed during free flow uroflowmetry and usual voiding pattern. If the voids do not corroborate, then the void during pressure-flow study cannot be

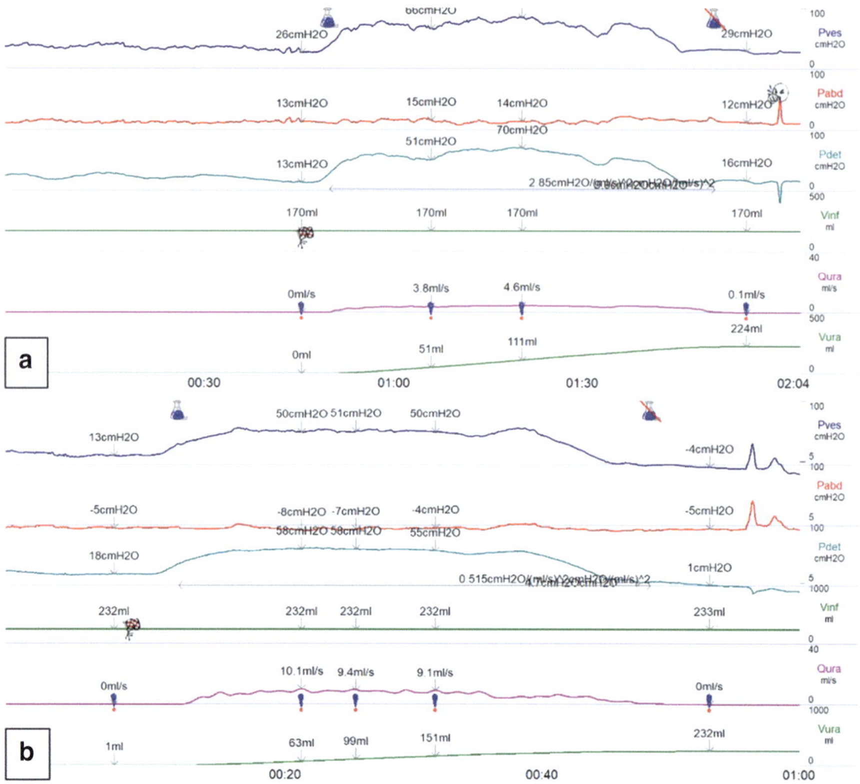

Fig. 10.34 (**a**) High-pressure-low-flow state in a 7-year-old follow-up child of PUV. He was found to have a meatal stenosis along with residual valves and very prominent bladder neck (**b**) Improvement in pressure-flow parameters after meatoplasty and incision of residual valves

regarded as "true." This kind of paradox can only become worse if the age of the child is lower. Hence, the smaller the child, the greater is the paradox in the voiding parameters (Figs. 10.41a, b and 10.42a, b).

The diagnosis of bladder outlet obstruction, therefore, needs to be considered extremely carefully in such cases. The authors prefer to use free flow on more than one occasion and a video clip of the child's standard voiding cycle at home (video taken against a dark background). Voiding parameters are useful in making the assessment of outlet obstruction only where the uroflow during voiding matches reasonably with a catheter-free uroflow of the child (preferably carried out before the investigation starts).

An MCUG correlation can reveal the true picture and rule-in or rule-out outflow tract obstruction in such cases with conflicting findings (Fig. 10.43).

In patients with gross VUR, a low-pressure-low-flow state may be noted as the voiding detrusor pressure gets dissipated into the ureters.

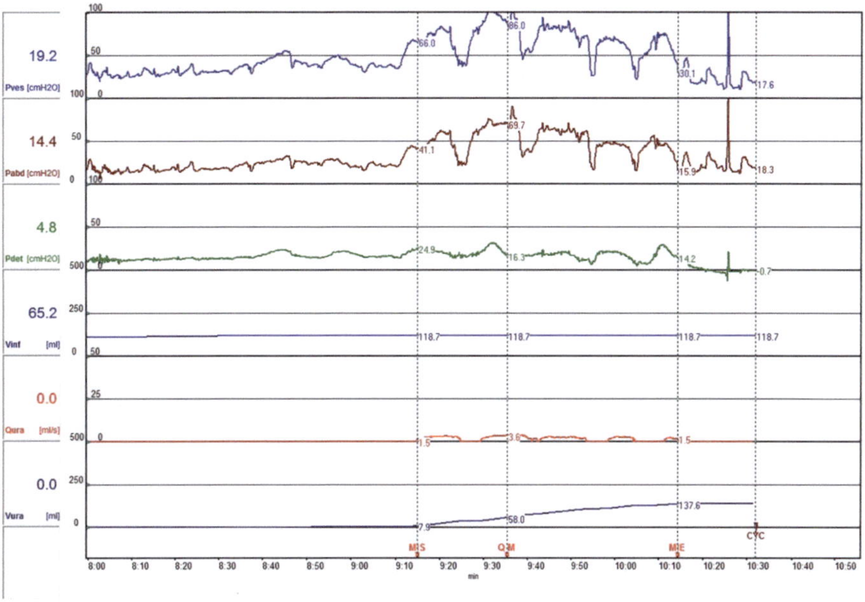

Fig. 10.35 Low pressure-low flow—8-year-old boy with neurogenic bladder. Slow interrupted flow due to detrusor underactivity; significant straining is seen during the void—Valsalva void. There was significant PVR after the void

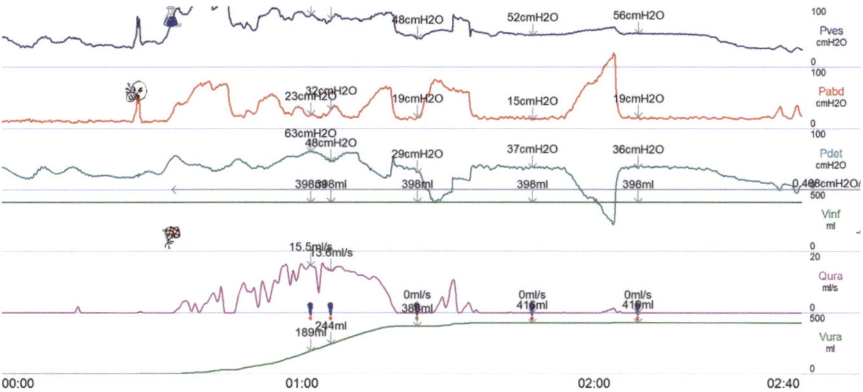

Fig. 10.36 A 15-year-old boy, follow-up case of PUV with bilateral HDUN, significant PVR, and poor uroflow suggestive of myogenic failure. Pressure-flow study shows normal detrusor contractility and “equivocal” pressure-flow relation (BOOI 30) which goes against the diagnosis of myogenic failure. So MCU was done. He has poor bladder neck opening for which he was started on alpha-blockers which resulted in marked improvement in flow pattern

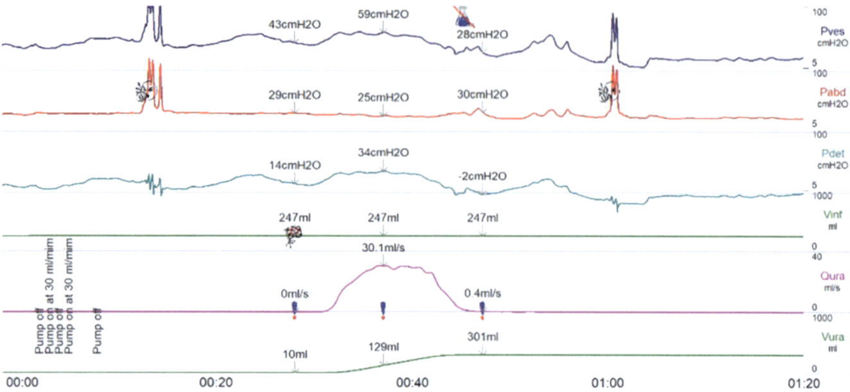

Fig. 10.37 Normal pressure and flow rate in a 10-year-old girl with urgency/urge incontinence/recurrent UTI. Filling phase showed severe detrusor overactivity. Voiding phase showed normal pressure-flow relation

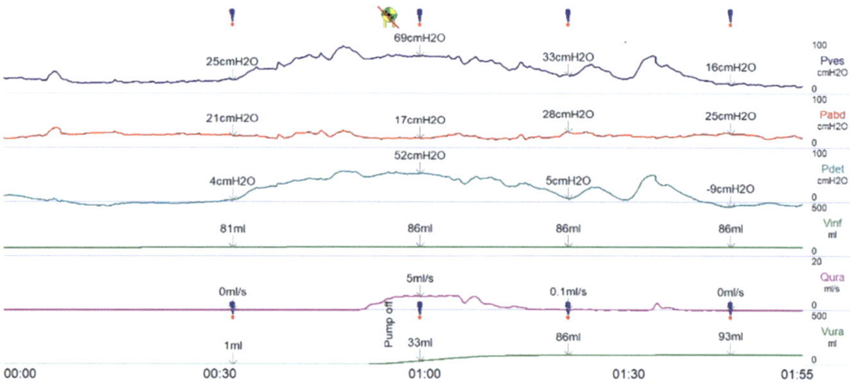

Fig. 10.38 High-pressure-low-flow obstructed void in a 5-year-old girl with short common channel urogenital sinus. She showed thick-walled small bladder on USG and significant overactivity in the filling phase

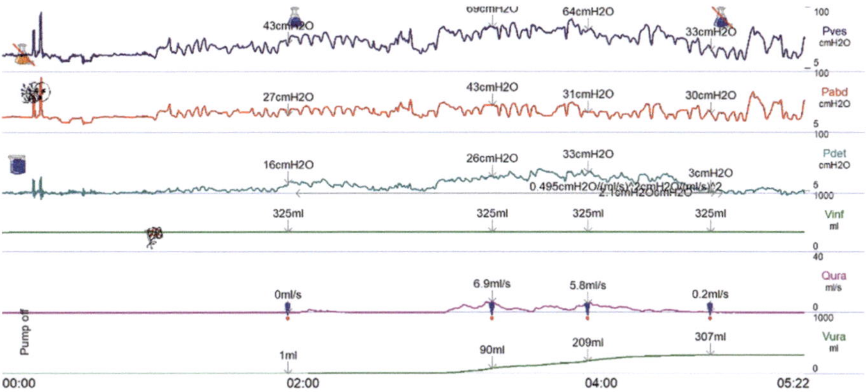

Fig. 10.39 Detrusor underactivity + obstruction in a 16-year-old girl with increased urinary frequency since last 3 years. During the filling phase, she was seen to have "sensory urgency" with no overactivity (not shown in the figure). Flow rates were very poor, but voiding pressures were normal, suggesting a combination of underactivity and mild outflow tract obstruction

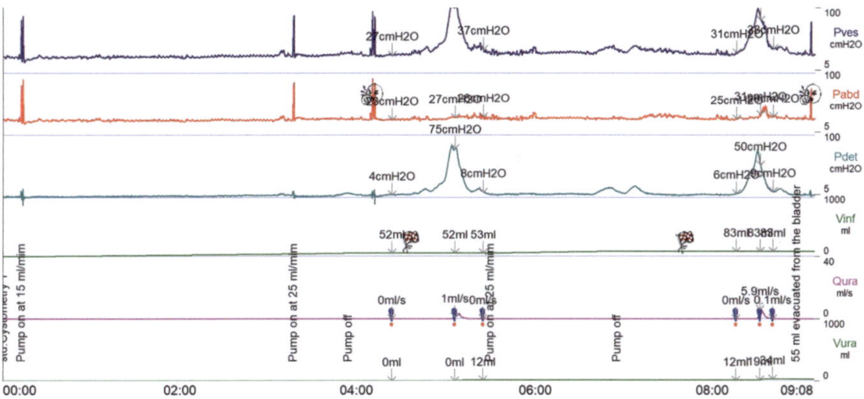

Fig. 10.40 Obstruction + underactivity in an 8-year-old girl with severe LUTS with recurrent UTI and significant PVR on USG. Voiding phase showed high-pressure detrusor contraction with poor flow (obstruction), but the contraction was short-lived (underactive) and resulted in significant PVR

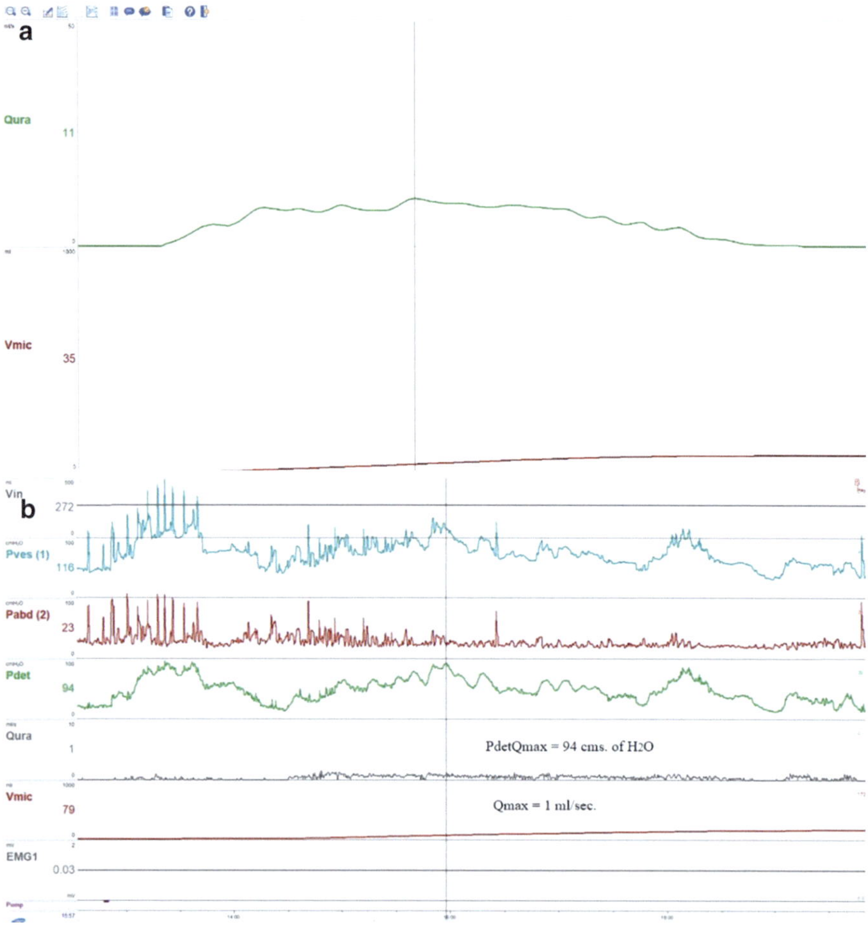

Fig. 10.41 (**a**) Uroflowmetry of a 5-year-old boy (investigated for a follow-up after PUV fulguration) shows a peak uroflow of 11 mls. per second over a volume of 105 ml (**b**) During voiding cystometry (with a 6F cystometry catheter in the urethra), he could only produce a flow rate of 1 ml per second with an abnormally high voiding pressure of 94 cms of H2O, being recorded. Thus, the voiding pattern during free flow uroflowmetry does not corroborate with the void during pressure-flow study and cannot be relied upon

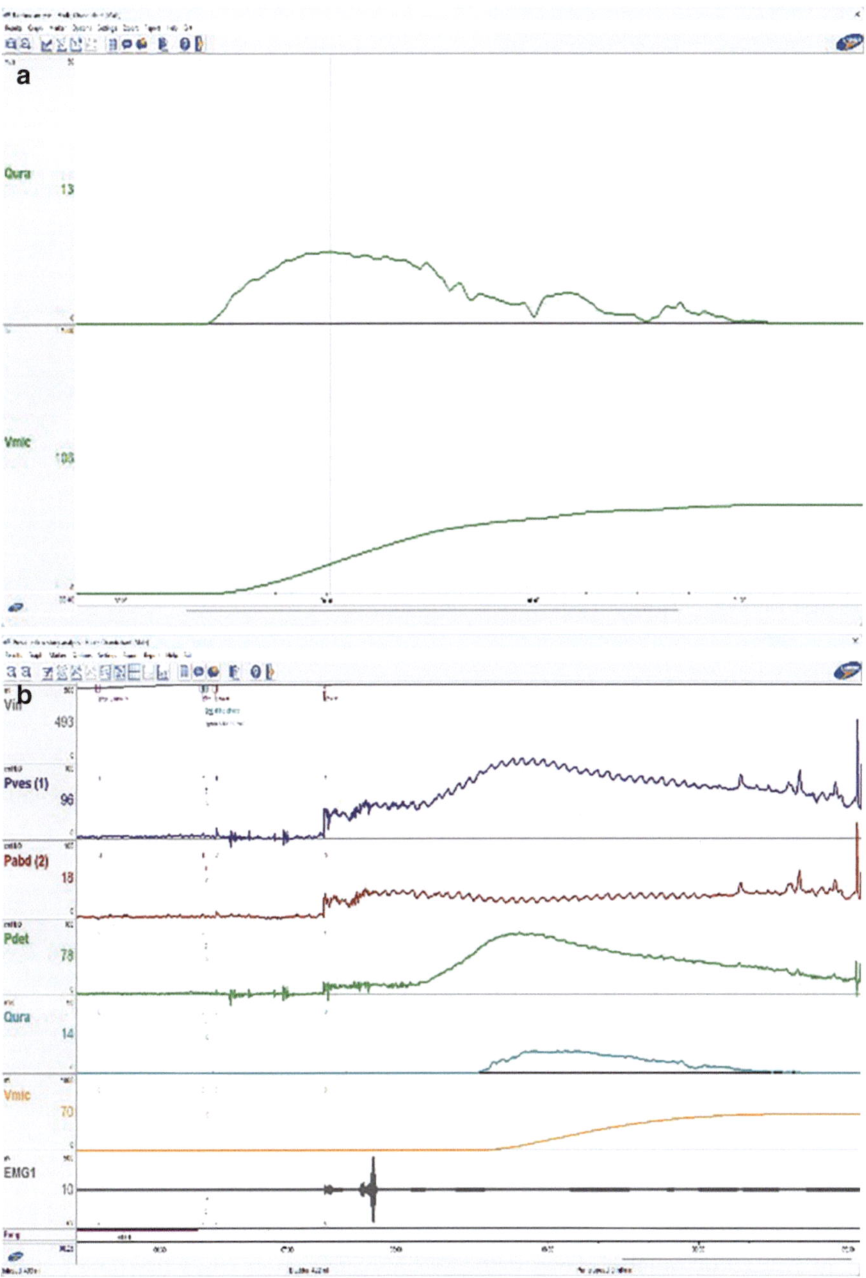

Fig. 10.42 Uroflow in a catheter free flow (**a**) and uroflow in a pressure-flow cycle (**b**) seem to match well in this 11-year-old boy being investigated for persistent nocturnal enuresis. This pressure-flow relationship therefore can be accepted for interpretation of the outflow function

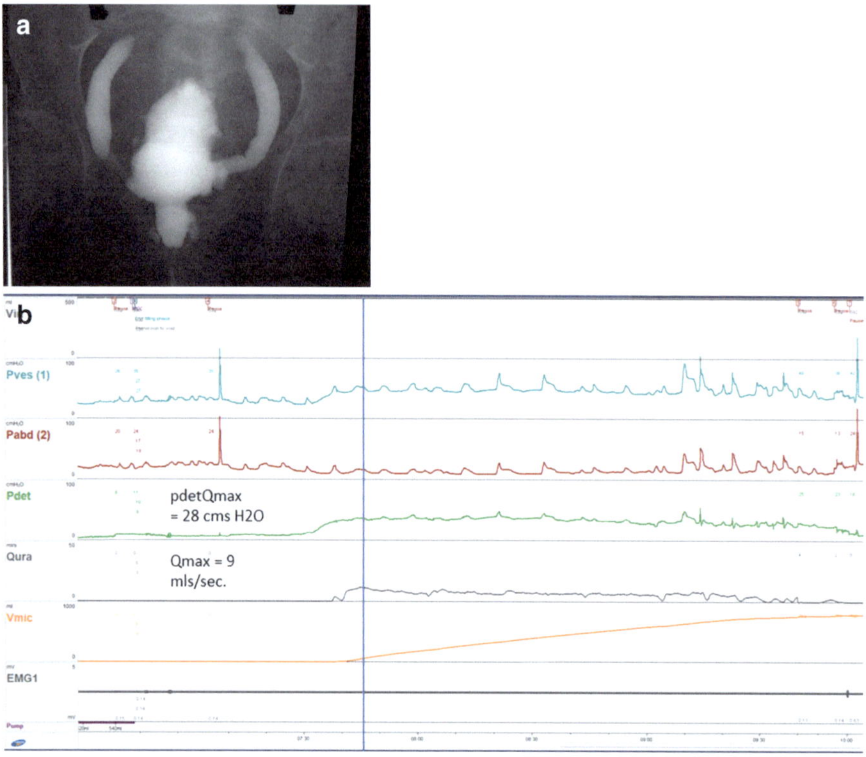

Fig. 10.43 (**a**) Gross VUR in a child (**b**) Voiding phase of UDS showing low-pressure-low-flow state in a child with gross bilateral VUR

Indirect Evidence of Dysfunctional Voiding

Dysfunctional voiding should not be assessed during flow phase of invasive urodynamics as there is urethra irritation during flow with catheter in the urethra which will lead to sphincteric contraction. But the pressure and flow pattern during invasive UDS can give indirect evidence of sphincteric contraction during the voids (Fig. 10.44). The spikes of rise in Pdet give us idea about the detrusor contractility.

After-Contraction

It is a wave of usually strong detrusor contraction seen when the flow ceases (Fig. 10.45). It probably represents voiding detrusor contraction which continues even after the bladder has emptied and sphincter has closed. There is no consensus as to what is the cause of such contractions, but we have seen such contractions only in children with overactive detrusors.

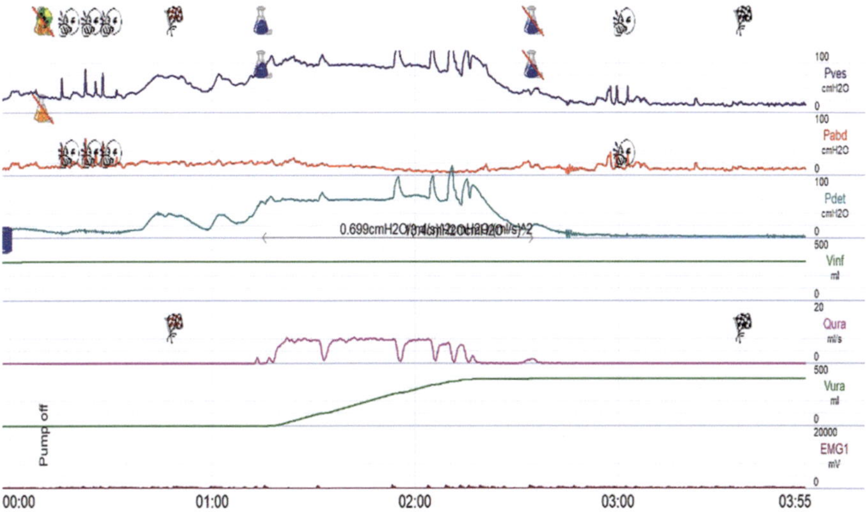

Fig. 10.44 Sudden dips in flow rates along with sudden spikes in detrusor wave in a 10-year-old child who had presented with interrupted urinary stream

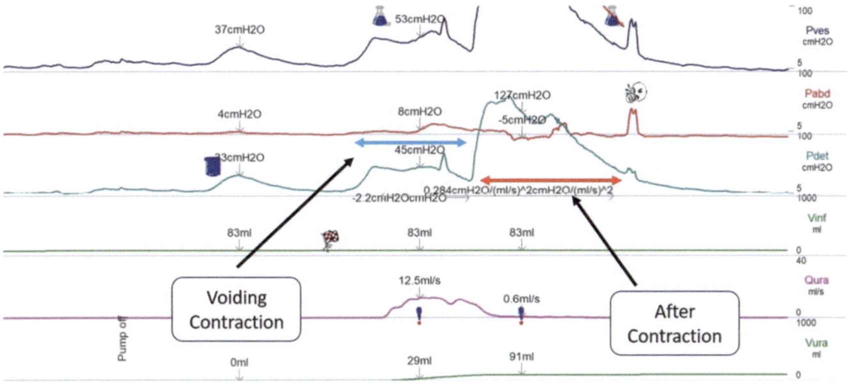

Fig. 10.45 Strong after-contraction in an 8-year-old girl with detrusor overactivity during the filling phase

Declarations

Competing Interests The author(s) has no competing interests to declare that are relevant to the content of this manuscript.

Ethics Approval The author(s) declares that this manuscript does not include primary research with human participants.

The author(s) declares that this manuscript does not include primary studies involving animals.

Suggested Reading

1. Abrams P. Bladder outlet obstruction index, bladder contractility index and bladder voiding efficiency: three simple indices to define bladder voiding function. BJU Int. 1999;84:14–5.
2. Abrams P, Artibani W, Cardozo L, et al. Reviewing the ICS 2002 terminology report: the ongoing debate. Neurourol Urodyn. 2009;28:287.
3. Austin PF, Bauer SB, Bower W, Chase J, Franco I, Hoebeke P, Rittig S, Walle JV, von Gontard A, Wright A, Yang SS, Nevéus T. The standardization of terminology of lower urinary tract function in children and adolescents: update report from the standardization committee of the International Children's Continence Society. Neurourol Urodyn. 2016;35(4):471–81. https://doi.org/10.1002/nau.22751. Epub 2015 Mar 14. PMID: 25772695.
4. Bauer SB, Nijman RJ, Drzewiecki BA, Sillen U, Hoebeke P. International Children's Continence Society Standardization Subcommittee. International Children's Continence Society standardization report on urodynamic studies of the lower urinary tract in children. Neurourol Urodyn. 2015;34(7):640–7. https://doi.org/10.1002/nau.22783. Epub 2015 May 21. PMID: 25998310.
5. Blaivas JG, Groutz A. Bladder outlet obstruction nomogram for women with lower urinary tract symptomatology. Neurourol Urodyn. 2000;19:553–64.
6. D'Ancona CD, Haylen BT, Oelke M, Herschorn S, Abranches-Monteiro L, Arnold EP, et al. An International Continence Society (ICS) Report on the terminology for adult male lower urinary tract and pelvic floor symptoms and dysfunction. Neurourol Urodyn. 2019; https://doi.org/10.1002/nau.23897.
7. Drake MJ, Doumouchtsis SK, Hashim H, Gammie A. Fundamentals of urodynamic practice, based on International Continence Society good urodynamic practices recommendations. Neurourol Urodyn. 2018;37(S6):S50–60. https://doi.org/10.1002/nau.23773.
8. Griffiths D, Hofner K, van Mastrigt R, et al. Standardisation of terminology in lower urinary tract function: pressure flow studies of voiding, urethral resistance and urethral obstruction. Neurourol Urodyn. 1997;6:1–18.
9. Guha Vaze P, Saha S, Sinha R, Banerjee S. Urodynamics in posterior urethral valve: pursuit of prognostication or optimisation. J Pediatr Urol. 2021;17(1):111.e1–8. https://doi.org/10.1016/j.jpurol.2020.11.008. Epub 2020 Nov 6. PMID: 33279434.
10. Nitti VW. Pressure flow urodynamic studies: the gold standard for diagnosing bladder outlet obstruction. Rev Urol. 2005;7(Suppl 6):S14–21.
11. Nitti VW, Tu LM, Gitlin J. Diagnosing bladder outlet obstruction in women. J Urol. 1999;161(5):1535–40. PMID: 10210391.
12. Vaze PG, Saha S, Sinha R. Change in Qmax in the presence of catheter during invasive urodynamics. J Indian Assoc Pediatr Surg. 2023a;28(5):445–6. https://doi.org/10.4103/jiaps.jiaps_99_23. Epub 2023 Sep 5. PMID: 37842214; PMCID: PMC10569282.
13. Vaze PG, Saha S, Sinha R. Voiding pressures in boys: Pdetmax versus PdetQmax - does it make a difference? J Indian Assoc Pediatr Surg. 2023b;28(4):282–7. https://doi.org/10.4103/jiaps.jiaps_51_23. Epub 2023 Jul 11. PMID: 37635896; PMCID: PMC10455708.
14. Wen JG, Djurhuus JC, Rosier PF, Bauer SB. ICS educational module: pressure flow study in children. Neurourol Urodyn. 2018;37:2311–4.

How to Report an *i*-UD Study

11

Poonam Guha Vaze

Proper reporting of an *i*-UDS is as important as proper performance of the study. It should be a conscious effort to include all the possible events/observations noted during performance of the study, which may be needed to understand the bladder behaviour, and should be recorded in the report. This is necessary so that the report makes sense if it is examined by a third person who has not performed the test or if the report is examined after a gap of few months or years.

The following table shows a few terms which are routinely used in the final report of an *i*-UDS, but there may be different possible reasons/explanations for the finding and hence different clinical implications. The table is presented as an example to advocate the need for detailed reporting.

Impression/ observation in final report	Possible variables responsible for the observation	Clinical implications
Small capacity	Filling may have been stopped at volumes < EBC because of one of the following reasons:	
	Patient reported severe urge in spite of normal pressures.	Probable functional bladder/sensory urgency
	Significant urine leak and bladder could not be filled any further.	Bladder outflow incompetence/repeat study with urethral occlusion
	Persistent pressure rise due to poor compliance	Denotes high-risk bladder
	Severe overactivity causing distress to the patient/leak	Bladder relaxants will be helpful.

P. G. Vaze (✉)
Neotia Bhagirathi Woman and Child Care Centre, Newtown, Kolkata, India

Department of Pediatric Surgery, Nilratan Sircar Medical College and Hospital, Kolkata, India

S. Saha, P. Guha Vaze (eds.), *Comprehensive Atlas of Practical Pediatric Urodynamics*, https://doi.org/10.1007/978-981-95-2709-0_11

Impression/observation in final report	Possible variables responsible for the observation	Clinical implications
Poor compliance	Pressure rise may be seen from early filling.	More risk of renal damage
	Pressure rise in later part of filling	If CIC/voided volumes can be limited in the normal pressure zone, risk of renal damage is lowered.
Detrusor overactivity (DO)	DO throughout filling	May have features of urgency/urge incontinence
	No urgency when there is DO	May leak urine unknowingly—'non-sensate loss'
	Pain during DO	May be responsible for intermittent suprapubic pain
	Overactivity appearing only on provocation	Child may be asymptomatic when asleep.
Leak observed during filling	Leak without any rise of detrusor pressures/straining	Weak bladder outlet/intermittent bladder neck relaxation
	Leak during straining in the absence of rise of detrusor pressure	Weak bladder outlet—may need bladder neck procedure
	Leak during overactivity	May benefit from anticholinergics
	Poor compliance with leak beyond a particular detrusor pressure in the absence of overactivity	May benefit from anticholinergics
Did not void during the study	Strong detrusor contractions are seen on attempted voiding but no flow is generated.	Outflow tract obstruction—MCU/video-UDS shows site of obstruction.
	No detrusor contraction is noted on attempted voiding	Shy bladder (in the setting of functional bladder) Neurogenic bladder
	Child refusing to void	Common in 2–5 years old children

A guideline was published from ICCS in 2015 for standardised performance and reporting of UDS. Another expert consensus was published in 2024 which enumerated 93 elements that should be included in any *i*-UDS report.

We usually record the following details in any i-UDS report:

1. History: Duration/symptoms pertaining to filling phase and voiding phase/enuresis/nocturia/incontinence with its elaboration/similar episode in the past/relevant past history/bowel habits/behavioural abnormalities
2. Investigations: Voiding diary/USG/MCUG/DTPA
3. Medications: Bladder relaxants/alpha blockers along with their doses; if stopped before the test, duration for which stopped
4. Uroflowmetry: We usually perform a uroflowmetry before catheter insertion and check the PVR after the catheter is inserted. Uroflowmetry findings are recorded.
5. Preparations for the *i*-UDS:

5.1. Details about urethral catheterisation: Route of insertion (per urethral/Mitrofanoff/ureterostomy/SPC/vesicostomy), size of catheter, type and number of catheter (double-lumen catheter or two feeding tubes), urethral sensation, any difficulty in catheterisation, PVR/volume of urine emptied after catheterisation
5.2. Details about abdominal pressure catheter: Type and size of catheter, route of insertion (per anally/stoma/nasogastric), anal tone, anal reflex/bulbocavernosus reflex
5.3. Any EMG used: Type of EMG electrode (patch/needle), any waterproof dressing used on the electrode
5.4. Posture of the patient during the test: Filling/voiding
5.5. Whether the child is irritable/calm during the study; whether the child is cooperative and able to obey commands
5.6. Documentation of cough impulse with appropriateness of cancelling out of vesical and abdominal waves
5.7. Fill rate: Whether fill rate had to be reduced because of poor compliance or severe overactivity

6. Filling phase:
   6.1. Capacity: Filled volume, voided volume, PVR, emptied volume if child does not void, reason for stopping filling (urge to void/pain/irritability of the child/high pressures/leak/> 150% EBC reached), EBC, observed bladder capacity as a percent of EBC
   6.2. Compliance: Pressures at intervals of 20–50 ml fill
   6.3. Overactivity: Spontaneous/provoked/provocative maneuvers used; phasic/tonic; intensity; any urgency/leak
   6.4. Leak: Time of leak, event during leak (spontaneous/during detrusor overactivity/on rise of abdominal pressure or Valsalva), detrusor pressure or abdominal pressure at point of leak (as applicable) and the bladder volume at which such leak is noted, amount of leak; in case of significant leak, if any urethral occlusion attempted; any leak through ureterostomy with time of appearance of such leak and whether it was kept occluded after that
   6.5. Sensation: Increased/normal/reduced/could not be assessed; any suprapubic/perineal/loin pain and time of appearance of such pain
   6.6. Rectal contractions
7. Voiding phase:
   7.1. Whether the patient could void?

      If the patient could not void—What event was noted when the patient tried to void; for example, strong detrusor contraction was noted but no flow recorded or no detrusor contraction was generated on attempted voiding.
   7.2. Number of voids assessed
   7.3. Posture of the child—Whether the child could not void in any particular position and void in another; difficulty in initiating void in supine/sitting position may be attributed to bladder neck dysfunction
   7.4. Whether voided in flowmeter

7.5. Initiation of void—On command/spontaneous void/during period of detrusor overactivity (terminal overactivity associated void)
7.6. Lag time—Between onset of detrusor contraction and beginning of flow
7.7. Qmax/Pdet at Qmax/Pdet Max/voided volume
7.8. Straining during void
7.9. Any malfunctioning of catheter during the void—Whether both catheters functioning after the voids (cough impulse after completion of void)
7.10. After-contraction
7.11. PVR
7.12. Any pain during voiding
7.13. EMG activity during voiding—Normal silencing/abnormal increase/artefactual
7.14. Whether the voiding pattern corroborates with usual voids of the patient
7.15. Impression about detrusor contractility—Normal/underactive
7.16. Impression about outflow tract obstruction—Obstructed/equivocal/unobstructed

8. Any video-fluoroscopic imaging used during the test
8.1. Type of contrast and contrast dilution that is used
8.2. Filling phase
8.2.1. Shape of the bladder
8.2.2. Outline
8.2.3. Any reflux/diverticulum
Time of appearance—Bladder volume and detrusor pressures
Grade of reflux—Change with bladder volume and during voiding
In cases of gross reflux—Increase in bladder size with filling vs increase in upper tract dilatation
8.3. Voiding phase
8.3.1. If patient unable to void—During attempted voiding, whether bladder neck remains closed or there is opening of bladder neck and contrast gets arrested in region of posterior urethra
8.3.2. Appearance of bladder neck and urethra during void
8.3.3. In cases of reflux—Completeness of emptying of bladder at end of void

9. Final impression
10. Can the UDS findings explain the clinical and radiological findings
11. Any possible confounding factors

Gross reflux can confound the filling phase and voiding phase parameters.

Rectal contractions can cause artefacts and detrusor pressures need to be read cautiously.

12. Comparison with previous UDS findings
13. Further plan

Declarations

Competing Interests The author(s) has no competing interests to declare that are relevant to the content of this manuscript.

Ethics Approval The author(s) declares that this manuscript does not include primary research with human participants.

The author(s) declares that this manuscript does not include primary studies involving animals.

Suggested Reading

1. Bauer SB, Nijman RJ, Drzewiecki BA, Sillen U, Hoebeke P, International Children's Continence Society Standardization Subcommittee. International Children's Continence Society standardization report on urodynamic studies of the lower urinary tract in children. Neurourol Urodyn. 2015;34(7):640–7. https://doi.org/10.1002/nau.22783. Epub 2015 May 21.
2. Meier KM, Mata C, Kaar JL, Rensing AJ, Dudley AG, Carrasco A Jr, Drzewiecki BA, VanderBrink BA, Streur CS, Bagli DJ, Chalmers DJ, Wilcox DT, Yerkes EB, Lau GA, Vricella GJ, Hecht SL, Copp HL, Pohl HG, Franco I, Ahn J, Wiener JS, Singer JS, Long CJ, Keays MA, Daugherty MR, Fuchs ME, Austin PF, Wu CQ, Zee RS, Misseri R, Tanaka ST, Bauer SB, Rove KO. Expert consensus on pediatric urodynamics reporting using modified Delphi technique. J Urol. 2024;212(1):165–74. https://doi.org/10.1097/JU.0000000000004000. Epub 2024 May 3.
3. Rosier PFWM, Schaefer W, Lose G, Goldman HB, Guralnick M, Eustice S, Dickinson T, Hashim H. International continence society good urodynamic practices and terms 2016: urodynamics, uroflowmetry, cystometry, and pressure-flow study. Neurourol Urodyn. 2017;36(5):1243–60. https://doi.org/10.1002/nau.23124. Epub 2016 Dec 5.
4. Rosier PFWM, Gammie A, Valdevenito JP, Speich J, Smith P, Sinha S, members of the ICS Working Group PFS23. ICS-SUFU standard: theory, terms, and recommendations for pressure-flow studies performance, analysis, and reporting. Part 2: analysis of PFS, reporting, and diagnosis. Neurourol Urodyn. 2023;42(8):1603–27. https://doi.org/10.1002/nau.25187. Epub 2023 May 4.

Video-UDS

12

Poonam Guha Vaze and Aniruddh Deshpande

Video-UDS is a technique where we perform MCUG and UDS at the same time for concomitant assessment of bladder anatomy and function.

Diluted contrast instead of saline is used as the infusate, and bladder is assessed by fluoroscopic images intermittently during filling and voiding.

Hardware Requirements

1. The UDS software have an optional upgrade to enable video-UDS after which it can be connected to the output port of the C-ARM or fluoroscopy machine. It enables the images captured by the C-ARM or fluoroscope to be transferred to the UDS machine and the images get stored along with the curves at their respective time frames.
2. C-ARM or fluoroscopy machine—C-ARM is a better option as it allows the patient to be screened in several positions—standing/sitting as well as lying down. Fluoroscopy machine usually allows the test to be performed in supine or standing position.

P. G. Vaze (✉)
Neotia Bhagirathi Woman and Child Care Centre, Newtown, Kolkata, India

Department of Pediatric Surgery, Nilratan Sircar Medical College and Hospital, Kolkata, India

A. Deshpande
Urology Unit, Department of Paediatric Surgery, Children's Hospital at Westmead, Westmead, NSW, Australia

Sydney Medical School, Faculty of Medicine and Health, University of Sydney, Sydney, NSW, Australia

S. Saha, P. Guha Vaze (eds.), *Comprehensive Atlas of Practical Pediatric Urodynamics*, https://doi.org/10.1007/978-981-95-2709-0_12

3. C-ARM-compatible dedicated bed for UDS provides the comfort of being able to perform in sitting position, and the voided volume can be assessed, which is not possible if the test is performed on the fluoroscopy table.

Indications

Broadly speaking, the paediatric urodynamic units follow two practice algorithms. In one group, video-UDS is selectively used, whilst in the other group, video-UDS is the standard of care.

1. In centres where availability of addition of 'video option' to routine UDS is limited, selective patients are subjected to video-UDS
   (a) To assess any underlying bladder dysfunction in patients with VUR where there is suspicion of bladder dysfunction from the history/MCU appearance of bladder or ongoing renal deterioration in absence of UTIs
   (b) Assessment of bladder function in presence of high-grade VUR where performing only UDS may have unreliable results due to misleading volume estimates and poor capture of rise in pressures
   (c) In an operated patient of PUV with persistent poor flow/upper tracts changes—to determine voiding pressures (whether persistent BOO or underactive bladder) and site of obstruction (bladder neck/sphincter/urethra)
2. Some centres perform video-UDS as standard of care and reserve cystometry only for very selected cases. The common additional indications for video-UDS in such units are:
   (a) Neurogenic bladders for baseline assessment, for interval increase in incontinence, for de novo upper tract dilatation or increased renal scarring
   (b) In select cases of complex urogenital malformations such as exstrophy, cloaca to assess bladder storage and emptying to refine treatment choices

Practical Points

1. We take a 500 ml NS bottle and empty out around 300 ml fluid from it through the pump tubing itself. We instil 100 ml (5 ampoules) of Urografin 76% in a sterile manner into the bottle and shake the bottle to mix the two fluids. The final contrast dilution remains around 1:3 and gives good quality images.
2. Before connecting the pump tubing to the patient, the pump is started to let out the contrast-free normal saline from the pump tubing and fill up the pump tubing with contrast solution.
3. UDS is then performed in the usual manner.
4. Fluoroscopic images are captured usually every 50–100 ml fill (depending on bladder capacity) and if there is any evidence of overactivity or urgency.
5. A Cine-Video can be recorded during voiding which can be assessed alongside the pressure changes during voiding.

At one of our centres, we not have the video-UDS upgrade to the UDS software. We perform the video-UDS in the fluoroscopy suite with the patient in supine position. We instil contrast as the infusate and start the UDS procedure. Whenever we capture fluoroscopic images, we mark the exact point by annotations on the curve. We record the void in supine position like a routine MCUG and mark the start and stop of void on the UDS tracing. We have found this method to be cost-effective and equally informative. We perform a second cycle of UDS with the child in sitting position without fluoroscopic visualisation to assess the voiding parameters appropriately.

We present a few case studies where video-UDS was performed and the findings helped in management of the children. First four cases show the use of video-UDS to assess the relation of bladder pressures and reflux which guides further management. Last three cases show the use of video-UDS as a substitute to performing UDS and MCU separately in cases where MCU would have been required in addition to UDS.

Case 1: Reflux During Overactivity

A 1.5-year-old girl had history of recurrent episodes of febrile UTI since the age of 2.5 months. She had no voiding symptoms—voided every 45 minutes to 1 hour in a good stream without straining. USG KUB showed normal bladder and upper tracts. MCU revealed a normal bladder with bilateral gr IV VUR with renal intraparenchymal reflux. Although there was no evidence to suggest any bladder dysfunction, video-UDS was performed to rule secondary VUR in light of severity of VUR—intraparenchymal reflux might represent reflux occurring under high pressure.

Video-UDS (Fig. 12.1) showed normal capacity bladder with normal compliance and detrusor overactivity. It was clearly demonstrated that the reflux appeared during periods of overactivity and immediately before voiding when detrusor pressures were above 30–50 cm H_2O. So even though there was no evidence to suggest bladder dysfunction in any other investigation, video-UDS suggested secondary VUR. She was started on anticholinergics—she did not have any further episodes of UTI in the next 6 months of follow-up.

Case 2: High-Pressure Void with Reflux

An 8-month-old female child presented with one episode of left pyelonephritis at the age of 7 months. USG KUB showed left upper polar pyelectasis. MCU revealed left gr III VUR with a normal bladder. She was thought to have primary VUR, but parents informed that she had some history of straining/making grunting sounds while passing urine. So a video-UDS was planned.

UDS (Fig. 12.2a) revealed a normal capacity bladder with detrusor overactivity just prior to voiding. Detrusor overactivity may be physiological finding at 7 months age, but in this child, during pre-void detrusor overactivity, pressures reached

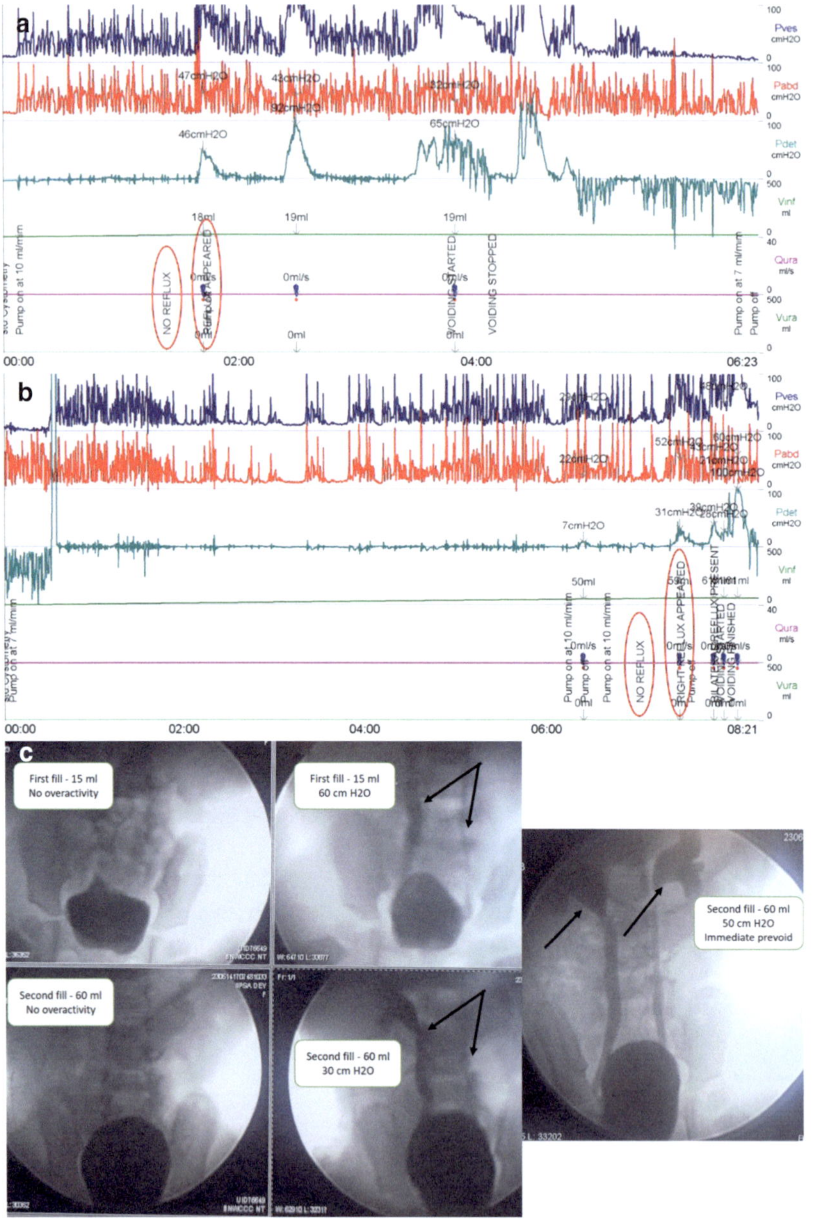

Fig. 12.1 (**a**, **b**, **c**) Two UDS tracings performed at the same sitting under video-fluoroscopic guidance. Both the studies have been performed in supine position on the fluoroscopy table with MCU and UDS being done simultaneously. Events like appearance of reflux and voiding have been added as annotations to the UDS tracing. Point of appearance of reflux has been highlighted as red oval. The first study (**a**) shows significant overactivity with voiding occurring at 19 ml volume. Second tracing (**b**) shows overactivity appearing after 50 ml volume with a normal bladder capacity. The corresponding fluoroscopic images show (**c**) that reflux (black arrow) is noted only during episodes of overactivity and during voiding

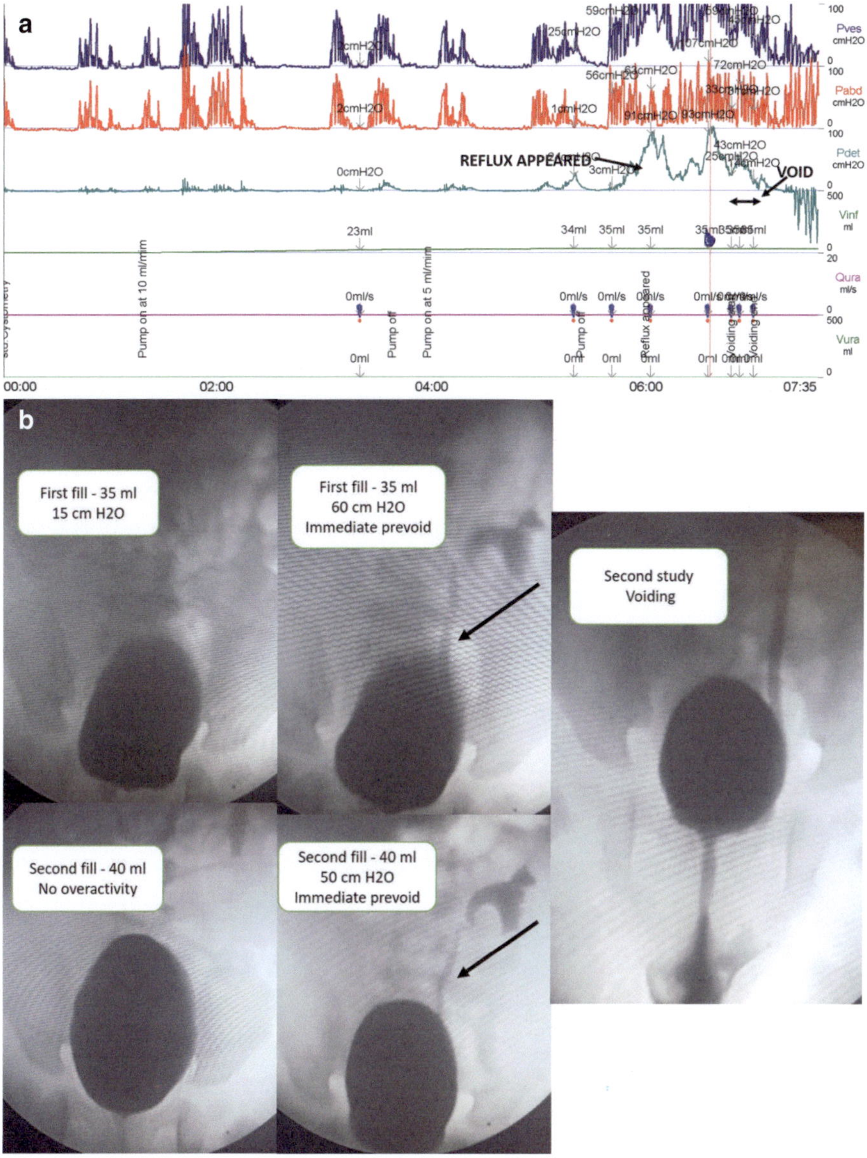

Fig. 12.2 (**a**) First of the two UDS studies performed under video-fluoroscopic screening showing mild detrusor overactivity appearing after 23 ml filling. overactivity increases in severity at 35 ml filling which corroborates with appearance of reflux on Video-fluoroscopic screening and is marked by an annotation. The patient voids during later part of the detrusor contraction (marked by an annotation) but the corresponding flow is not recorded as the study is done in supine position. (**b**) Video-fluoroscopic screening images obtained during the two cycles are shown and labelled appropriately. Upper two images were obtained during the first study where at 35 ml volume, reflux is seen when detrusor pressure increases to 60 cm H2O. Lower set of images show video-fluoroscopic images during the second study when reflux is seen at 40 ml volume when detrusor pressures reach 50 cm H2O

80–90 cm H_2O. Detrusor pressures during voiding were variable—probably due to physiological dysfunctional voiding. Video-fluoroscopic screening (Fig. 12.2b) showed that reflux appeared (black arrow) during the pre-void overactivity and during voiding at detrusor pressures of 50–60 cm H_2O. So she was started on alpha blockers and low-dose anticholinergics and continued on constipation management. She didn't have any further UTIs. Repeat video-UDS at 2 years of age revealed mild detrusor overactivity with transient left gr II VUR during voiding. Renal function remained stable on scintigraphy.

Case 3: Small Bladder with Gross VUR

A 2.7-year-old female child had history of poor, interrupted urinary stream since beginning with recurrent episodes of UTI. USG revealed bilateral gross HDUN (antero-posterior diameters of both pelves were 30 and 37 mm) with thick-walled UB. MCU revealed small bladder with bilateral gross gr V VUR. UDS was contemplated because of abnormal voiding history. Video-UDS was performed as it was presumed that findings of UDS would be confounded by gross VUR.

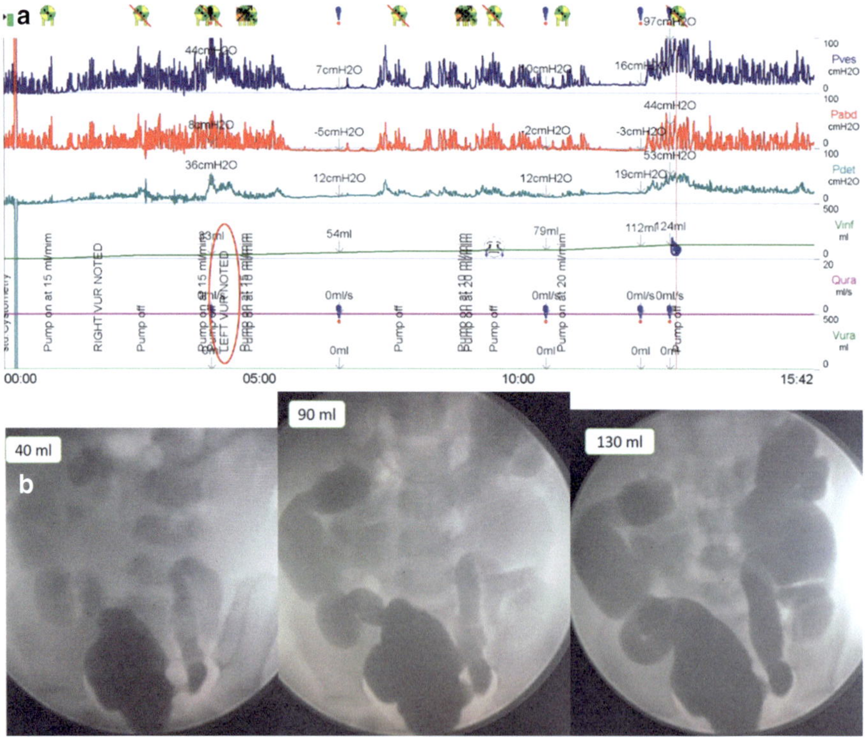

Fig. 12.3 (**a**) UDS tracing showing appearance of left VUR marked by red oval. (**b**) Fluoroscopic images showing bladder to be almost similar in size and the contrast filling up the upper tracts

During UDS (Fig. 12.3a), bladder could be filled up to 120 ml which would otherwise signify a large capacity bladder, but video-fluoroscopic screening (Fig. 12.3b) suggested that the bladder was elongated in shape with irregular outline, did not increase in size after 40 ml fill and rest all of the fluid got accommodated in the upper tracts, thus proving it to be a small capacity bladder. Compliance was reduced (19 cm H_2O at 120 ml) and intermittent severe DO was noted with pressures reaching 30–50 cm H_2O. She leaked a few drops of urine at detrusor pressures of 50 cm H_2O. Right VUR was noted from beginning of fill. Left VUR was noted at 40 ml fill during period of DO. At 120 ml, the upper tracts were hugely distended and appeared tense. She did not void during the study.

The overall UDS and MCU findings were suggestive of high-pressure, small capacity bladder, probably neurogenic in aetiology. She underwent unilateral loop ureterostomy.

Case 4: Stable Bladder with Gross VUR

A 16-year-old girl, follow-up case of LSMMC repair at neonatal period, underwent bilateral Deflux injections at the age of 5 years and 10 years, bilateral ureteric reimplantation at the age of 12 years. She could not pass urine on her own and performed CIC whenever she felt the urge to pass urine—CIC volumes were around 500–600 ml. She had intermittent bilateral flank pain in the last 2 years.

USG revealed bilateral moderate HDUN with cortical thinning and thick-walled trabeculated bladder. Creatinine was 1.69. MCU revealed bilateral gr V VUR into grossly dilated ureters.

UDS (Fig 12.4a) suggested that the bladder was stable and large capacity (600 ml), but fluoroscopic screening (Fig 12.4b) revealed that the bladder did not increase in size after 350 ml fill and the contrast was accommodated in the upper tracts. Bladder was elongated/irregular in shape. Right VUR was noted at 70 ml fill, and left VUR at 200 ml fill. She complained of flank pain at 500–600 ml volume when upper tracts were severely full (marked by 'crying' sign on UDS tracing).

This shows that although UDS shows that the bladder is stable and large capacity, video-UDS suggests that the bladder was non-distensible, probably stiff, which may have resulted in persistence/recurrence and severity of reflux even after so many anti-reflux procedures. As the bladder could not accommodate the urine, upper tracts took up the brunt.

Case 5: Locating Cause of Bladder Outflow Obstruction

A 12-year-old boy presented with history of poor urinary stream with increased frequency of micturition noted since last 1 year with one episode of UTI. USG showed thick-walled trabeculated bladder. He had undergone cystoscopy elsewhere which did not reveal any PUV.

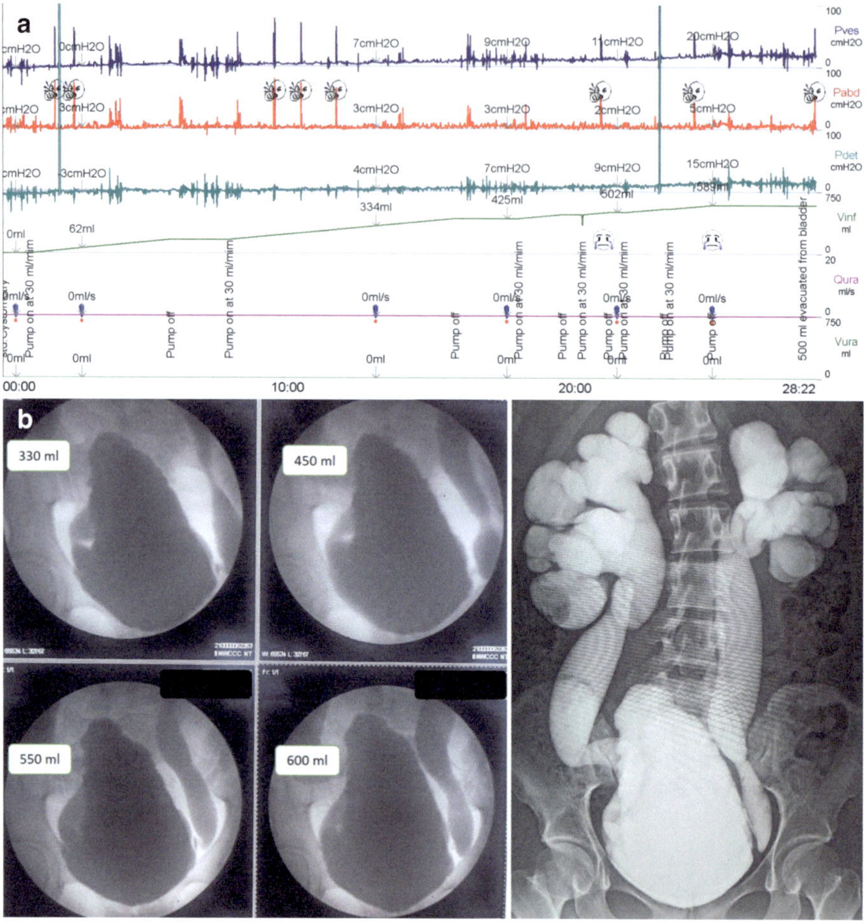

Fig. 12.4 (**a**) UDS tracing showing a stable bladder till 600 ml fill. Flank pain is reported at 500–600 ml fill marked by 'cry' sign. (**b**) Video-fluoroscopic images showing no change in bladder size from 300–600 ml fill

Uroflowmetry (Fig. 12.5a) revealed plateau-shaped curve with mild increase in EMG activity. He was suspected as having an underactive bladder as increased EMG activity in a single-channel EMG may have been caused by component of abdominal straining. Video-UDS was performed to rule out any anatomical outflow tract obstruction. UDS showed a stable bladder during filling (Fig. 12.5b). During attempted voiding, strong waves of detrusor contraction were noted, but no flow was recorded which suggested anatomical outflow tract obstruction (Fig. 12.5c). Fluoroscopic screening showed presence of probable anterior urethral valve (Fig. 12.5d) which was missed at the previous surgery.

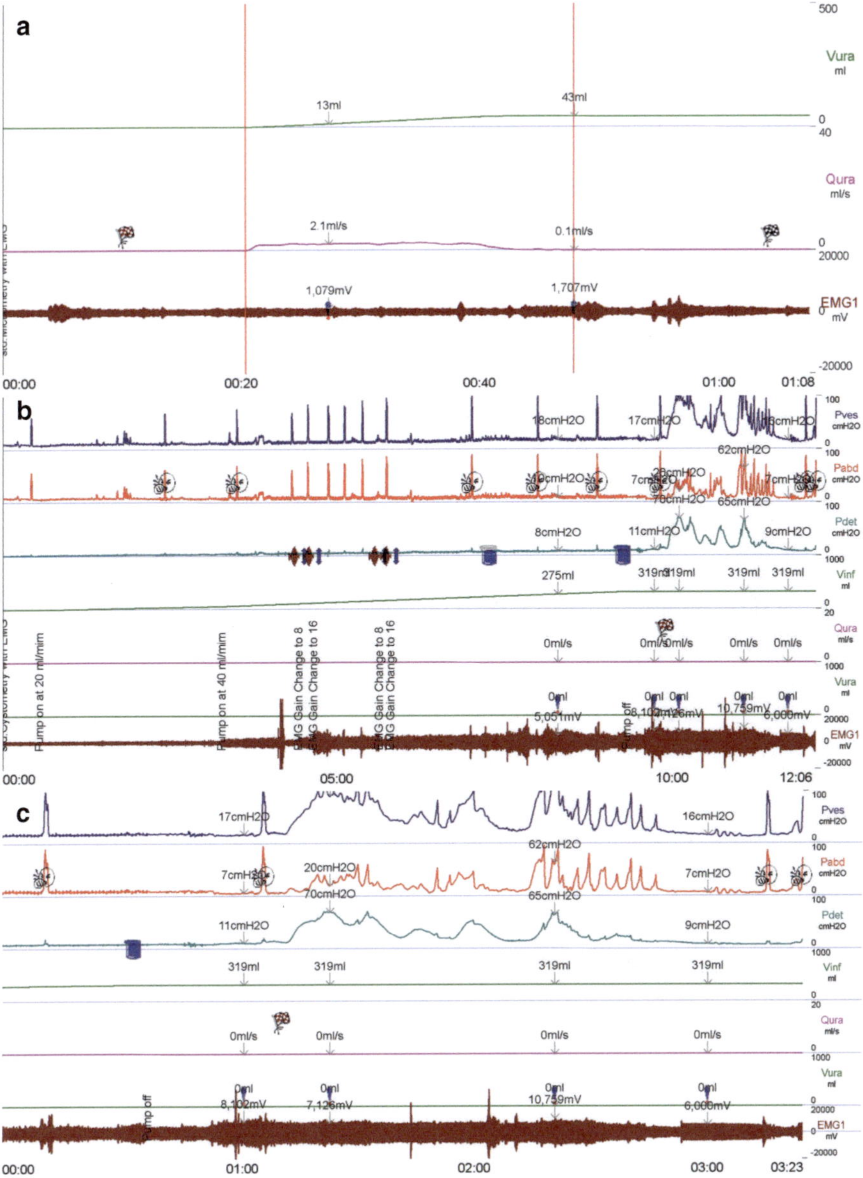

Fig. 12.5 (**a**) Uroflowmetry showing plateau shaped curve with some increase in EMG activity during voiding. (**b**) Full tracing of UDS showing stable bladder during filling. (**c**) Voiding phase of UDS tracing shown in an expanded form. Strong waves of detrusor contraction are seen with pressures reaching 65–70 cm H2O but no flow was produced. (**d**) Video-Fluoroscopic image during attempted voiding showing probable anterior urethral valve

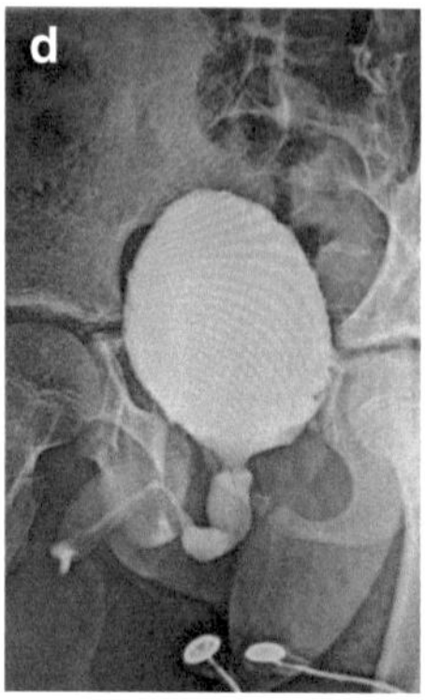

Fig. 12.5 (continued)

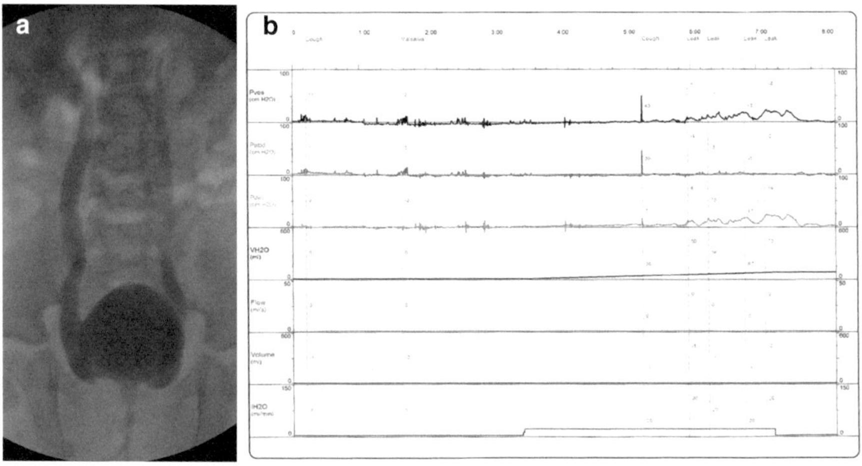

Fig. 12.6 (**a**) Video-fluoroscopic image showing a small capacity bladder with bilateral VUR. (**b**) UDS tracing showing detrusor overactivity from early fill

Case 6: Follow-Up Case of Exstrophy with Reflux

This 4-year female child had a few episodes of febrile UTI following closure of exstrophy bladder in her infancy. There were DMSA changes in her left kidney. She was stable with clean intermittent catheterisation and night-time drainage. When she had a fresh episode of febrile UTI at 4 years of life, video-urodynamic (Fig 12.6 a, b) assessment was planned.

Filling was started at 10 ml/min. At around 40 ml of filling, she developed reflux into her dilated right ureter and pelvicalyceal system and into the left renal system at around 60 ml of filling when she started leaking as well. The detrusor pressure was 10–12 cm H_2O when the leak started. There was evidence of sustained detrusor contraction throughout the study with impaired drainage. The study was stopped and bladder drained with complete rapid emptying of bladder and the upper tracts.

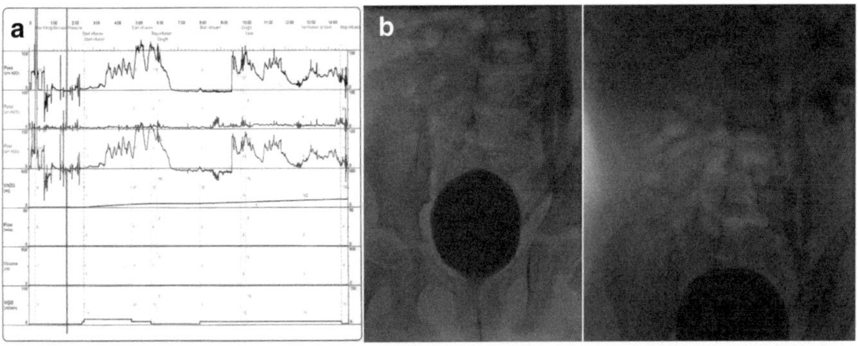

Fig. 12.7 (**a**) UDS tracing showing strong detrusor contractions with pressures reaching 100 cm H2O (**b**) Video-Fluoroscopic images showing small bladder with left VUR into a partially duplex system

Though low-pressure reflux, the UTI may be related to the reflux per se and the colonisation of the bladder.

Case 7: Neurogenic Bladder with Reflux and Partial Duplication

A 3-year child with h/o lumbosacral lipomyelomeningocele (repaired in infancy) presented with recurrent febrile UTI (6 monthly interval). She was wet throughout the day and night. CIC was being performed twice a day. She could void 45 ml urine on her own with postvoid CIC volumes of 60–70 ml. Maximum amount of postvoid residual was 110 ml.

Video-urodynamic study (Fig 12.7) was conducted with a start fill rate of 20 ml/min which was immediately reduced to 10 ml/min due to reactive detrusor overactivity. She had evidence of bladder instability with sustained detrusor contractions with high pressure intermittently throughout the study. At around 30–40 ml of filling, reflux into both the moieties of left partially duplicated ureter were seen. She leaked intermittently and the leak point pressure was 50–100 cm water. On voiding command, she was unable to express more than 10–20 ml of urine. PVR was 85 ml.

This was a girl with neurogenic poorly compliant unsafe bladder with a high leak point pressure. Anticholinergics, clean intermittent catheterisation with night-time drainage and bowel management should be advised before any consideration is given to management of VUR.

Declarations

Competing Interests The author(s) has no competing interests to declare that are relevant to the content of this manuscript.

Ethics Approval The author(s) declares that this manuscript does not include primary research with human participants.

The author(s) declares that this manuscript does not include primary studies involving animals.

Suggested Reading

1. Arunachalam P, et al. Video-urodynamic studies under anesthesia in children – Is it worthwhile? J Pediatr Urol. 2020;16:S5.
2. Glazier DB, Murphy DP, Fleisher MH, Cummings KB, Barone JG. Evaluation of the utility of video-urodynamics in children with urinary tract infection and voiding dysfunction. Br J Urol. 1997;80(5):806–8. https://doi.org/10.1046/j.1464-410x.1997.00447.x. PMID: 9393308.
3. Hoebeke P, Van Laecke E, Van Camp C, Raes A, Van De Walle J. One thousand video-urodynamic studies in children with non-neurogenic bladder sphincter dysfunction. BJU Int. 2001;87(6):575–80. https://doi.org/10.1046/j.1464-410x.2001.00083.x. PMID: 11298061.
4. Spinoit AF, Decalf V, Ragolle I, Ploumidis A, Claeys T, Groen LA, Van Laecke E, Hoebeke P. Urodynamic studies in children: standardized transurethral video-urodynamic evaluation. J Pediatr Urol. 2016;12(1):67–8. https://doi.org/10.1016/j.jpurol.2015.08.025. Epub 2015 Nov 27. PMID: 26638696.
5. Van Batavia JP, Fischer K, Moran M, Kerr J, Messina A, McClatchy K, Berry A, Weiss D, Long C, Zderic SA. Can videourodynamics shape management in refractory pediatric lower urinary tract dysfunction? J Pediatr Urol. 2025;21(2):276–82. https://doi.org/10.1016/j.jpurol.2024.05.018. Epub 2024 May 25. PMID: 38845245; PMCID: PMC11586459.
6. Wyndaele M, Rosier PFWM. Basics of videourodynamics for adult patients with lower urinary tract dysfunction. Neurourol Urodyn. 2018;37(S6):S61–6. https://doi.org/10.1002/nau.23778. PMID: 30614055.

Ambulatory Urodynamics and Newer Technologies for Lower Urinary Tract Assessment in Children

13

Aniruddh Deshpande, Bandar AlSahn,
and Kiarash Taghavi

Background

Urodynamics in pediatric patient align closely with adult practices in many ways, but with important nuances. Urodynamic studies provide vital insights into bladder function. There are several types of urodynamic studies used in children to evaluate bladder function and lower urinary tract abnormalities, including uroflowmetry, bladder diary, pressure-flow studies, and electromyography, each providing specific insights into different aspects of urinary physiology. They assess bladder filling dynamics, compliance, capacity, pressures, detrusor-sphincter dyssynergia, detrusor overactivity (DO), and post-void residual volume. When cystometrography (CMG) is combined with fluoroscopy, it also detects vesicoureteric reflux and congenital/acquired anomalies of the bladder, bladder neck, and urethra.

In patients with known lower urinary tract dysfunction stemming from congenital or acquired neurological deficits or severe obstructive uropathy, formal urodynamic studies are essential for establishing bladder pressures. Common pediatric

A. Deshpande (✉)
Urology Unit, Department of Paediatric Surgery, Children's Hospital at Westmead, Westmead, NSW, Australia

Sydney Medical School, Faculty of Medicine and Health, University of Sydney, Sydney, NSW, Australia

B. AlSahn
Urology Unit, Department of Paediatric Surgery, Children's Hospital at Westmead, Sydney, Australia
e-mail: Bandar.alsahn@health.nsw.gov.au

K. Taghavi
Department of Paediatric Urology, Monash Children's Hospital, Melbourne, Australia

Department of Paediatrics, Monash University, Melbourne, Australia

S. Saha, P. Guha Vaze (eds.), *Comprehensive Atlas of Practical Pediatric Urodynamics*, https://doi.org/10.1007/978-981-95-2709-0_13

conditions associated with neurogenic bladder include spinal dysraphism, sacrococcygeal teratoma, sacral agenesis, transverse myelitis, and spinal cord injury. Lower urinary tract dysfunction can also result from severe obstructive processes, such as posterior urethral valves, urethral atresia, or large ectopic ureteroceles. Studies examining the utility of CMG in pediatric patients with lower urinary tract symptoms (in the absence of other neurological signs or symptoms) have shown that significant information is rarely obtained to justify invasive testing [1–3]. Urodynamic studies may be performed at baseline, because of clinical or radiological changes, as surveillance (protocolized) in patients with known disease, repeated to reestablish baseline measures before medical or surgical therapies, or conducted to rule in or rule out specific bladder dysfunction patterns. Many congenital conditions affecting lower urinary tract function can lead to altered function over time, necessitating repeat urodynamic studies [4–6]. Generally, formal urodynamic testing should be reserved for patients in whom a new or abnormal result will influence treatment options.

Why Ambulatory Urodynamics?

Urodynamics encompasses a range of techniques used to assess the lower urinary tract, from clinical assessments and uroflowmetry to videocystometrography (V-CMG) [7]. The goal of urodynamic studies is to detail and document a child's bladder physiology or pathological patterns during storage and voiding phases [8]. Urodynamic testing should provide the best available information to directly influence the management of lower urinary tract disorders in children, whether functional or structural.

Reproducibility of the current armamentarium of urodynamic studies may be limited, and consistent study techniques are challenging due to various factors. For example, interpreting simple uroflow curves is hindered by significant interobserver variability (0.21–0.64) [9]. Moreover, a recent multicenter North American study on pediatric neurogenic bladder (UMPIRE study) found only 50% agreement regarding bladder evaluation using CMG [10]. Specifically, the assessment of bladder risk category and the risk of subsequent upper tract damage varied significantly between institutions. Despite its limitations, CMG remains the current gold standard for defining lower urinary tract disorders in children, including those with complex urological and neurological conditions [10]. Despite its shortcomings (non-physiological quality and propensity for artefact), many significant clinical decisions are currently based on CMG, with far-reaching consequences for the child [11, 12]. For instance, the largely irreversible decision to proceed with augmentation cystoplasty carries risks such as a >20% chance of bladder urolithiasis, long-term risk of malignancy, and a potentially life-threatening risk of bladder rupture/perforation. Additionally, if the child ultimately requires renal transplantation, the combination of immunosuppression and the increased bacterial load following augmentation cystoplasty can make recurrent urinary tract infections highly problematic. Similarly, the formation of a catheterizable channel has a high complication rate (>50%) [13].

New technologies, such as Ambulatory Urodynamic Monitoring (AUM) and Telemetric Ambulatory Urodynamic Monitoring, are currently in development. These techniques allow for real-time physiological evaluation as the child moves freely, with the study continuing remotely and often without the need for catheterization [14]. It remains to be seen how effectively these technologies will evolve (in the short-and medium-term) to address and mitigate the challenges related to reproducibility and variability in reporting associated with videocystometry.

Catheter-Based Ambulatory Urodynamic Studies

Catheter-based AUM utilizes traditional pressure catheters (urethral/bladder and rectal) connected to portable data loggers. This technology enables children to move relatively freely during natural bladder filling cycles over extended periods, ranging from several hours to days. The key advantages of this approach include its ability to capture bladder physiology during normal daily activities and routines, potentially revealing symptom triggers missed within the confines of the clinic (Fig. 13.1). Prolonged observation over multiple natural filling and voiding cycles increases the likelihood of detecting intermittent pathological events, such as incontinence episodes [15]. Furthermore, remote monitoring features—such as Bluetooth-enabled systems like LUNA™ (Fig. 13.2) connected to flowmeters and digital diaries—may eliminate the need for continuous practitioner supervision during the study [16].

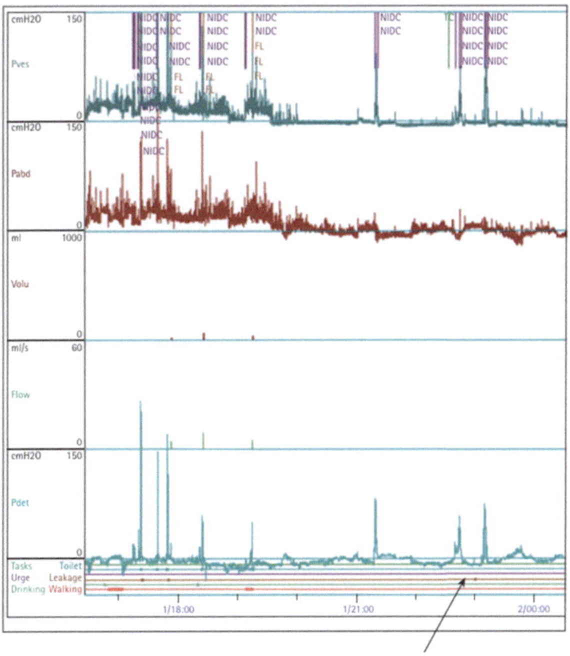

Fig. 13.1 Ambulatory urodynamic tracing in a child with neurogenic bladder showing detrusor overactivity with no rise in storage pressures

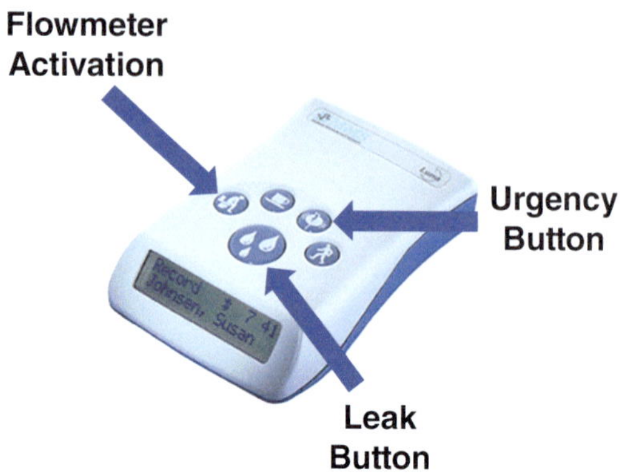

Fig. 13.2 Example of the portable recording unit of Ambulatory Urodynamic Device

However, the current catheter-based AUM in children continue to face significant challenges. Since they involve indwelling catheters, it is invasive and can cause discomfort. Additionally, the presence of the catheter may affect bladder function, potentially influencing measurements like detrusor leak point pressure (DLPP) [17]. Accurately tracking dynamic bladder volume continuously remains a major unsolved challenge, typically relying on imperfect patient voiding diaries or intermittent ultrasound scans [17]. The generation of hours of continuous pressure tracings without easily labelled events creates significant "data smog," complicating interpretation, although machine learning algorithms show promise in automating analysis (demonstrating sensitivities and specificities around 84–86% for detecting detrusor overactivity in pilot studies) [15]. The accuracy of the study also depends heavily on diligent patient or parent input for event logging (e.g., incontinence, urgency episodes), introducing potential inaccuracies. Air-charged catheters allow longer recordings without loss of accuracy. Practical considerations include likely higher costs compared to conventional CMG and the perception, noted by the International Children's Continence Society (ICCS), that it remains time-consuming and impractical for widespread routine pediatric use [16, 18]. Notably, studies suggest AUM detects detrusor overactivity more frequently than CMG but often fails to show the characteristic progressive pressure rise ("hypocompliance") commonly observed in the artificial CMG setting, raising fundamental questions about the nature and clinical significance of this traditional metric derived from nonphysiological testing [19] (Figs. 13.1 and 13.2). Although recording real-time bladder events is a desirable goal, it is unlikely that catheter-based techniques will be used in the future for this purpose.

Bioimpedance Techniques and Near-Infrared Spectroscopy

Bioimpedance and near-infrared spectroscopy (NIRS) represent noninvasive approaches aiming to indirectly estimate bladder volume or detect detrusor contractions. Bioimpedance techniques measure changes in electrical impedance across the abdominal wall or within pelvic tissues as the bladder fills with urine [20–22].

While bench studies and theoretical models suggest potential for high accuracy (error rates potentially below 5%), clinical application in children has been hampered by poor real-world accuracy, significant susceptibility to motion artefact, and variability introduced by individual anatomical differences and fluctuations in urine composition affecting conductivity [21, 22]. Near-infrared spectroscopy (NIRS) utilizes the absorption characteristics of near-infrared light passing through tissues to infer changes in bladder volume [20–22]. A fundamental limitation of NIRS is its assumption that the optical properties of surrounding pelvic organs remain constant, which may not hold true physiologically. Like bioimpedance, NIRS is highly susceptible to motion artefact and interference from other tissues, limiting its reliability. Currently, neither bioimpedance nor NIRS has demonstrated sufficient accuracy, robustness, or reliability to serve as a standalone method for comprehensive clinical urodynamic diagnosis in the pediatric population. Their development warrants further significant refinement and rigorous clinical validation studies.

Telemetric Ambulatory Urodynamic Monitoring Through Implantable Devices

Telemetric Ambulatory Urodynamic Monitoring (TAUM) signifies a paradigm shift toward catheter-free, prolonged physiological monitoring. This approach utilizes miniaturized implantable sensors that measure and wirelessly transmit pressure data [23].

A. Intravesical Devices: These compact devices, such as the investigational "Bladder Pill," are designed to float freely within the bladder lumen. Insertion is typically performed cystoscopically; however, current prototype dimensions (15–21 French) are designed for adult urethras and cystoscopes. They measure intravesical pressure relative to an internal vacuum-sealed reference chamber [23]. The primary advantages include being the least surgically invasive TAUM option, allowing for truly natural bladder filling and unrestricted activity, and enabling onboard data storage and/or transmission facilitating home monitoring. Significant disadvantages and risks include the potential for expulsion during voiding, the possibility of causing bladder outlet obstruction (a critical concern in small pediatric bladders), the risk of device encrustation from prolonged urine exposure, and accuracy typically limited to around ±2.5 cm H_2O. Downsizing these devices for safe and effective use in children remains unexplored. Sampling rates are adjustable (e.g., 0.5 Hz for capturing rapid events like contractions down to 0.003 Hz for long-term trend monitoring) [24].
B. Intradetrusor Devices: These sensors are implanted within the substance of the detrusor muscle wall, either via advanced cystoscopy techniques (creating a detrusor pocket) or open surgery. Being embedded within the bladder wall protects them from direct urine exposure, significantly reducing the risk of encrustation. Their main advantage is this protected position. However, the disadvantages and risks are substantial. The implantation procedure requires

creating a detrusor pocket. A significant risk, observed in animal models, is erosion of the sensor through the detrusor muscle into the bladder lumen or the perivesical space. Miniaturizing the device sufficiently for implantation through pediatric cystoscopes while maintaining adequate power and wireless communication capabilities presents a major engineering challenge. Crucially, like intravesical devices, they do not directly measure abdominal pressure, relying instead on complex signal processing algorithms for correction. General anesthesia is mandatory for both insertion and removal [24–27].

C. A third category, transdetrusor devices, involves percutaneous elements traversing the abdominal and bladder wall to measure intravesical pressure directly; some designs incorporate a second sensor for concurrent abdominal pressure measurement. Sizes under investigation range from 4 to 14 Fr. External components allow for larger batteries and storage capacity but create a permanent percutaneous tract with associated infection risks [24]. Onboard data storage and wireless transmission are key advantages, enabling prolonged home monitoring. Real-time data transmission, however, typically requires the external receiver/charger to be in very close proximity (2–12 cm) to the implanted sensor, which is problematic in patients with obesity and limits practicality in active children. The choice of power source (internal battery vs. external charging) significantly impacts device size and functional lifespan [24–27]. For pediatric application, the primary hurdle is device size relative to small bladder volumes and narrow urethral size. Insertion and removal almost invariably require general anesthesia. Significant risks include surgical complications (bleeding, infection), device migration, erosion (especially for intradetrusor types), device failure, and the potential to induce artifactual detrusor overactivity due to the foreign body. Long-term safety and efficacy data in children are currently lacking.

Ultrasound-Based UDS

Ultrasound technology offers several noninvasive pathways for bladder assessment, moving beyond simple volume estimation.

A. Proof of Principles: Studies have explored various ultrasound-derived metrics and their merits. Increased bladder wall thickness (BWT) has been traditionally associated with bladder outlet obstruction, or detrusor overactivity. However, establishing consistent normative pediatric data and reliable diagnostic thresholds remains challenging [20–22]. Ultrasound Bladder Vibrometry (UBV) is an emerging technique measuring low-frequency vibrations of the bladder wall. A pilot study demonstrated the ability to detect detrusor overactivity using time-stamped UBV measurements, achieving 70% sensitivity and 75% specificity, though accuracy was limited by irregular and relatively large sampling intervals [28]. Refinement, particularly implementing denser and more regular temporal sampling, is needed to enhance its diagnostic capability.

Shear Wave Elastography (SWE) quantitatively measures tissue stiffness by assessing the speed of shear waves propagating through the bladder wall. It has shown promise in effectively predicting detrusor overactivity and hypocompliance in children with neurogenic bladders (specificity 83%, $p < 0.05$), reflecting underlying pathological changes in detrusor smooth muscle elasticity [29]. Color Doppler ultrasound, applying the Bernoulli principle to estimate urinary flow velocity proximal to the bladder neck, has been explored for identifying bladder outlet obstruction in adults, but results across studies have been inconsistent and its utility in children requires further validation [30].

B. Wearable Bladder Technology: Commercially available devices like SENS-U kids and DFree utilize miniaturized ultrasound transducers worn on the suprapubic abdomen. They estimate bladder volume by measuring bladder dimensions (typically length/depth, not direct volume) and applying algorithmic calculations [31]. Their primary advantages are noninvasiveness and the potential for convenient home bladder volume monitoring, empowering patients and families (e.g., studies show home pressure/volume tracking correlating well with CMG for predicting high detrusor pressures and hydronephrosis) [31]. However, significant limitations exist. They measure linear dimensions, not direct volume, relying on geometric assumptions. Current error rates for volume estimation using standard ultrasound techniques range from 14% to 22%, inherent to the challenge of approximating the highly variable bladder shape (round, ellipsoid, cuboid, triangular) using simple geometric models. Accuracy diminishes significantly with smaller bladder volumes and is often compromised in patients with obesity. While SENS-U successfully detected a "full bladder" in 90% of children in one study, pediatric data for DFree is lacking [31, 32]. Future improvements may stem from multi-probe systems, advanced machine learning algorithms for data interpretation and artefact rejection, and the development of more sophisticated volume estimation models that better account for individual bladder morphology.

Summary and Future Considerations

The advancement of pediatric ambulatory urodynamics hinges on sustained, close collaboration between clinicians, biomedical engineers, and data scientists. Key priorities for the future include refining noninvasive techniques to improve the accuracy, reliability, and practicality of bioimpedance, NIRS, and especially ultrasound-based methods (wearable tech, SWE, UBV) through enhanced sensor design, multimodal integration, and sophisticated machine learning algorithms for robust data analysis and artefact rejection. Concurrently, substantial effort is needed in the miniaturization of implantable TAUM devices and the development of novel biomaterials to ensure long-term biocompatibility, safety, and reliability within the unique constraints of pediatric anatomy. Advanced signal processing and machine learning algorithms are crucial automatic event detection (contractions, incontinence), effectively removing artefact, and intelligently integrating diverse data streams (pressure, estimated volume, EMG, flow). Seamless integration with home monitoring and telemedicine platforms, leveraging Bluetooth and cloud technology for effortless data upload and remote clinician review, will improve functionality and accessibility. Developing intuitive user interfaces and automated alerts (e.g., prompting catheterization based on real-time pressure/volume thresholds) could significantly improve management. Research must focus on defining and validating the clinical significance of novel parameters derived from natural-fill studies against meaningful long-term outcomes like preservation of renal function and achievement of social continence.

Rigorous, standardized validation of new technologies against clinical outcomes in pediatric populations and the development of consensus protocols for performing and interpreting AUDS are paramount. Exploring the potential for permanently implanted devices in high-risk neurogenic bladder patients, enabling continuous pressure monitoring and potentially closed-loop therapeutic interventions (analogous to continuous glucose monitors and insulin pumps in diabetes), represents a futuristic but compelling direction. Ultimately, a major goal is the development of accurate, noninvasive, or minimally invasive triaging tools capable of reliably identifying low-risk children, thereby sparing them the burden and risks of invasive conventional CMG. The trajectory points toward less invasive, more reliable, and patient-centric urodynamic evaluation, promising better individualized management strategies for children with complex lower urinary tract disorders.

Acknowledgments The authors would like to acknowledge that parts of this chapter are similar to their manuscript published recently (Paediatric urodynamic studies: emerging technologies and new frontiers—Tayla Fay, Aniruddh V. Deshpande, Thomas Blanc, Chris Kimber, Kiarash Taghavi, 2025).

The authors would like to acknowledge that Fig. 13.1 has been adapted from the publication Ambulatory urodynamic studies (UDS) in children using a Bluetooth-enabled device—Deshpande—2012—BJU International—Wiley Online Library.

Declarations

Competing Interests The author(s) has no competing interests to declare that are relevant to the content of this manuscript.

Ethics Approval The author(s) declares that this manuscript does not include primary research with human participants.

The author(s) declares that this manuscript does not include primary studies involving animals.

References

1. Hoebeke P, Van Laecke E, Van Camp C, Raes A, Van De Walle J. One thousand video-urodynamic studies in children with non-neurogenic bladder sphincter dysfunction. BJU Int. 2001;87:575–80.
2. Kaufman MR, DeMarco RT, Pope JC, Scarpero HM, Adams MC, Trusler LA, et al. High yield of urodynamics performed for refractory nonneurogenic dysfunctional voiding in the pediatric population. J Urol. 2006;176:1835–7.

3. Soygür T, Arikan N, Tokatli Z, Karaboga R. The role of video-urodynamic studies in managing non-neurogenic voiding dysfunction in children. BJU Int. 2004;93:841–3.
4. De Gennaro M, Capitanucci ML, Capozza N, Caione P, Mosiello G, Silveri M. Detrusor hypocontractility in children with posterior urethral valves arises before puberty. Br J Urol. 1998;81:81–5.
5. De Gennaro M, Capitanucci ML, Mosiello G, Caione P, Silveri M. The changing urodynamic pattern from infancy to adolescence in boys with posterior urethral valves. BJU Int. 2000;85:1104–8.
6. Koff SA, Mutabagani KH, Jayanthi VR. The valve bladder syndrome: pathophysiology and treatment with nocturnal bladder emptying. J Urol. 2002;167:291–7.
7. Brown ET, Krlin RM, Winters JC. Urodynamics: examining the current role of UDS testing. What is the role of urodynamic testing in light of recent AUA urodynamics and overactive bladder guidelines and the VALUE study? Curr Urol Rep. 2013;14:403–8.
8. Drzewiecki BA, Bauer SB. Urodynamic testing in children: indications, technique, interpretation and significance. J Urol. 2011;186:1190–7.
9. Kanematsu A, Johnin K, Yoshimura K, Okubo K, Aoki K, Watanabe M, et al. Objective patterning of uroflowmetry curves in children with daytime and nighttime wetting. J Urol [Internet]. 2010;184:1674–9. Available from: https://pubmed.ncbi.nlm.nih.gov/20728134/.
10. Yerkes EB, Cheng EY, Wiener JS, Austin JC, Tu DD, Joseph DB, et al. Translating pediatric urodynamics from clinic into collaborative research: lessons and recommendations from the UMPIRE study group. J Pediatr Urol [Internet]. 2021;17:716–25. Available from: https://www.jpurol.com/article/S1477-5131(21)00271-0/fulltext.
11. Tarcan T, Bauer S, Olmedo E, Khoshbin S, Kelly M, Darbey M. Long-term follow up of newborns with myelodysplasia and normal urodynamic findings: is follow up necessary? J Urol [Internet]. 2001;165:564–7. Available from: https://www.sciencedirect.com/science/article/abs/pii/S0022534705667675.
12. Swithinbank LV, Woodward MN, O'Brien M, Frank JD, Nicholls G, Abrams P. Pediatric urodynamics: baseline audit and effect on management. J Pediatr Urol [Internet]. 2005;1:27–30. Available from: https://www.sciencedirect.com/science/article/abs/pii/S1477513104000063#preview-section-references.
13. Chang Y, Yanf SSD, Chuangg YC, Shen JH, Lin CC, Li C. Automatic classification of uroflow patterns via the grading-based approach. J Inform Sci Eng [Internet]. 2022:38. Available from: https://www.airitilibrary.com/Publication/alDetailedMesh?docid=10162364-202203-202202170001-202202170001-463-477.
14. Ha JS, Lee YS, Han SW, Kim SW. The relationship among flow index, uroflowmetry curve shape, and EMG lag time in children. Neurourol Urodyn. 2020;39:1387–93.
15. Hobbs KT, Choe N, Aksenov LI, Reyes L, Aquino W, Routh JC, et al. Machine learning for urodynamic detection of detrusor overactivity. Urology. 2022;159:247–54.
16. Deshpande AV, Craig JC, Caldwell PHY, Smith GHH. Ambulatory urodynamic studies (UDS) in children using a Bluetooth-enabled device. BJU Int. 2012;110:38–45.
17. Rosen J, Johnson L, Joseph DB. Radiation exposure in pediatric videourodynamics: an evaluation of safety in comparison to voiding cystourethrogram. J Pediatr Urol. 2024;20:745.e1–6.
18. Bauer SB, Nijman RJM, Drzewiecki BA, Sillen U, Hoebeke P. International Children's Continence Society standardization report on urodynamic studies of the lower urinary tract in children. Neurourol Urodyn. 2015;34:640–7.
19. Radley SC, Rosario DJ, Chapple CR, Farkas AG. Conventional and ambulatory urodynamic findings in women with symptoms suggestive of bladder overactivity. J Urol. 2001;166:2253–8.
20. Shin S, Moon J, Kye S, Lee K, Lee YS, Kang HG. Continuous bladder volume monitoring system for wearable applications. IEEE Xplore; 2017. p. 4435–8.
21. Schlebusch T, Nienke S, Leonhardt S, Walter M. Bladder volume estimation from electrical impedance tomography. Physiol Meas. 2014;35:1813–23.
22. Jo HG, Park BH, Joung DY, Jo JK, Hoh JK, Choi WY, et al. Forward-looking ultrasound wearable scanner system for estimation of urinary bladder volume. Sensors (Basel). 2021;21:5445.

23. Jourand P, Puers R. The BladderPill: an in-body system logging bladder pressure. Sens Actuators A Phys. 2010;162:160–6.
24. Wright DN, Züchner M, Annavini E, Escalona MJ, Hammerlund Teige L, Whist Tvedt LG, et al. From wires to waves, a novel sensor system for in vivo pressure monitoring. Sci Rep. 2024;14:7570.
25. Melgaard J, Rijkhoff NJM. Detecting the onset of urinary bladder contractions using an implantable pressure sensor. IEEE Trans Neural Syst Rehabil Eng. 2011;19:700–8.
26. Karam R, Bourbeau D, Majerus S, Makovey I, Goldman HB, Damaser MS, et al. Real-time classification of bladder events for effective diagnosis and treatment of urinary incontinence. IEEE Trans Biomed Eng. 2016;63:721–9.
27. Clausen I, Tvedt LGW, Hellandsvik A, Rognlien DKW, Glott T. An in vivo MEMS sensor system for percutaneous measurement of urinary bladder. In: Annual International Conference of the IEEE Engineering in Medicine and Biology Society; 2017. p. 1857–60.
28. Rosen DP, Husmann DA, Mynderse LA, Kelly TF, Alizad A, Fatemi M. Detrusor overactivity assessment using ultrasound bladder vibrometry. Physiol Meas. 2021;42:105012.
29. Sarkarian M, Arjomandi A, Musapour I, Hanafi MQ. Can bladder shear wave elastography be an alternative method for detection of neurogenic bladder instead of urodynamic study? J Family Med Prim Care. 2020;9:921–4.
30. Ozawa H, Igarashi T, Uematsu K, Watanabe T, Kumon H. The future of urodynamics: non-invasive ultrasound videourodynamics. Int J Urol. 2010;17:241–9.
31. van Leuteren PG, Klijn AJ, de Jong T, Dik P. SENS-U: validation of a wearable ultrasonic bladder monitor in children during urodynamic studies. J Pediatr Urol. 2018;14:569.e1–6.
32. Kocher NJ, Damaser MS, Gill BC. Advances in ambulatory urodynamics. Curr Urol Rep. 2020;21:41.

14 Bedside Urodynamics

Santosh Karmarkar and Sushma Achugatla

Urodynamic studies (UDS) collect physiological data on lower urinary tract function during bladder filling and emptying. Video urodynamics (video UDS) is the gold standard for the diagnosis. It has the advantage to recognize pathological changes in the lower urinary tract like abnormal bladder neck configuration, reflux, diverticulae, and pathological bladder shape. Evaluation of neurogenic bladder by using machine urodynamics is widely followed worldwide. But it is an expensive and cumbersome test that is not easily available and when available not easy to perform and interpret, especially in young children.

Bedside urodynamics (bedside UDS) (a term we have used for assessing urodynamics of the lower urinary tract without the use of a UDS machine) can be done easily and is inexpensive.

Bedside urodynamics can also be termed as *simple manual cystometry (SMC)*, which entails manual measurement of pressure-volume relationship of the bladder without the use of any UDS machine. It is the mainstay of investigation for bladder storage function and is a method of measuring the cystometric parameters. Bedside UDS when performed along with fluoroscopy and voiding cystourethrogram (VCUG) is the best alternative to video UDS.

Not many such bedside UDS studies have been reported in literature. Only readily available reports are an abstract published in Cerebrospinal Fluid Research 2007 and a recent paper by Sarin et al.

The main differences between bedside UDS and conventional UDS is given below in Table 14.1.

S. Karmarkar (✉) · S. Achugatla
Lilavati Hospital and Research Centre, Bandra Reclamation, Mumbai, India

S. Saha, P. Guha Vaze (eds.), *Comprehensive Atlas of Practical Pediatric Urodynamics*, https://doi.org/10.1007/978-981-95-2709-0_14

Table 14.1 Machine UDS versus simple manual cystometry/bedside UDS

Simple cystometry (without UDS machine)	Machine UDS
Equipment and costs	
No requirement for a costly UDS machine. Only fluoroscopic facilities required	Costly equipment along with costly accessories and consumables required
Procedure performance costs are minimal.	The costs for performing the UDS are usually high.
Technique and expertise required	
Simple technique which can be easily mastered and is easily reproducible. Interpretation is easier.	Requires years of experience to perform the test and obtain consistent results. Also, interpretation requires more experience.
Comfort of patient	
Requires less time, only one catheter introduced, no electrodes used—thus more comfortable	Many catheters are placed and electrodes applied. It takes much longer, thus causing greater discomfort
Interpretation of results	
Interpretation is relatively easy (although sphincter activity cannot be interpreted directly).	Interpretation is difficult and requires more experience. (Sphincter activity can be interpreted directly.)

Cystometric parameters assessed: One can easily assess the following cystometric parameters by bedside UDS:

1. Random resting bladder pressure
2. Post-void residual volume
3. Bladder capacity
4. Effective leak point pressure
5. Comment on compliance and hyperreflexia

Technique of Performing the Bedside UDS

Simple manual cystometry is a simple single-channel cystometry.

Cystometry consists of catheterization with infant feeding tube of appropriate size for the age. The end of the catheter is connected to an infusion drip tubing set held vertical up to a height of about 50–75 cms, and readings are recorded from the level of symphysis pubis to the level of the urine in the catheter. The markings on the infant feeding tube are useful for these readings.

How Is It Done

- Under strict aseptic conditions, once the catheter is inserted, urine flow can be visualized into the tube. This marking on the infant feeding tube at this instance is recorded as random resting bladder pressure.
- The bladder is completely emptied with the catheter.

The bladder is then filled slowly with warm saline (at room temperature) mixed with diluted dye (that is used for VCUG) by infusion drip with a filling speed of 10 to 20 ml per minute (at filling rate of 10% of the expected bladder capacity per minute). As the filling is continued, the same can be observed under fluoroscopy. The filling is continued until the child has a strong desire to void occurs, or the bladder is seen to be full on fluoroscopy, or until urethral leakage occurs, or until bladder pressure exceeds 40 cm H_2O (the height of the water column is more 40 cm). The filling rate and volume may have to be modified in cases of high-grade VUR.

Thus, one could assess the pressure changes in bladder with changes in the level of the water column (correlating with the markings labelled on the infant feeding tube).

- At the point when the filling is stopped, one can record the bladder capacity (amount of fluid infused) and leak point pressure if there is a leak. The pressure at which the leak was seen is measured as effective leak point pressure.
- Bedside UDS ends here, and the catheter is removed. The patient is then asked to void if the child is able to initiate and maintain voiding.
- After voiding, the catheter is reintroduced and post-void residual volume is to be measured. This can also be checked under fluoroscopy.

Definition and Assessment of Cystometric Parameters in Simple Cystometry

- Random/resting bladder pressure: This is the baseline detrusor pressure. The height of the column of urine from level of pubic symphysis into the catheter in cm as recorded with markings labelled on the infant feeding tube. (Resting bladder pressure is considered as safe when it is less than 20 cm of water.)
- Sensation of bladder fullness: If felt by the patient
- Bladder capacity: Cystometric capacity is the bladder volume at the end of the filling cystometrogram, as per the criteria mentioned above.

  The estimated bladder capacity is calculated using the following formula:

  Age-based capacity may be estimated by formulas proposed by *Koff*

  For children, less than 2 years – volume in ml = weight in kgs × 7

  For children older than 2 years – volume in ml = 30 (age in years + 2)

  Bladder capacity is considered adequate if it is more than two-third of the expected capacity.
- Effective leak point pressure: Detrusor leak point pressure is defined as the lowest detrusor pressure at which urine leakage occurs in the absence of either a detrusor contraction or increased abdominal pressure. Leak point pressure of 40 cms or more is considered as normal.
- Post-void residual volume is defined as the volume of fluid remaining in the bladder immediately after a voluntary void (if possible, in many NGB cases, voiding may not be possible).

  Note: The leak point pressure measured by this technique is termed effective leak point pressure because it is the effective pressure generated in the bladder, which is the detrusor pressure plus the intra-abdominal pressure. In the bedside technique, no additional rectal catheter is inserted to measure pressure.

- Compliance and hyperreflexia

  As regards compliance and hyperreflexia, a correct judgment can usually be made based on the shape of the bladder and resting bladder pressures (see comment below).

Our Experience of Using Bedside UDS

As mentioned earlier, a voiding cystourethrogram (VCUG) under fluoroscopy is done along with bedside UDS in all our patients. The shape and outline of the urinary bladder, presence of trabeculations, presence/absence of vesicoureteric reflux, and morphology of the bladder neck and urethra are observed during the VCUG bedside UDS procedure. These findings are useful in interpreting UD features such as capacity, compliance, hyperreflexic bladder, etc.

We have performed a clinical prospective interventional study comparing bedside UDS versus machine UDS (mainly the cystometry) in our institute that involved 31 children of age less than 18 years with neurogenic bladder due to different causes and who had not undergone any previous surgery on their urinary tracts. The results of both the methods were not known (blinded) to other team. The results were compared by a senior consultant and the principal investigator. The results were compared and summarized as a match or a mismatch—as per Table 14.2 below.

As regards compliance and hyperreflexia, a judgment was made based on the shape of the bladder and resting bladder pressures. Though there was a mismatch in about 40% of cases for these parameters, they were not consequential for deciding the management, especially in NGB. Most management decisions can be made by knowing capacity and leak point pressure and the dry interval.

Thus, it can be stated that both bedside UDS (SMC) and machine UDS (EFC) can be used for the urodynamic evaluation in children (Fig. 14.1).

Some of the VCUG images of our patients during bedside UDS (Fig. 14.2).

Table 14.2 Comparison of two important UDS parameters in both the methods and results summarized

Parameter	Matching	Mismatching
Maximum bladder capacity	25/31	6/31
Effective leak point pressure	24/31	7/31

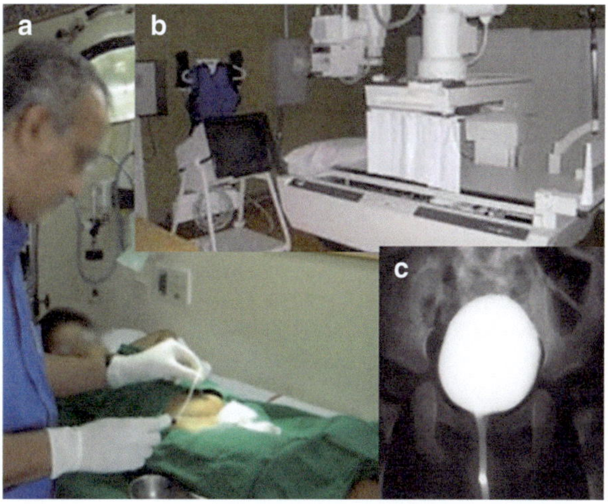

Fig. 14.1 Performing simple cystometry/bedside UDS in our center. (**a**) Performing simple manual cystometry. (Source: one of our study patients). (**b**) Setup of fluoroscopy room for performing VCUG in the department of radiology. (**c**) VCUG showing voiding phase with smooth-walled bladder and normal urethra. (Source: one of our study patients)

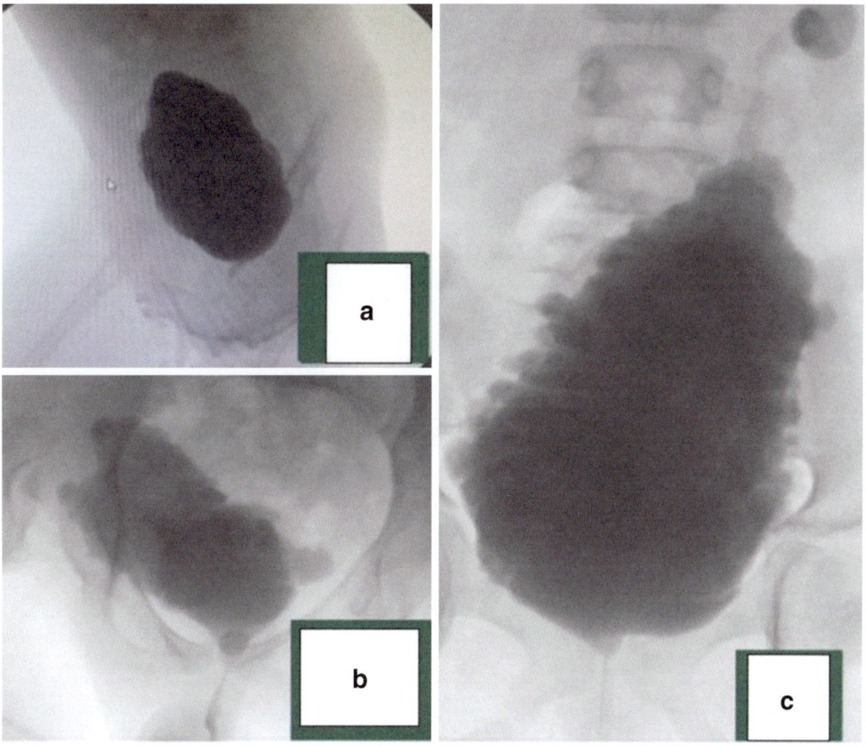

Fig. 14.2 VCUG. (**a**) shows mildly crenated bladder. (**b**) Severe trabeculated bladder with irregular shape. (**c**) shows moderately crenated bladder with classical Christmas tree-shaped bladder. (Source: some of our study patients)

Declarations

Competing Interests The author(s) has no competing interests to declare that are relevant to the content of this manuscript.

Ethics Approval The author(s) declares that informed consent to participate in the study and for the publication of the case report/data and/or photographs was obtained from all individual participants/legal guardians of participants. Ethics Committee for Biomedical & Health Research (EC-BHR)

Regn. No. EC/NEW/INST/2020/504

LILAVATI HOSPITAL & RESEARCH CENTRE

Meeting No.06/20 dated 17" July 2020

The author(s) declares that this manuscript does not include primary studies involving animals.

Suggested Reading

1. Szabó L, Lombay B, Borbás É, Bajusz I. Videourodynamics in the diagnosis of urinary tract abnormalities in a single center. Pediatr Nephrol. 2004;19:326–31.
2. Jiang YH, Chen SF, Kuo HC. Role of videourodynamic study in precision diagnosis and treatment for lower urinary tract dysfunction. Tzu-Chi Med J. 2020;32(2):121.
3. Bangar A, Karmarkar S. Simple clinical and bedside urodynamic evaluation is sufficient for successful management decisions in spina bifida patients with urinary incontinence and the machine urodynamics are not necessary. Cerebrospinal Fluid Res. 2007;4(S1):S21.
4. Rahul SK, Sarin Y. Bedside Cystometry against that of urodynamic study in diagnosing bladder functional abnormalities in children. 2024;1:278–83. https://doi.org/10.5281/zenodo.13893756.
5. Tanaka H, Matsuda M, Moriya K, Mitsui T, Kitta T, Nonomura K. Ultrasonographic measurement of bladder wall thickness as a risk factor for upper urinary tract deterioration in children with myelodysplasia. J Urol. 2008;180:312–6.
6. McGuire EJ, Woodside JR, Borden TA, Weiss RM. Prognostic value of urodynamic testing in myelodysplastic patients. J Urol. 1981;126(2):205–9.
7. Campbell-Walsh Urology: Pediatric Urology.

i-UDS in Infants

15

Poonam Guha Vaze

Infants rarely present with unusual voiding problems which are similar to the presentation of BBD or NNNB in older children. Most common presentations include:

1. Increased urinary frequency
2. Straining/crying while passing urine
3. Recurrent UTI with normal MCU findings or VUR
4. Features suggestive of BOO without any anatomical evidence of BOO

These cases mandate the assessment of bladder function to plan the further treatment which is usually accomplished by 4-hour voiding observation. *i*-UDS may be needed if there are diagnostic dilemmas.

We have performed *i*-UDS in infants in the following circumstances:

1. Known case of neurogenic bladder
2. Follow-up cases of PUV with persistent post-fulguration upper tract changes/UTI/dribbling
3. Cases where functional bladder problem is suspected from history (frequent micturition, straining/crying while passing urine, poor urinary stream) which causes significant distress to baby/parents or recurrent UTI
4. UTI with vesicoureteric reflux where bladder dysfunction is suggested based on history/MCU appearance of bladder

P. G. Vaze (✉)
Neotia Bhagirathi Woman and Child Care Centre, Newtown, Kolkata, India

Department of Pediatric Surgery, Nilratan Sircar Medical College and Hospital, Kolkata, India

S. Saha, P. Guha Vaze (eds.), *Comprehensive Atlas of Practical Pediatric Urodynamics*, https://doi.org/10.1007/978-981-95-2709-0_15

Challenges faced while performing i-UDS in an infant are as follows:

1. Size of catheter—Urodynamics can be performed in infants using the standard 6 Fr double-lumen catheter and per-rectal 5 Fr gloved feeding tube.
2. Positioning the baby—We usually position the baby at the edge of the table on the mother's lap so that the urine falls into the uroflowmetry jar. Study can also be performed in the supine position and the episodes of passage of urine marked by annotations on the curve.
3. Irritability of the child—Young children become irritable when held in a fixed position. We use distractors like toys/cartoon videos to keep them engaged.
4. Obeying commands—We cannot expect young babies to obey commands. Rather, we observe their response—change of facial expressions/activity in response to bladder fill. These children usually pass urine spontaneously whenever they feel the urge.
5. Checking cough impulse—Working of both the catheters can be ascertained whenever the child cries/is irritable or by gentle suprapubic pressure (as the baby cannot cough on command).
6. Length of catheter to be introduced—In infants, catheter should be introduced till 10–12 cm in boys and 5–8 cm in girls to prevent artefacts when bladder collapses.
7. Fill rate should be kept low (5 ml/min). We have had to keep the fill rate at 1–2 ml/min in two patients who were voiding after every 3–4 ml filling.
8. Lack of standard reference values—UDS findings which are deemed abnormal in older children may be normally seen in infants like:
   (a) Overactivity can be a normal finding in infants.
   (b) Voiding frequency and voided volumes are variable.
   (c) Voids may be partial with significant PVR.
   (d) Voiding detrusor pressures may be normally very high.
   (e) Physiological dysfunctional voiding is the rule—detrusor sphincter coordination matures by 2 years of age.

Interpretation of i-UDS findings in infants:

It is very difficult to differentiate 'physiological' abnormality due to infancy from 'true' abnormality due to disease process. In other words, labelling a UDS finding in an infant as abnormal is challenging.

The dictum we follow is that we interpret the UDS findings in light of the symptomatology and other radiological findings of the patient and ascertain whether the urodynamic parameters can explain the other findings.

Babies usually fall asleep after initial half of the study; thus, they allow bladder behaviour to be assessed when the child is irritable as well as when they are calm.

Babies pass urine spontaneously whenever the bladder is full or whenever there is a wave of involuntary detrusor contraction. It is impossible to differentiate between voluntarily generated void and overactivity-induced void in young children. In infants, overactivity is seldom seen as isolated waves of detrusor contraction. It usually manifests as voiding at volumes much smaller than the capacity expected for their weights. Occasionally, these voids are preceded by detrusor contractions of smaller amplitudes. We usually repeat two or three voiding filling-voiding cycles to confirm the finding. This finding of voiding at smaller volumes when corroborated with the usual voiding behaviour and added history of UTIs clinches the diagnosis of 'pathological' detrusor overactivity.

As physiological dysfunctional voiding is the norm in infants, detrusor pressures have been shown to be highly variable and even pressures of 120 cm H_2O have been reported to be normal. We have seen that although Pdetmax may be very high, PdetQmax is usually around 40–50 even in infants. If an infant has history of significant crying/straining during micturition with poor urinary stream and we find high voiding detrusor pressures, we can call it as probable voiding dysfunction. This provides us evidence to start alpha-blockers or even injecting botox at bladder neck/sphincter even if there is no PVR on USG.

We have compiled a list of seven cases where UDS was performed in infants due to one of the various indications stated earlier. All the studies were performed without sedation. The cases represent that excellent UDS curves can be generated in infants. UDS can provide valuable information which can guide management planning.

In many of these cases, the USG did not show any significant changes in the bladder although UDS showed significant findings. This shows that changes in bladder behaviour can be picked up early on *i*-UDS whereas structural changes take time to appear.

Case 1

A 6-month-old female child presented with frequent micturition and significant straining while passing urine. Increased voiding frequency was confirmed on 4-hour voiding observation (3–4 voids per hour). USG showed normal bladder and upper tracts. MCU showed small capacity bladder with no VUR. She had history of constipation and had been started on stool softeners. UDS was performed when symptoms persisted after adequate management of constipation.

UDS revealed spontaneous voids at small bladder volumes (15–20 ml)—probable detrusor overactivity with voiding at variable detrusor pressures (40–60 cm H_2O) (Fig. 15.1a and b).

The child was started on low-dose anticholinergics and alpha-blockers following which the child became comfortable. Dose of anticholinergic was titrated to have a voiding frequency of 1–2 times per hour.

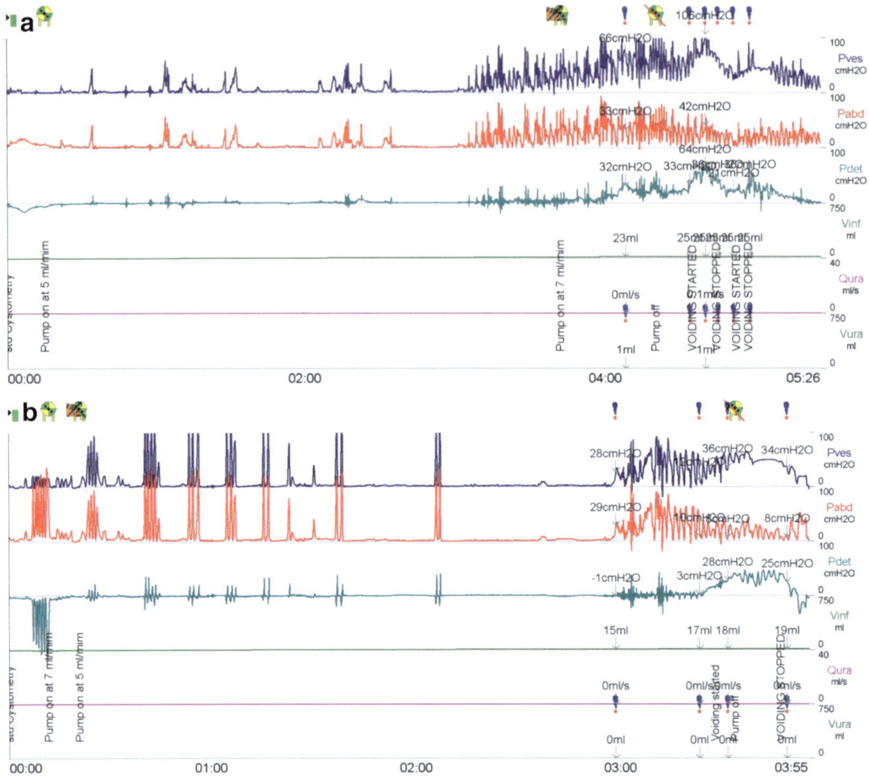

Fig. 15.1 (**a**) First UDS cycle—void at 20 ml volume in an interrupted stream. (**b**) Second UDS cycle, voiding at 17 ml with slow and prolonged void

Case 2

An 11-month-old boy, follow-up case of PUV fulgurated at the age of 1 month, underwent check cystoscopy done at the age of 7 months. He passed urine well in good stream with history of occasional dribbling. USG showed bilateral mild HDUN with normal bladder wall thickness. He was on oxybutynin 1.25 mg twice a day during the study.

UDS was performed to check for any significant overactivity or poor compliance as a cause of dribbling.

The child fell asleep during the study without any sedation. UDS showed large capacity stable bladder with normal voiding pressures (Fig. 15.2a and b). The dose of anticholinergics was reduced after the study.

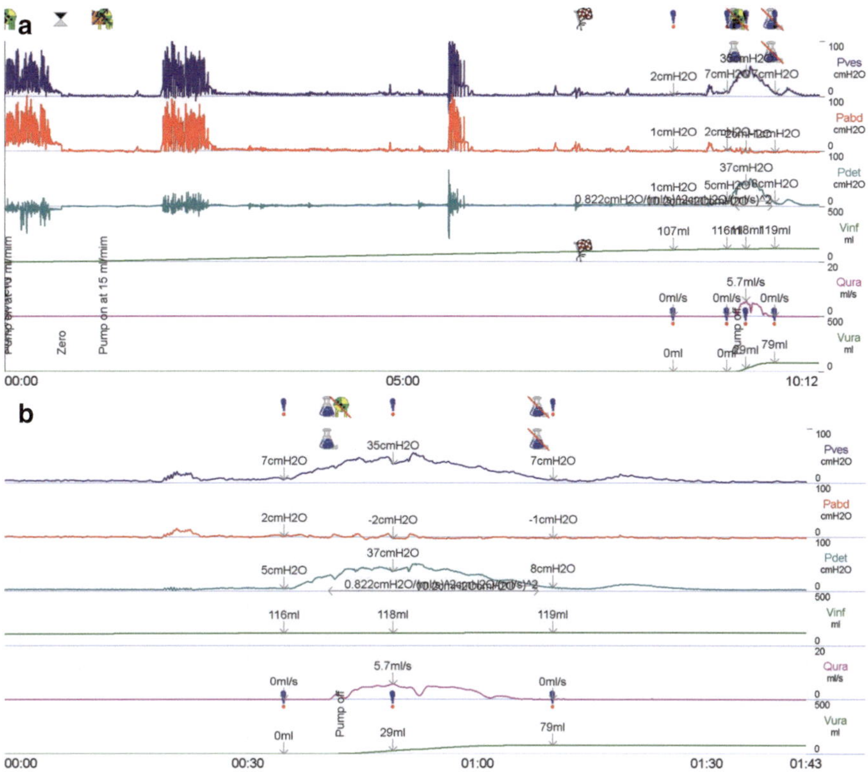

Fig. 15.2 (**a**) Full urodynamic trace showing stable bladder with normal compliance and no overactivity. Bladder capacity was 120 ml (EBC 60 ml). (**b**) Voiding phase of the study—expanded—normal voiding pressures and flow rates

Case 3

A 6-month-old baby boy had two episodes of culture-proven UTI. He had history of frequent micturition (2–4 times per hour) with variable urinary stream. USG showed normal bladder and upper tracts. MCU showed small capacity bladder with normal bladder neck and urethra.

UDS was performed to assess any bladder dysfunction as the cause of recurrent UTI. The child voided variable amounts of urine every 10 ml fill. Some prevoid overactivity was noted. Detrusor pressures during actual periods of void were around 30–50 cm H_2O (Fig. 15.3a). He fell asleep during the study (Fig. 15.3b). When asleep, he tolerated a fill of 20 ml. As soon as he woke up, detrusor overactivity was noted with some leak followed by voiding contraction and void.

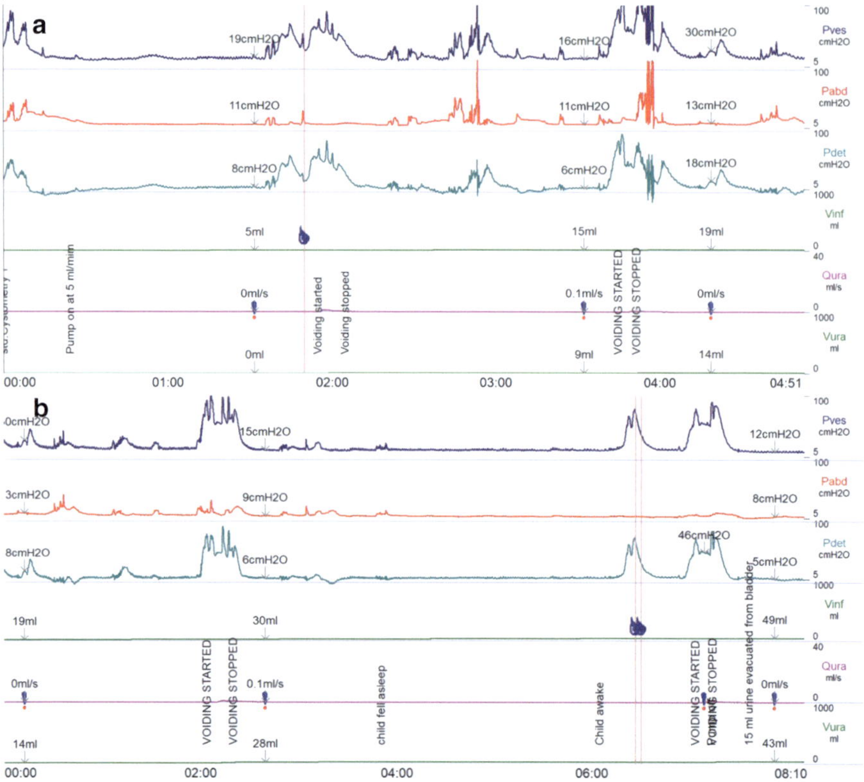

Fig. 15.3 (**a**) First half of the study showing two voids and one overactivity in between. The voids have been represented by 'leak/drop' sign or text annotations. (**b**) Second half of the study when the child fell asleep

He was started on anticholinergics based on history of two episodes of UTI, clinical findings of increased frequency and urodynamic findings of detrusor overactivity. He had no further UTIs in the subsequent 6 months follow-up.

Case 4

An 8-month-old female baby had history of two episodes of UTI. USG showed normal bladder with left mild HDN. Parents did not notice any abnormal voiding behaviour.

MCU (Fig. 15.4a) showed smooth round-walled bladder which became elongated on attempt to void and appearance of left Gr V VUR. There was poor visualisation of urethra with significant PVR. MRI spine was normal.

Urodynamics (Fig. 15.4b) was performed as the bladder appeared abnormal during voiding with high-grade reflux that appeared only during voiding.

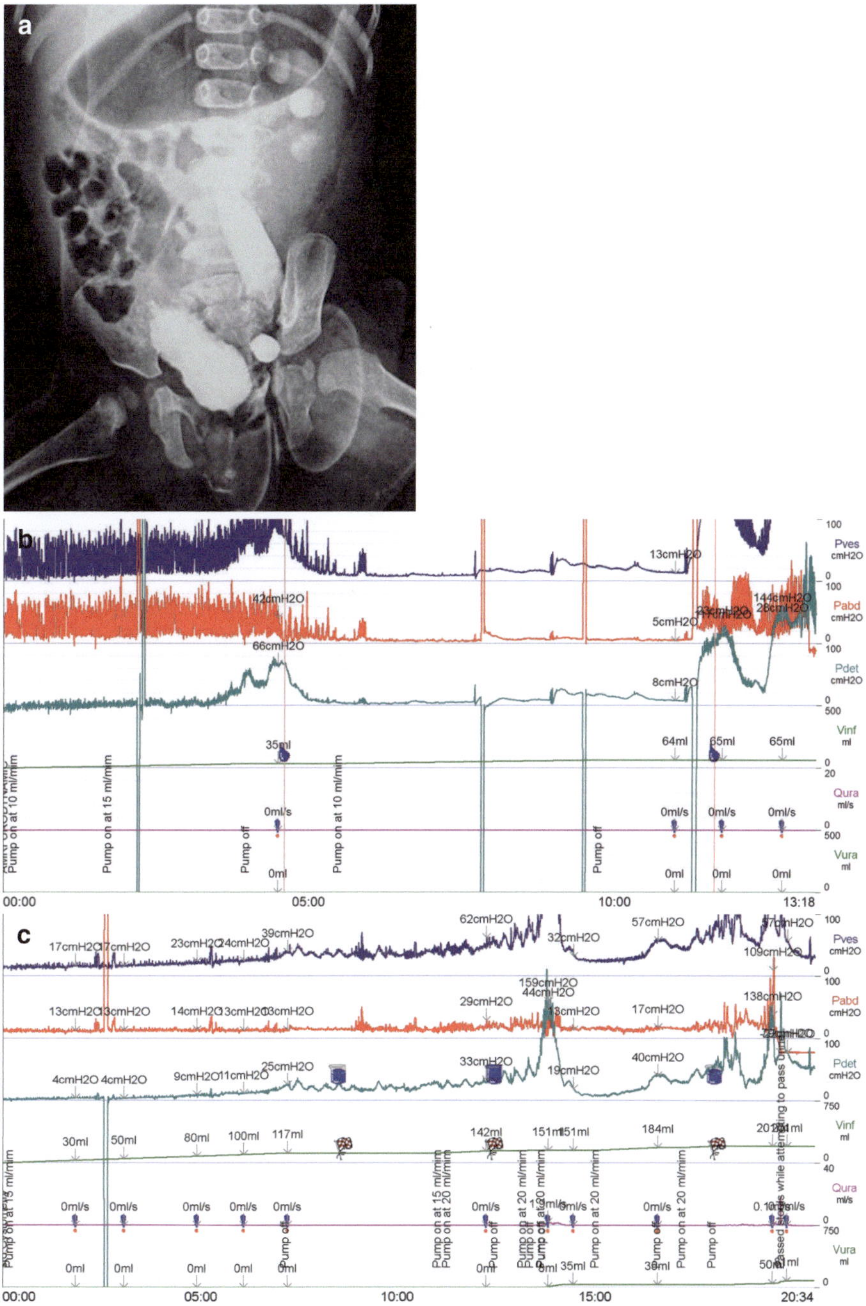

Fig. 15.4 (**a**) MCU images showing filling phase and voiding attempt (**b**) UDS tracing showing strong detrusor contractions (60–120 cm H_2O) at volumes of 35 ml and 60 ml fill along with leak/void of urine (showed by 'leak/drop' sign). (**c**) Repeat study at 2.5 years showing improved capacity, reduced compliance, detrusor overactivity, very high voiding pressures and poor flow rates

Voids/leaks have been marked as 'leak/drop' as the study was done in supine position. The child was irritable in beginning and terminal part of the study and fell asleep in the mid part. After bladder was filled to volumes of 30–40 ml, waves of strong detrusor contraction were noted with pressures of 60–140 cm H_2O, when she was seen to void/leak 10–20 ml. There was a PVR of 20–30 ml after the voids.

Based on the MCU and UDS findings, she was thought to have high voiding pressures with significant PVR (obstructed voiding, probably due to bladder neck dysfunction), and the high voiding pressures were responsible for appearance of reflux during voiding. She was started on anticholinergics, alpha-blockers and CIC.

Repeat study was done at 2.5 years (Fig. 15.4c) which revealed an overactive bladder with reduced compliance and very high voiding pressures, thus confirming the previous UDS findings, and she was labelled as having non-neurogenic-neurogenic bladder.

Case 5

An 8-month-old male baby, follow-up case of giant right-sided hutch diverticulum with recurrent episodes of UTI—underwent excision with ureteric reimplant at the age of 6 months. He continued to have repeated episodes of UTI after the surgery. He passed urine in robust stream at frequent intervals. Repeat MCU suggested resolution of diverticulum with new onset Gr I reflux on the contralateral side.

UDS was done at 8 months of age to ascertain cause of repeated UTI. UDS (Fig. 15.5) showed spontaneous voiding after every 10–20 ml fill –probable voiding due to overactivity contractions with mildly raised voiding detrusor pressures and complete emptying of bladder.

MRI spine showed normal study. He was started on anticholinergics with night-time catheter drainage. He did not have any further UTIs in the following 1 year.

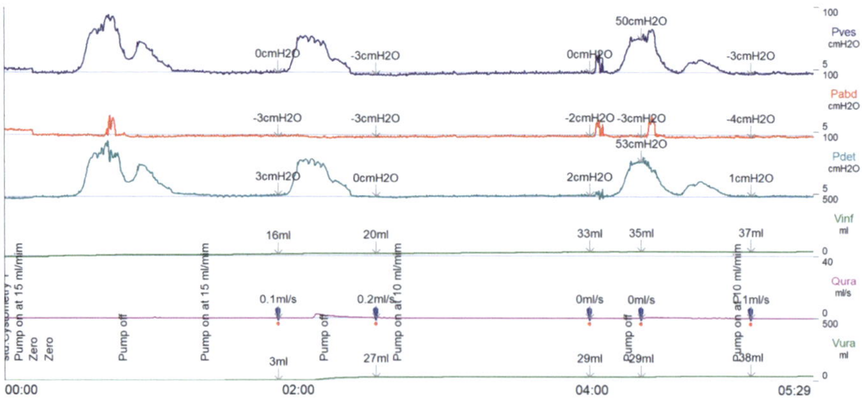

Fig. 15.5 UDS tracing showing detrusor contractions after every 10–20 ml fill associated with voids. The episodes of void are not very apparent on the tracing due to the small voided volumes, but the Vura is seen to rise from 3 to 27 to 38 ml after respective voids

Case 6

A 6-month-old male boy had history of crying and severe straining during micturition with variable urinary stream and recurrent UTI for which he had been on catheter drainage since the last 2 months. USG showed normal bladder with left mild HDUN. MCU (Fig. 15.6a) showed small irregular bladder with very prominent bladder neck.

He underwent cystoscopy which ruled out PUV. He was started on alpha-blockers but developed another episode of UTI.

UDS was performed at 6 months of age to assess bladder behaviour and impact of the prominent bladder neck on voiding. UDS (Fig. 15.6b) revealed small capacity

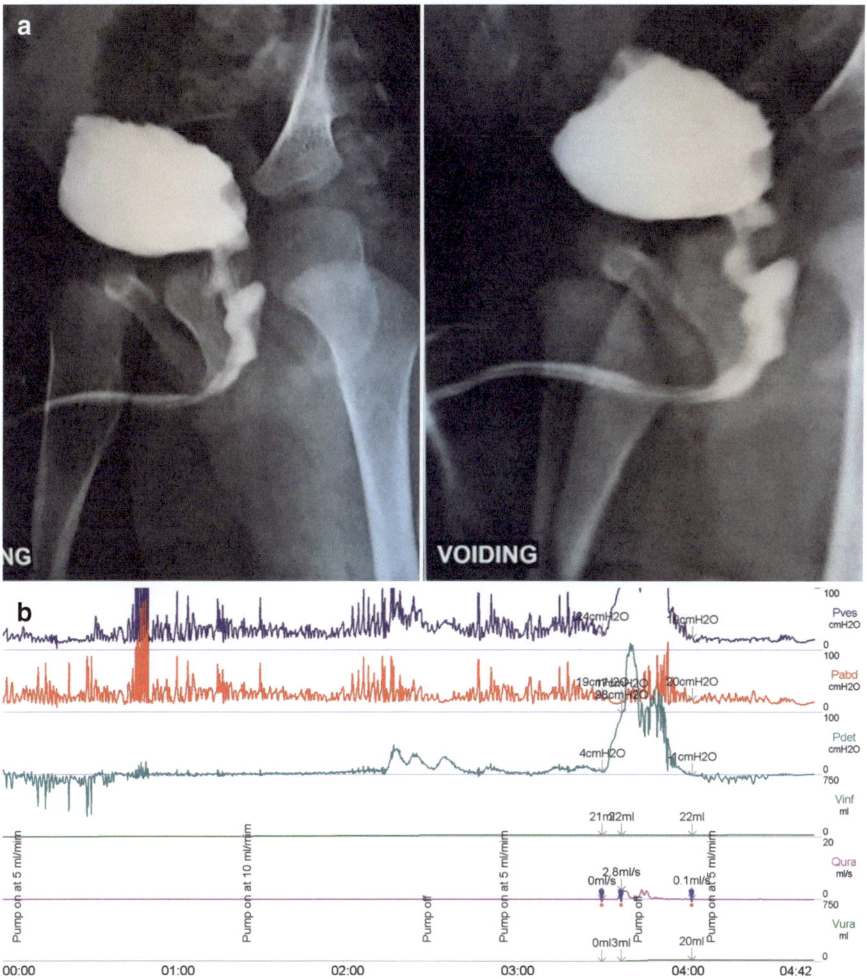

Fig. 15.6 (**a**) MCU showing very prominent bladder neck impression. (**b**) UDS tracing showing waves of detrusor overactivity followed by a very strong detrusor contraction associated with passage of urine in a weak stream

bladder (20 ml) with detrusor overactivity and very high detrusor pressures (200 cm H_2O) during voiding with very poor flow but complete emptying of bladder.

He underwent cystoscopy with superficial bladder neck incision along with botox injection at bladder neck/sphincter. His urinary stream improved significantly after the surgery and he did not have any further UTIs at 1 year follow-up.

Case 7

A 6-month-old female child with history of lumbosacral meningomyelocele repair at the age of 1 month presented with history of constant irritability and increased frequency of micturition with crying/straining while passing urine. USG KUB showed normal bladder and upper tracts. MCU showed normal capacity rounded bladder, but the baby could not void during the study (Fig. 15.7a).

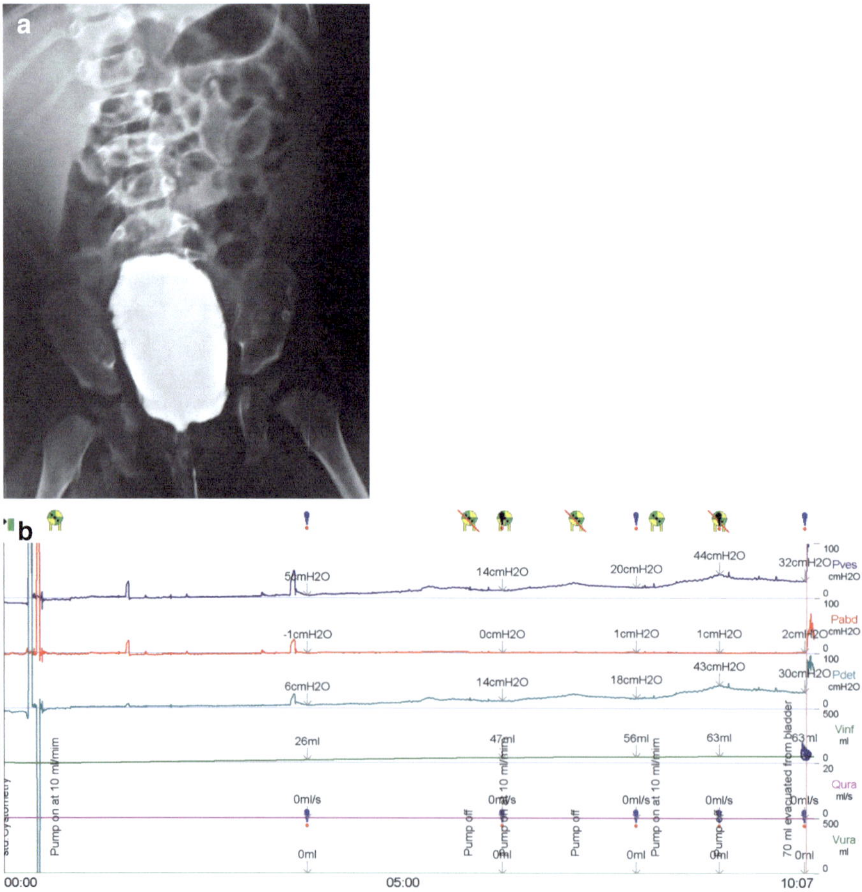

Fig. 15.7 (**a**) MCU image (**b**) UDS tracing showing normal capacity badder with significantly reduced compliance

UDS (Fig. 15.7b) showed a normal capacity bladder; filling was continued till urine leak/voiding was documented. Mild overactivity was noted but leak appeared long after Pdet of 40 cm H_2O was reached.

So, although the USG was normal, this child had a high-risk bladder. She was started on CIC for bladder emptying and anticholinergics to reduce detrusor pressures. Child improved clinically and her irritability disappeared.

Declarations

Competing Interests The author(s) has no competing interests to declare that are relevant to the content of this manuscript.

Ethics Approval The author(s) declares that this manuscript does not include primary research with human participants.

The author(s) declares that this manuscript does not include primary studies involving animals.

Suggested Reading

1. Al Mosawi AJ. Identification of nonneurogenic neurogenic bladder in infants. Urology. 2007;70(2):355–6; discussion 356–7. https://doi.org/10.1016/j.urology.2007.04.049. PMID: 17826506.
2. Guerra L, Leonard M, Castagnetti M. Best practice in the assessment of bladder function in infants. Ther Adv Urol. 2014;6(4):148–64. https://doi.org/10.1177/1756287214528745. PMID: 25083164; PMCID: PMC4054507.
3. Ichino M, Igawa Y, Seki S, Ishizuka O, Nishizawa O. Natural history and etiology of high pressure voiding in male infants. J Urol. 2007;178(6):2561–5; discussion 2565–6. https://doi.org/10.1016/j.juro.2007.08.048. Epub 2007 Oct 22. PMID: 17945306.
4. Ichino M, Igawa Y, Seki S, Iijima K, Ishizuka O, Nishizawa O. The nature of high-pressure voiding in small boys and its relation with the influence of a transurethral catheter. Neurourol Urodyn. 2008;27(4):319–23. https://doi.org/10.1002/nau.20493. PMID: 17701987.
5. Jayanthi VR, Khoury AE, McLorie GA, Agarwal SK. The nonneurogenic neurogenic bladder of early infancy. J Urol. 1997;158(3 Pt 2):1281–5. https://doi.org/10.1097/00005392-199709000-00163. PMID: 9258195.
6. Shapiro E. Urodynamics in children. Rev Urol. 2012;14(1–2):36–8. PMID: 23173000; PMCID: PMC3502051.
7. Sillén U. Bladder function in healthy neonates and its development during infancy. J Urol. 2001;166(6):2376–81. https://doi.org/10.1016/s0022-5347(05)65594-2. PMID: 11696790.
8. Wen JG, Yeung CK, Chu WC, Shit FK, Metreweli C. Video cystometry in young infants with renal dilation or a history of urinary tract infection. Urol Res. 2001;29(4):249–55. https://doi.org/10.1007/s002400100194. PMID: 11585280.

i-UDS in VUR

16

Poonam Guha Vaze

The role of *i*-UDS in patients with VUR is controversial.

Conventional teaching says that the role of *i*-UDS in children with VUR is limited as the results of *i*-UDS are unreliable in such kids. If *i*-UDS is contemplated in such children, video-UDS would be recommended rather than conventional *i*-UDS. As the availability of video-UDS is limited, *i*-UDS is usually not offered to these patients.

We have performed *i*-UDS in patients with VUR and have made the following observations:

1. In children with low-grade VUR or high-grade VURs with not much dilatation of upper tracts, the *i*-UDS findings are fairly reliable.
2. In the presence of VUR, there will be some overestimation of bladder capacity, compliance and PVR and underestimation of overactivity and voiding detrusor pressures.
3. If there is significant overactivity, reduced compliance or high voiding pressures, it manifests even in the presence of gross VUR.
4. In a patient with gross VUR, if we find abnormal bladder dynamics, we consider it significant; that is, presence of abnormal UDS findings in the presence of gross VUR has a strong positive predictive value for abnormal bladder dynamics.

P. G. Vaze (✉)
Neotia Bhagirathi Woman and Child Care Centre, Newtown, Kolkata, India

Department of Pediatric Surgery, Nilratan Sircar Medical College and Hospital, Kolkata, India

S. Saha, P. Guha Vaze (eds.), *Comprehensive Atlas of Practical Pediatric Urodynamics*, https://doi.org/10.1007/978-981-95-2709-0_16

5. In a patient with gross VUR, if the bladder appears stable on *i*-UDS, video-UDS may be contemplated to check whether the fluid that is infused is expanding the bladder or the upper tracts only, because of which the bladder appears to be stable. In other words, finding of normal UDS parameters in the presence of gross VUR has a poor negative predictive value. In many such cases when we perform video-UDS, we observe that the volume infused actually fills up the upper tracts preferentially with the bladder practically remaining same in size. After the upper tracts become sufficiently full, true bladder pressures become apparent—detrusor pressures start rising or overactivity appears.
6. In patients with VUR, normal appearance of bladder on MCU and USG may be deceptive, and these children may have significant overactivity. These children stop having UTIs once they are started on bladder relaxants.
7. Chances of post-procedure UTI is higher in patients with VUR—we keep the catheter draining for a few minutes after the end of procedure so that the refluxed fluid drains out completely to reduce the incidence of post-procedure UTI.

We present few cases of VUR of varying severity with their corresponding UDS findings.

Case 1: Primary VUR

A 3.9-year-old girl presented with recurrent episodes of UTI. USG showed bilateral mild pelvicalyceal system fullness with bilateral mild ureteric dilatation. MCU showed bilateral Gr IV VUR (Fig. 16.1a).

Uroflowmetry showed a normal bell-shaped curve with a voided volume of 130 ml which was appropriate for her age (Fig. 16.1b). UDS showed a stable normal capacity bladder with normal compliance and no overactivity. Voiding parameters were also normal (Fig. 16.1c).

As the upper tract dilatation was not significant, refluxed volume did not seem to be large enough to confound the UDS findings. So this was considered as a case of primary VUR with no bladder dysfunction.

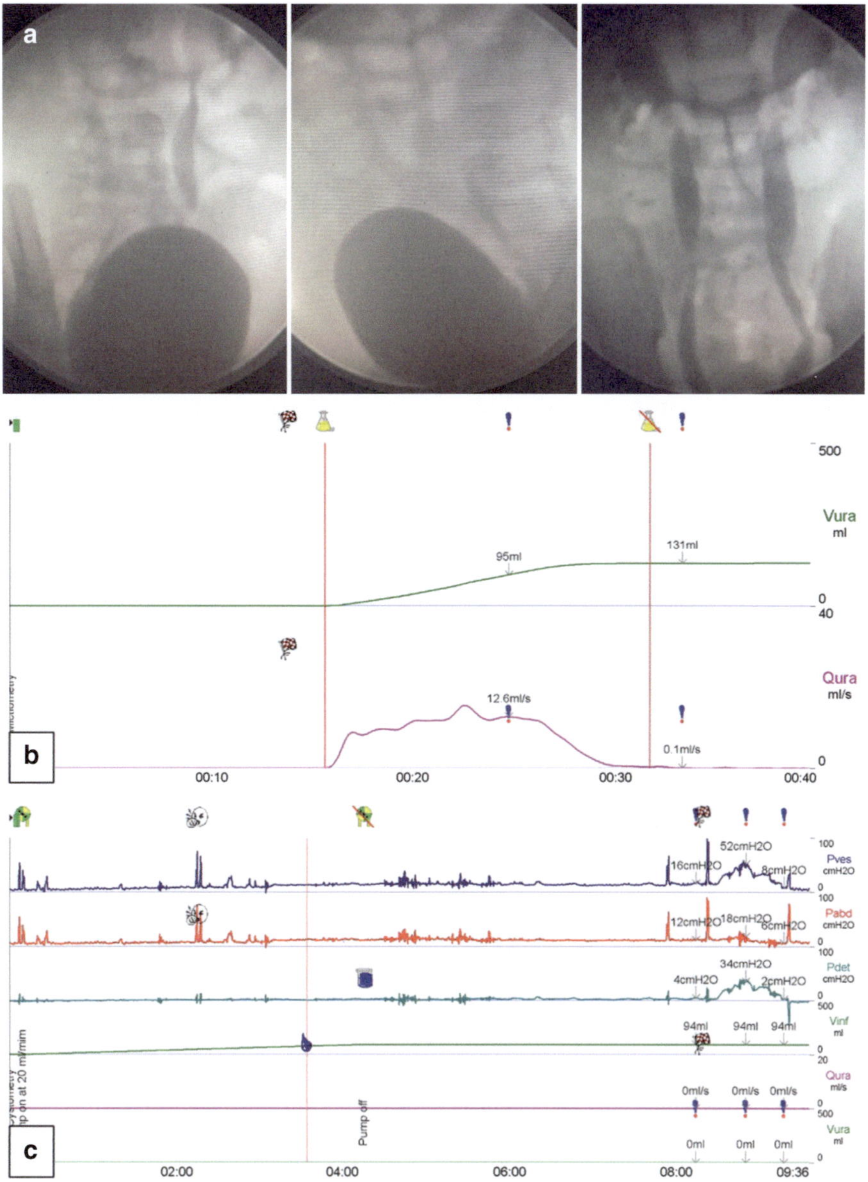

Fig. 16.1 (**a**) MCU showed bilateral Gr IV VUR. (**b**) Uroflowmetry showed a normal bell-shaped curve with a voided volume of 130 ml, which was appropriate for her age. (**c**) UDS showed a stable normal capacity bladder with normal compliance and no overactivity. Voiding parameters were also normal

Case 2: VUR with DO

A 5-year-old girl had recurrent episodes of UTI since 3 years of age. She did not have any urinary symptoms during the episodes of UTI. She complained of intermittent mild urgency with wetting of pants during the daytime when child was engrossed in activities and primary enuresis. She had history of constipation for which she was started on laxatives. USG revealed small scarred right kidney with mild HDN and mild ureteric dilatation on the right side. MCU revealed a normal-looking bladder with right Gr IV and left Gr I VUR, but no much dilatation of upper tracts (Fig. 16.2a).

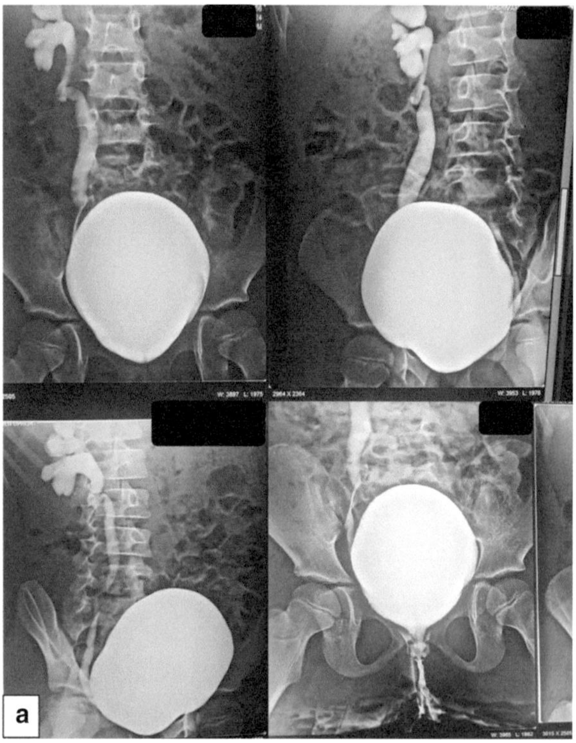

Fig. 16.2 (**a**) MCU revealed a normal looking bladder with right Gr IV and left Gr I VUR (**b**) Uroflowmetry revealed a normal bell-shaped curve with good flow rates, but some increase in EMG activity during voiding. (**c**) UDS revealed severe detrusor overactivity during filling with normal voiding parameters with urgency noted during episodes of detrusor overactivity

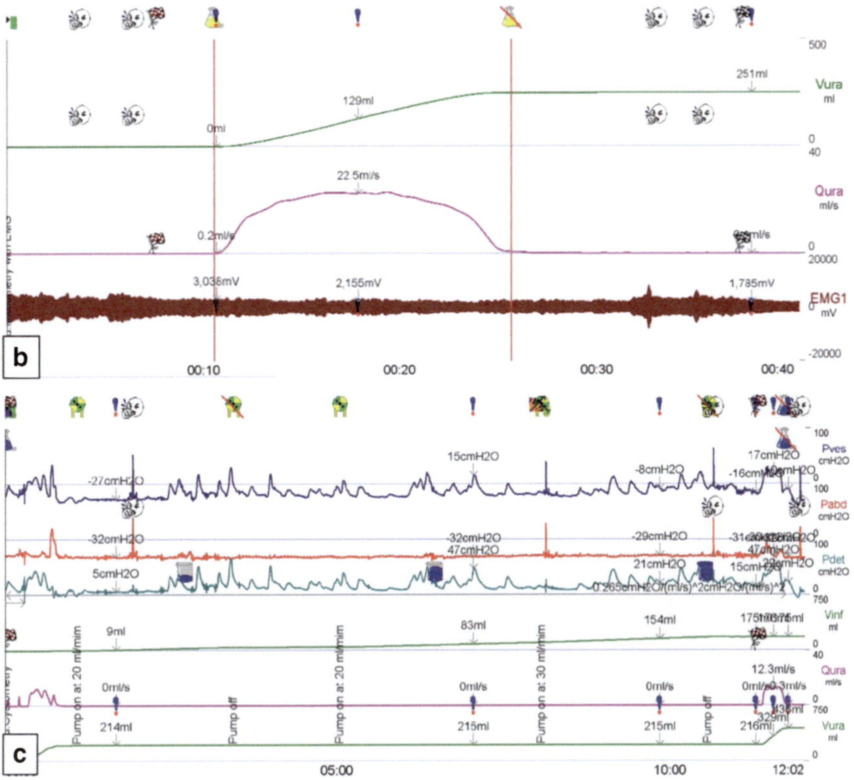

Fig. 16.2 (continued)

Voiding diary revealed 8–10 voids per day with usual voided volumes of 150–220 ml which was appropriate for her age.

Uroflowmetry revealed a normal bell-shaped curve with good flow rates but some increase in EMG activity during voiding (Fig. 16.2b).

UDS was performed after proper management of constipation to rule out any bladder dysfunction. UDS revealed severe detrusor overactivity during filling with normal voiding parameters (Fig. 16.2c). So this patient had detrusor overactivity which was not apparent in any of the other investigations. She requires stabilisation of bladder before correction of reflux.

Case 3: Gross VUR with DO

A 3-year-old female child presented with recurrent episodes of febrile UTI since the age of 6 months with poor weight gain and failure to thrive. Her voiding history and continence was appropriate for age with no enuresis. USG revealed bilateral mild HDN with bilateral ureteric dilatation but normal bladder.

MCU revealed bilateral gross VUR with significant dilatation of upper tracts with normal-looking bladder (Fig. 16.3a).

Uroflowmetry revealed a bell-shaped curve with normal flow rates and voided volume (Fig. 16.3b).

UDS revealed severe detrusor overactivity during filling phase with normal voiding pressure and flow rates (Fig. 16.3c). In spite of gross bilateral VUR, UDS revealed severe detrusor overactivity which suggests significant detrusor dysfunction. Managing the VUR without addressing the DO may result in recurrence of VUR.

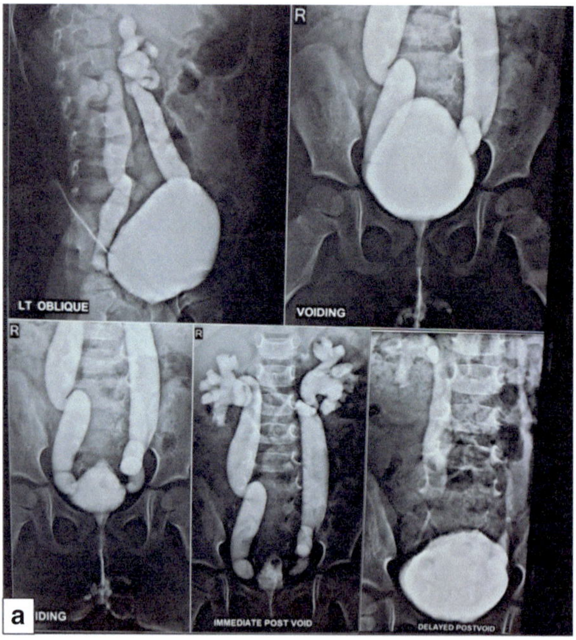

Fig. 16.3 (**a**) MCU revealed bilateral gross VUR with significant dilatation of upper tracts with normal looking bladder. (**b**) Uroflowmetry revealed a bell-shaped curve with normal flow rates and voided volume. (**c**) UDS revealed severe detrusor overactivity during filling phase with normal voiding pressure and flow rates. She reported urge to void at around 90 ml fill

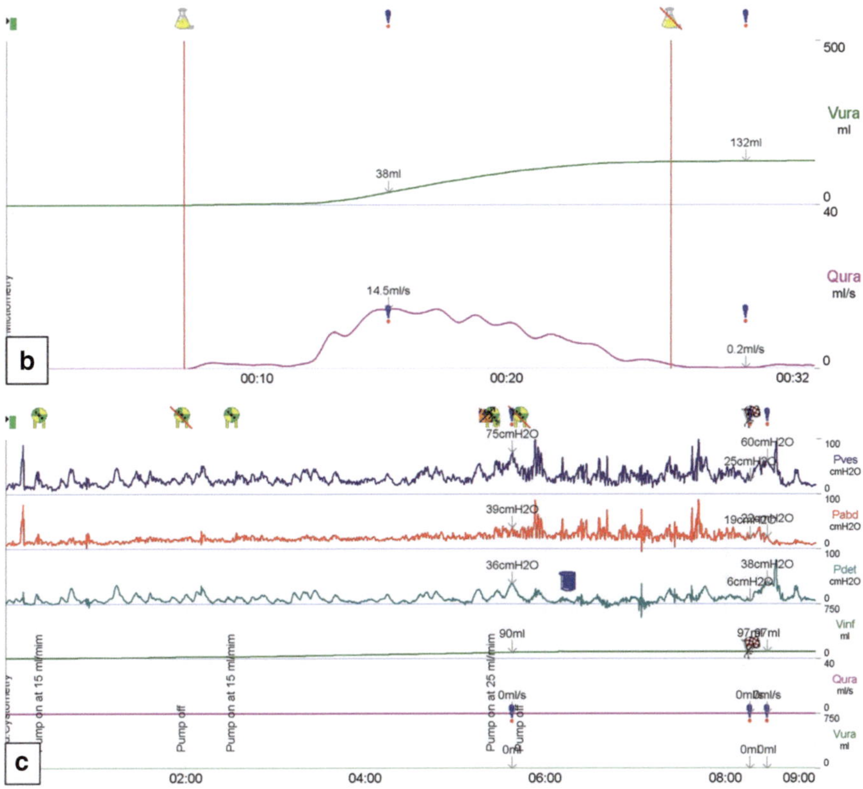

Fig. 16.3 (continued)

Case 4: VUR with BOO

A 6.5-year-old male child, FUC of PUV, had undergone fulguration at 4 months of age and circumcision after 3 months. He had h/o straining while passing urine before the surgery which improved after the surgery. He presently passed urine in good stream and had no wetness of pants during the day. He had wetness of pants at night. USG showed right Gr I HDN, left Gr III HDUN and thickened trabeculated UB wall with significant PVR.

MCU (Fig. 16.4a) showed prominent bladder neck with narrowing in region of PUV with right Gr IV VUR, but there was not much dilatation of the upper tracts.

Uroflowmetry (Fig. 16.4b) showed suboptimal flow rates with a plateau-shaped curve.

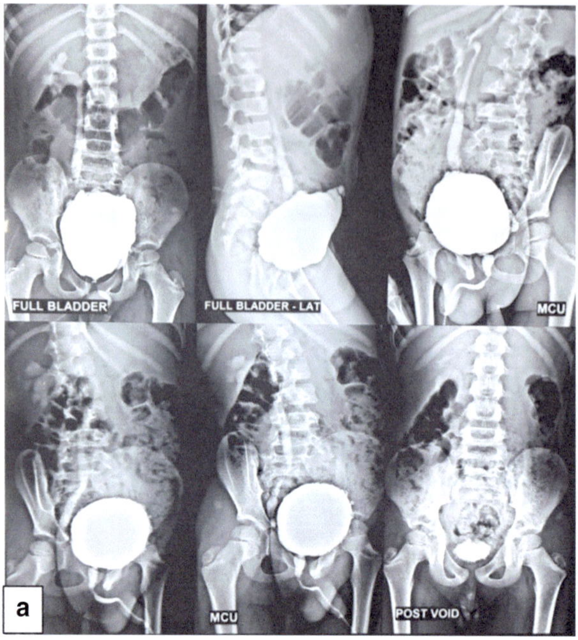

Fig. 16.4 (**a**) MCU showed prominent bladder neck with narrowing in region of PUV with right Gr IV VUR, but there was not much dilatation of the upper tracts. (**b**) Uroflowmetry showed sub-optimal flow rates with a plateau shaped curve. (**c**) UDS (full study) showed mild overactivity in the filling phase with mildly reduced compliance (14 cm H2O at 140ml). (**d**) Voiding phase of the UDS (in an expanded form) showed very high voiding pressures with very poor flow rates (4.6ml/sec at 70 cm H2O), suggestive of BOO

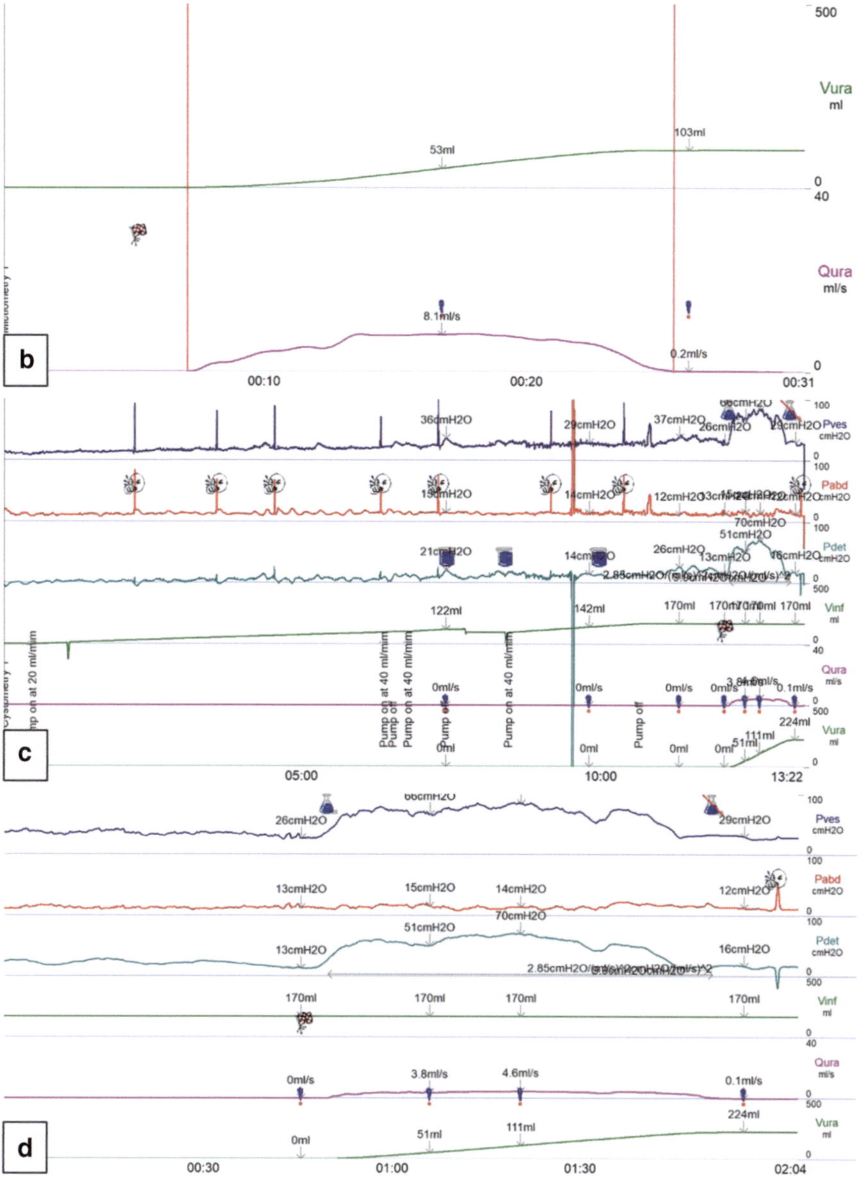

Fig. 16.4 (continued)

UDS showed mild overactivity in the filling phase (Fig. 16.4c) with mildly reduced compliance. Voiding phase showed very high voiding pressures with very poor flow rates suggestive of BOO (Fig. 16.4d). Corroborating the MCU and UDS findings, in this child, persistent BOO may be caused by bladder neck hypertrophy or residual valves.

Findings of abnormal bladder dynamics in the presence of VUR indicated actual bladder dysfunction.

Case 5: Gross VUR with BOO

A 4.7-year-old male child, had been diagnosed as a case of bilateral gross VUR with recurrent UTI in infancy, was detected as having PUV on cystoscopy and underwent fulguration of valves in infancy. The child was lost to follow up after the surgery. He had been well in between with no episodes of UTI. At 4.7 years age, the child had persistent relatively poor urinary stream with enuresis. USG revealed normal bladder with bilateral mild to moderate HDUN.

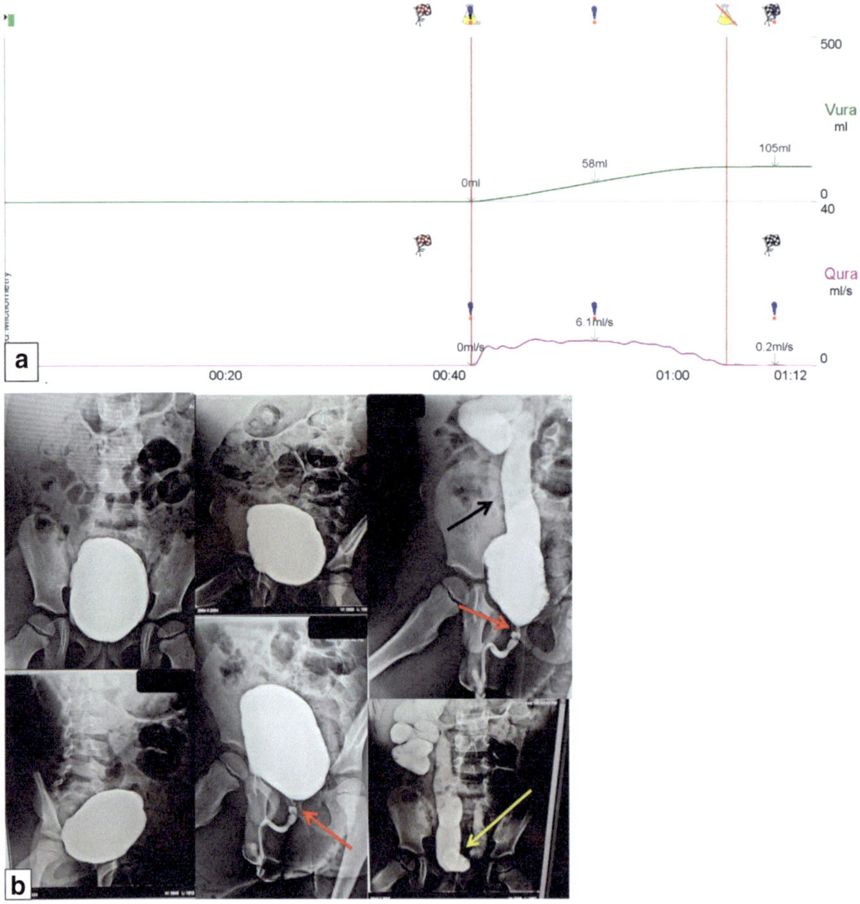

Fig. 16.5 (**a**) Uroflowmetry showed a poor stream with suboptimal flow rates (105 ml at 6 ml/sec) generating a plateau-shaped curve. (**b**) MCU showed normal-looking bladder with left gross VUR only during voiding (black arrow), very poor opening of bladder neck (red arrow), normal appearance of urethra and complete emptying of bladder at the end of the void (yellow arrow). (**c**) UDS (full study) revealed a normal capacity bladder (178ml) with mild overactivity after 50 ml fill. The study shows a voiding detrusor contraction at the end but flow is not recorded as the study is performed in supine position (**d**) Voiding phase of another cycle of UDS performed in sitting position reveals very poor flow rates with the voiding pressures being very high (4.7ml/sec at 80 cm H2O), suggestive of BOO

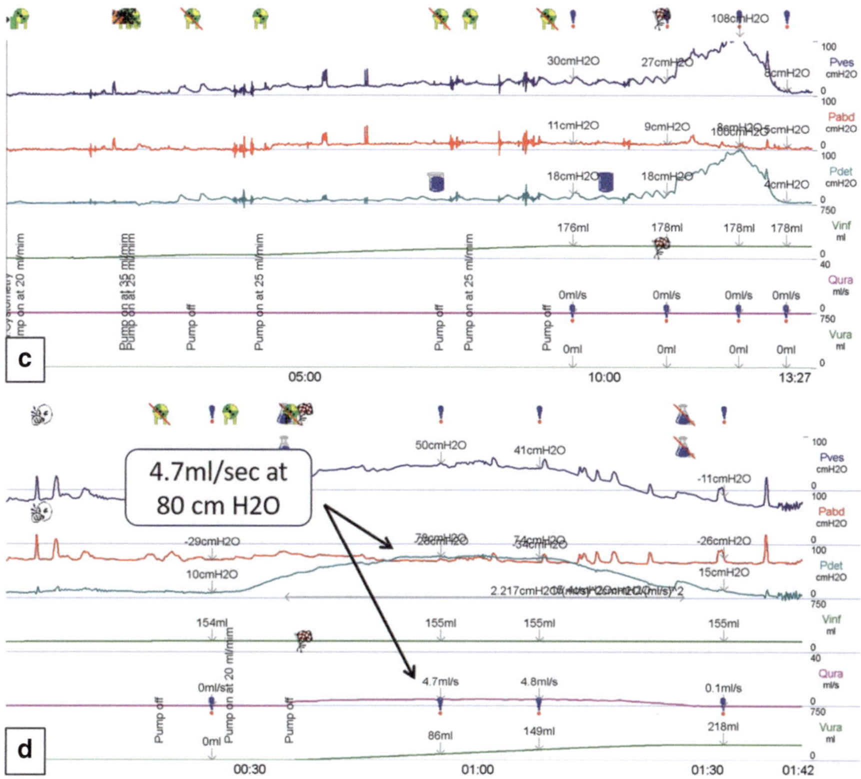

Fig. 16.5 (continued)

Uroflowmetry showed a poor stream with suboptimal flow rates (105 ml at 6 ml/sec) generating a plateau-shaped curve (Fig. 16.5a).

MCU was done to rule out any residual urethral obstruction. MCU (Fig. 16.5b) showed normal-looking bladder with left gross VUR only during voiding (black arrow), very poor opening of bladder neck (red arrow), normal appearance of urethra and complete emptying of bladder at the end of the void (yellow arrow).

UDS was performed to assess the bladder behaviour. UDS revealed a normal capacity bladder with mild overactivity after 50 ml fill (Fig. 16.5c). During voiding, the flow rate was very poor with the voiding pressures being very high (Fig. 16.5d) suggestive of BOO. In the presence of such high-grade VUR during voiding, we would expect to have underestimation of voiding detrusor pressures. Presence of high-pressure voiding in the face of such high-grade VUR shows that there is significant element of BOO—the reflux observed during voiding may in fact be secondary to the BOO. MCU appearance of bladder along with UDS finding of BOO suggests probable bladder neck dysfunction as the cause of BOO.

Case 6: Gross VUR with Poor Compliance

A 7-year-old male child, follow-up case of high type of anorectal malformation with presacral mass, underwent staged repair of ARM and presacral mass excision. All stages were completed by the age of 4 years. He had history of continuous dribbling of urine, urgency and urge incontinence and passed 40–50 ml urine voluntarily when prompted to. He did not have any episodes of UTI.

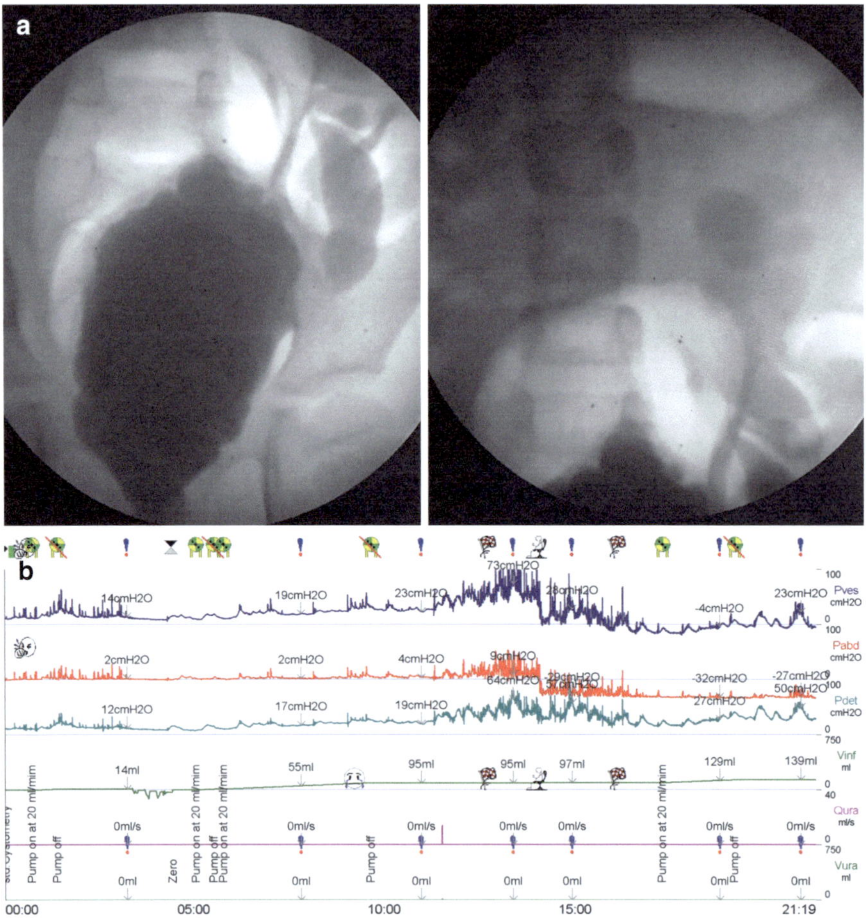

Fig. 16.6 (**a**) MCU showed an elongated bladder with grossly irregular outline suggestive of neurogenic bladder with gross left-sided VUR. (**b**) UDS was performed in supine position during initial part of the study. Filling is stopped at around 95 ml as the patient reported suprapubic pain (as marked by 'cry' sign). He is asked to void in supine position (red chequered flag). When he is not able to void, he is made to sit up ('sitting' sign) and voiding command is given again (red chequered flag). When he attempts to void only valsalva manoeuvre is seen (evidenced by increased deflections in both rectal and vesical tracings), overactivity is seen to increase but no flow is recorded. Pump is started again to check whether he can void at larger bladder volumes. Pump is turned off as detrusor overactivity and detrusor pressures increase

USG KUB showed thick-walled trabeculated bladder with significant PVR, left partial duplication with HDUN and right normal kidney.

MCU (Fig. 16.6a) showed an elongated bladder with grossly irregular outline suggestive of neurogenic bladder with gross left-sided VUR. Funnelling of the bladder neck was seen during filling, but it was not seen to open up during attempted voiding. Patient could not void during the study.

UDS (Fig. 16.6b) was performed in supine position during initial part of the study. When the bladder was full, he was asked to pass urine. When he could not pass urine, he was made to sit up ('sitting' sign on UD tracing, marked by black arrow) and the rest of the study was performed in sitting position. The study showed a small capacity bladder (130 ml) with reduced compliance (19 cm H_2O at 90 ml) and mild overactivity. When the patient was asked to void, he could not void during the study; on attempted void, only Valsalva manoeuvre was seen. No detrusor contraction was noted.

Case 7: Gross VUR with Unreliable UDS Findings

A 12-year-old male child, follow-up case of LSMMC repair in infancy, presented with neurogenic bladder-bowel and difficulty in passing urine with recurrent UTIs. He had been started on CIC at the age of 9 years. On CIC, he had been dry with no leaks in between CICs and no UTIs. USG showed bilateral gross HDUN with thinning of parenchyma and creatinine was 1.2 mg%.

MCU showed bilateral gross VUR with bladder appearing to be small (Fig. 16.7a).

UDS showed a normal capacity stable bladder (Fig. 16.7b).

Due to severity of VUR, finding of stable bladder on UDS was not reliable and a video-UDS was performed. During video-UDS, it was noted that the bladder did not expand in size after 100 ml fill and all the instilled contrast got accommodated in the dilated upper tracts (Fig. 16.7c), thus making the finding of 'stable' bladder unreliable.

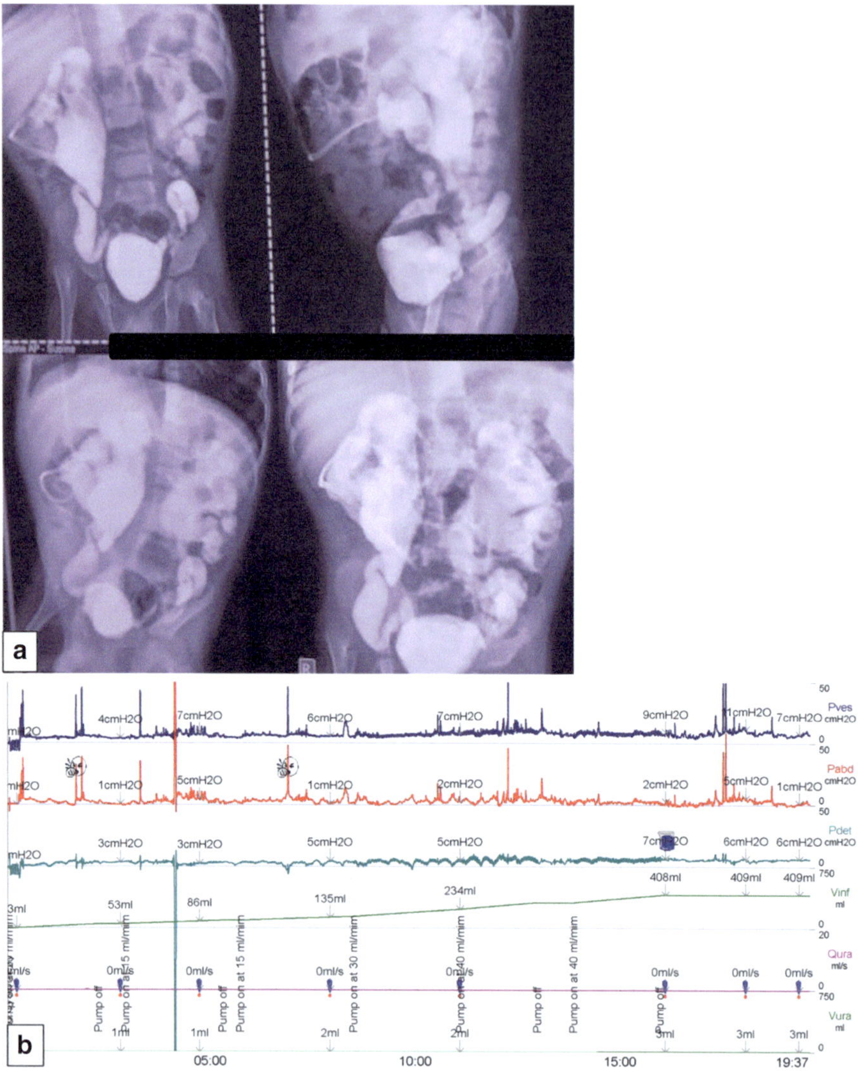

Fig. 16.7 (**a**) MCU showed bilateral gross VUR with bladder appearing to be small. (**b**) UDS showed a normal capacity stable bladder-detrusor pressure of 7 cm H2O at 400 ml when he reported urge to pass urine. (**c**) During video-UDS, it was noted that the bladder did not expand in size after 100 ml fill, and all the instilled contrast got accommodated in the dilated upper tracts

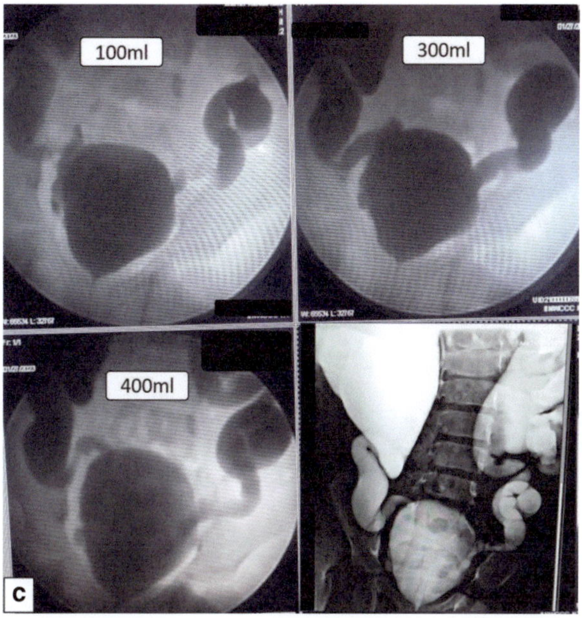

Fig. 16.7 (continued)

Declarations

Competing Interests The author(s) has no competing interests to declare that are relevant to the content of this manuscript.

Ethics Approval The author(s) declares that this manuscript does not include primary research with human participants.

The author(s) declares that this manuscript does not include primary studies involving animals.

Suggested Reading

1. Altobelli E, Buscarini M, Nappo SG, Nguyen HT, Caione P. Urodynamics investigation on children with vesicoureteral reflux identifies overactive bladder and poor compliance in those with voiding dysfunction. Pediatr Surg Int. 2011;27(5):517–22. https://doi.org/10.1007/s00383-010-2822-z.
2. Batinic D, Miloševic D, Topalovic-Grkovic M, Nizic L, Vrljicak K, Batinic D, Turudic D. Vesicoureteral reflux and urodynamic dysfunction. Urol Int. 2013;90(4):480–3. https://doi.org/10.1159/000345713. Epub 2012 Dec 22.
3. Chandra M, Maddix H. Urodynamic dysfunction in infants with vesicoureteral reflux. J Pediatr. 2000;136(6):754–9.
4. Izquierdo RM, Luque Mialdea R. Valoración de la función del tracto urinario inferior en el paciente pediátrico portador de reflujo vesicoureteral primario [Evaluation of the lower urinary tract function in pediatric patients with primary vesicoureteral reflux]. Arch Esp Urol. 2008;61(2):191–207. Spanish.

5. Podesta ML, Castera R, Ruarte AC. Videourodynamic findings in young infants with severe primary reflux. J Urol. 2004;171(2 Pt 1):829–33; discussion 833. https://doi.org/10.1097/01.ju.0000108126.23417.17.
6. Sharifiaghdas F, Narouie B, Mirzakhanlouei A, Ahmadzade M, Rouientan H, Dadpour M. Evaluation of the results of urodynamic studies in patients with vesicoureteral reflux. Urologia. 2024;91(1):183–8. https://doi.org/10.1177/03915603231198556. Epub 2023 Sep 26.
7. Sillén U, Hellström AL, Hermanson G, Abrahamson K. Comparison of urodynamic and free voiding pattern in infants with dilating reflux. J Urol. 1999;161(6):1928–33.
8. Sjöström S, Bachelard M, Sixt R, Sillén U. Change of urodynamic patterns in infants with dilating vesicoureteral reflux: 3-year followup. J Urol. 2009;182(5):2446–53. https://doi.org/10.1016/j.juro.2009.07.057. Epub 2009 Sep 17.

i-UDS in Neurogenic Bladder

17

Poonam Guha Vaze

Neurogenic bladder (NB) can be caused due to abnormal neural innervation of the bladder at any point from the cerebral cortex to the level of peripheral nerves in the pelvis which can manifest as a wide spectrum of abnormal bladder behaviour.

The common causes of NB in children are as follows:

1. Spina bifida
2. Tethered cord
3. Anorectal malformation
4. Cerebral palsy
5. Post pelvic surgery like sacrococcygeal teratoma
6. Sequelae of transverse myelitis

Of these causes, the most commonly encountered scenario is of spina bifida where there is lower motor neuron bladder with varied severity depending on the degree of bladder denervation.

There are several classifications of bladder dysfunction in NB, discussion of which is outside the purview of this book.

P. G. Vaze (✉)
Neotia Bhagirathi Woman and Child Care Centre, Newtown, Kolkata, India

Department of Pediatric Surgery, Nilratan Sircar Medical College and Hospital, Kolkata, India

S. Saha, P. Guha Vaze (eds.), *Comprehensive Atlas of Practical Pediatric Urodynamics*, https://doi.org/10.1007/978-981-95-2709-0_17

Aims of Performing *i*-UDS in Children with NB

Performing *i*-UDS in children with NB is intended to further the general aim of

- Safeguarding the upper tracts
- Keeping the child dry/socially continent

Each child with NB has a different bladder behaviour due to the varied aetiology as well as completeness of the neural insult. So the management options for each child have to be planned individually after proper characterisation of the bladder dysfunction. Figure 17.1 mentions the basic clinical questions that need to be answered when managing a child with NB, the information obtained from a well-performed *i*-UDS and its usefulness in guiding management.

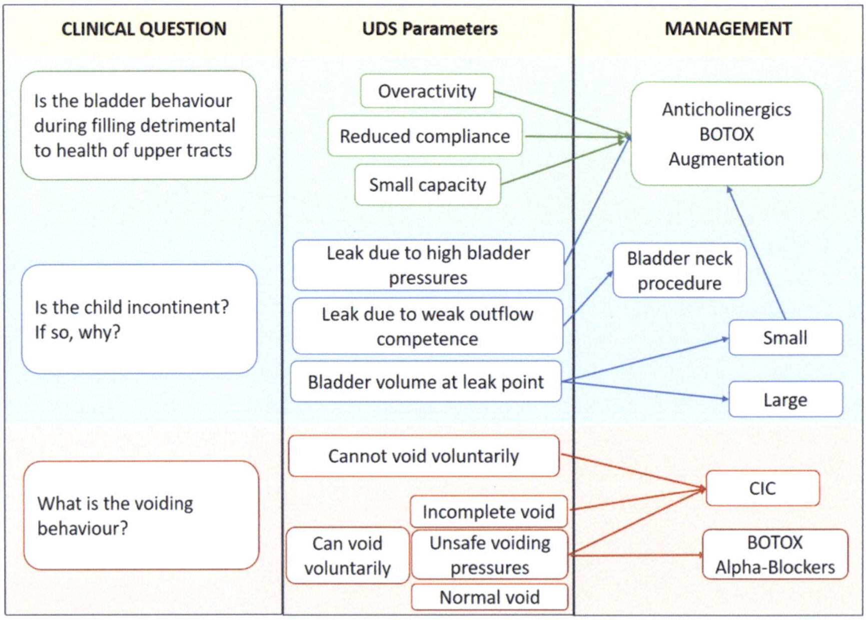

Fig. 17.1 Basic clinical questions in children with NB, their explanations from UDS and further management

Challenges in Performing *i*-UDS in Children with NB

1. *Positioning*—Children may have neurological deficit of the lower limb and contractures of the hip where positioning of the child may become difficult. If possible, the test should be done in sitting position so that the voided/leaked volume can be documented. If needed, the study may be performed in the supine position with a recording of the points of leak and approximate volume of leak by means of appropriate annotations.
2. *Urinary leakage*—Many children with neurogenic bladder may have weak bladder outflow. The infused fluid starts leaking out shortly after filling is started. In such children, it may be necessary to occlude the urethra to allow bladder filling to proceed so that the storage parameters can be assessed. If urethra is occluded during the study, filling has to be stopped if there is significant overactivity, persistent rise of pressure (> 20–40 cm H_2O) or if the child shows features of discomfort or pain. In boys, it is possible to occlude the urethra by compressing the penis. In girls, it is difficult. The urethral meatus may be occluded by digital pressure if the child has non-sensate perineum, or Foley's balloon inflation by the side of the double-lumen catheter may be attempted (but it usually results in peri-catheter leak of urine).
3. *Difficult catheterisation*—In a few children, the sphincter may be very overactive and obstruct the passage of catheter. Instilling lubricating jelly liberally and patiently waiting for a give-way to appear at the point of resistance usually solve the problem.
4. *Urethral sensation*—Most children with neurogenic bladder due to spina bifida have a non-sensate urethra. But children with other aetiologies of NB may have sensate urethra (e.g., transverse myelitis). Children with sacral agenesis tend to have hypersenstitive urethras and may not allow catheterisation/CIC.

Points to Be Noted in the *i*-UDS in NB

Properly performed *i*-UDS study gives a complete insight into bladder function and guides management plan accordingly.

While performing a urodynamic study in a child with NB, we should have definite questions which we want the *i*-UDS study to answer:

1. *What are the filling phase parameters?*

   (a) *Capacity*

   Filling is stopped if there is significant leak, baseline detrusor pressure is >40 cm H_2O, child complains of discomfort/pain or usual CIC volumes/EBC is reached.

   Small capacity bladder needs bladder relaxants (anticholinergics or beta-3 receptor agonists)/Botox/augmentation cystoplasty sequentially depending on the degree of fibrosis in the bladder and response to interven-

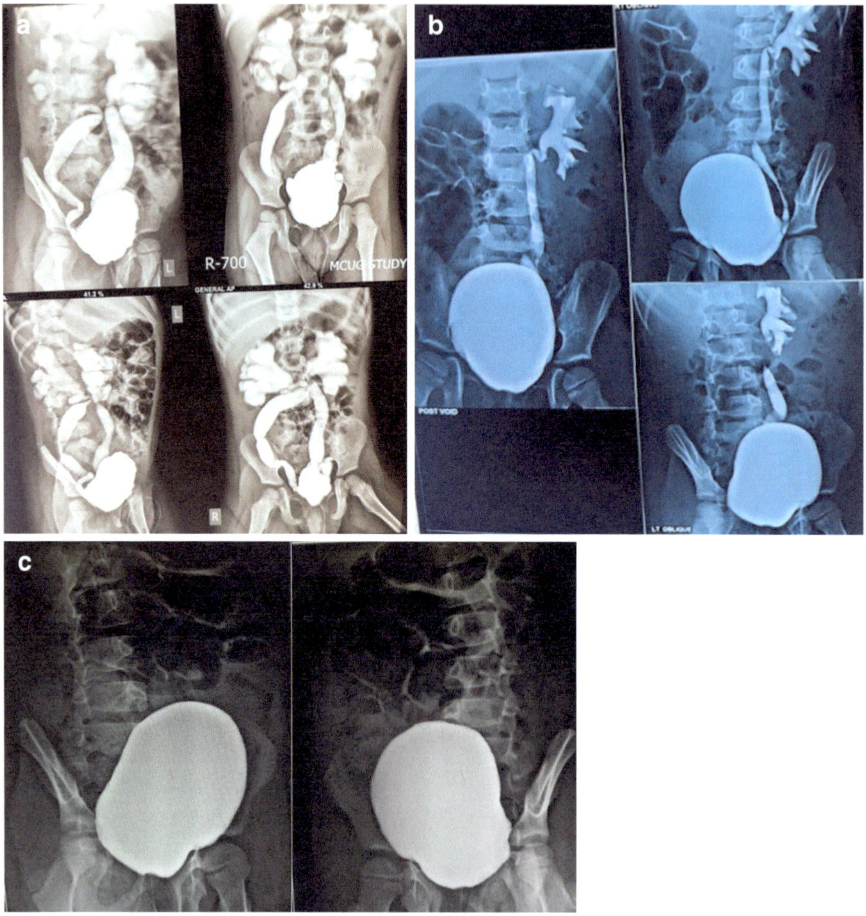

Fig. 17.2 (**a**–**c**) Sequential MCUs in a child with history of LSMMC showing initial small bladder with bilateral Gr V VUR (**a**) which later improves to a normal-looking bladder with no VUR when the bladder pressures and capacity are normalised after appropriate anticholinergic therapy (**b**, **c**)

tion. As the bladder capacity improves, bladder and upper tract changes tend to improve (Figs. 17.2 and 17.3a, b).

The aim should be to achieve a bladder capacity so that CIC may be performed every 3–4 hourly during the day. Small bladder volumes would necessitate night-time catheter drainage.

(b) *Compliance*

NB may often show poor compliance. Classically, end fill detrusor pressures of >40 cm H_2O has been said to be detrimental to upper tracts. It has been later documented in animal and human studies that detrusor pressure of >20 cm H_2O has higher sensitivity in predicting upper tract changes. Our

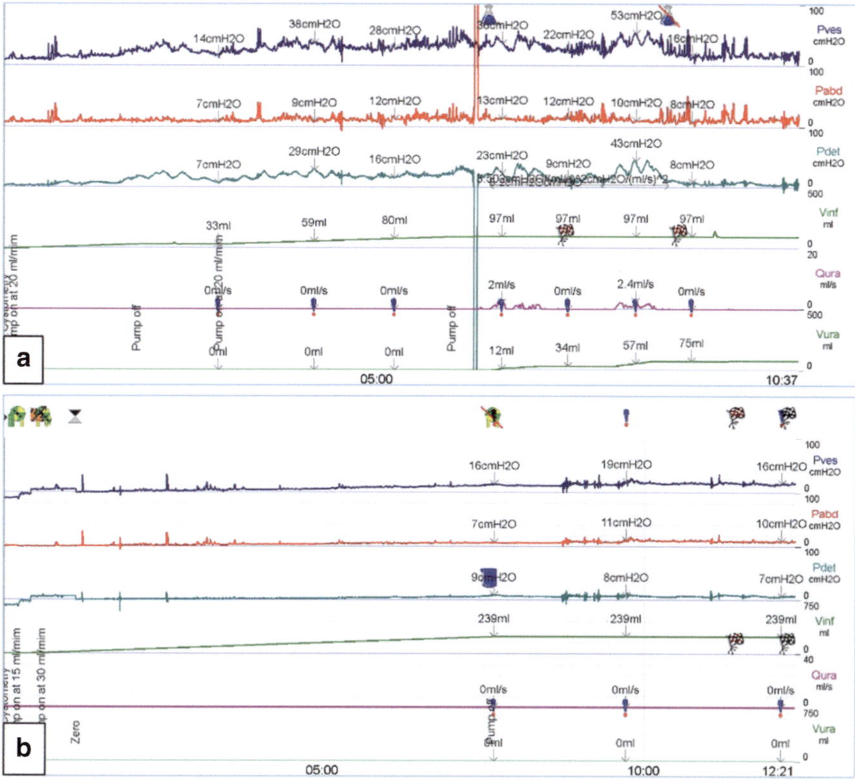

Fig. 17.3 (**a**, **b**) A 3-year-old girl (same patient as in Fig. 17.2), known case of LSMMC operated at neonatal age, presented with continuous urinary dribbling and recurrent UTI. USG showed bilateral HDUN with thick-walled UB. MCU showed bilateral Gr V VUR. Initial UDS (**a**) performed at 3 years of age showed a small capacity bladder with significant overactivity and reduced compliance. She was started on anticholinergics and CIC and CIC volumes were monitored. Doses of anticholinergics were modified accordingly. After 3 years follow-up, her UDS (**b**) revealed a stable bladder with normal capacity. Clinically, she was dry with no UTIs in the last 3 years and MCU showed resolution of reflux

current practice is to try to reduce end fill pressures to <10–15 cm H_2O. We have observed that upper tract changes reverse and even gross reflux disappears (Figs. 17.4 and 17.5) and the incidence of UTIs decreases if detrusor pressure can be lowered to this level. If baseline bladder pressure is high, night-time catheter drainage of bladder is required.

Many patients have high-pressure bladder although the capacity is normal. These patients also need anticholinergics to manage their bladder pressures in spite of the capacity being normal (Fig. 17.6a and b).

When we talk about safe bladder pressures, we aim to achieve safe pressures at the usual CIC volumes of the child and not the EBC volume. As the frequency of bladder emptying is determined by frequency of CIC and not

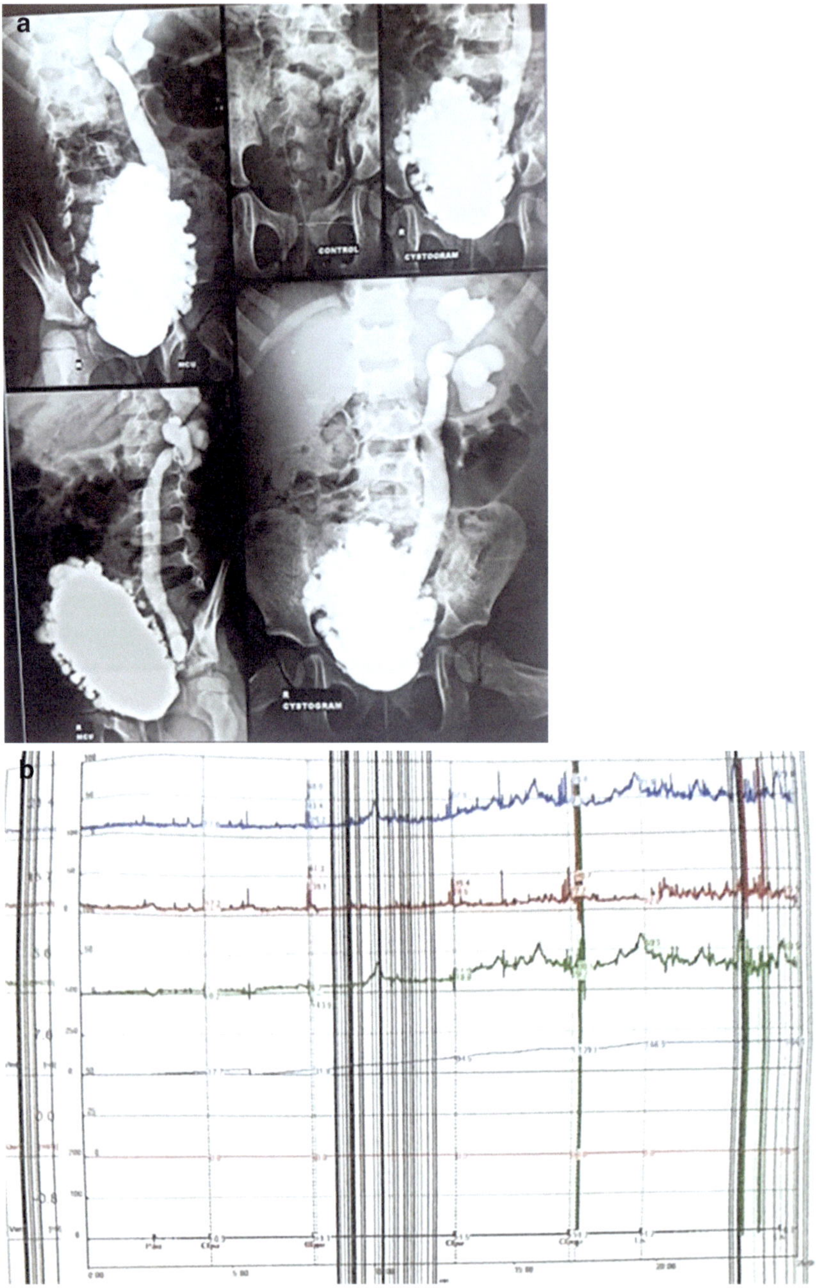

Fig. 17.4 (**a–d**) A 6-year-old girl with NB with urinary incontinence and recurrent UTI. MCU (**a**) showed bilateral grade 5 VUR with trabeculated bladder wall and diverticuli. UDS (**b**) showed a normal capacity bladder, but there was significant overactivity and significantly reduced compliance. She was started on anticholinergics and CIC. At 2 years follow-up, MCU (**c**) shows improvement in bladder appearance and absence of reflux. UDS (**d**) shows stable good/large capacity bladder with normal compliance

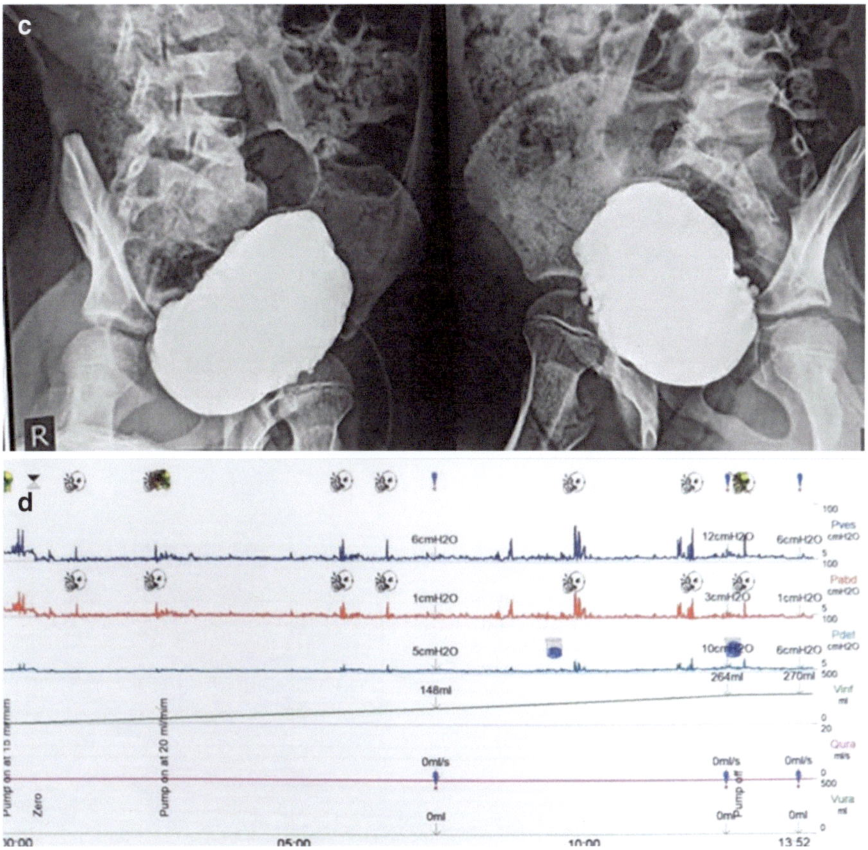

Fig. 17.4 (continued)

the sense of bladder fullness, any excess fluid intake results in bladder overdistension and the CIC volumes often exceed the calculated EBC. Thus, we should promote the maintenance of CIC diaries and aim to have end fill detrusor pressures of <10–20 cm H_2O at those volumes (Fig. 17.7).

(c) *Overactivity*

Overactivity is a common finding in patients with NB which may or may not have associated urgency/pain. We have observed that patients with even mild overactivity may present with recurrent UTIs which improve after addition of anticholinergics.

Many patients demonstrate leak in the presence of DO—detrusor overactivity-associated leak. In such cases, once medical management is initiated, we monitor the frequency of leak in between CICs which is an indirect indicator of persistence of overactivity. Absence of leak signifies that detrusor pressure is constantly below the pressure at which overactivity-associated leak manifests.

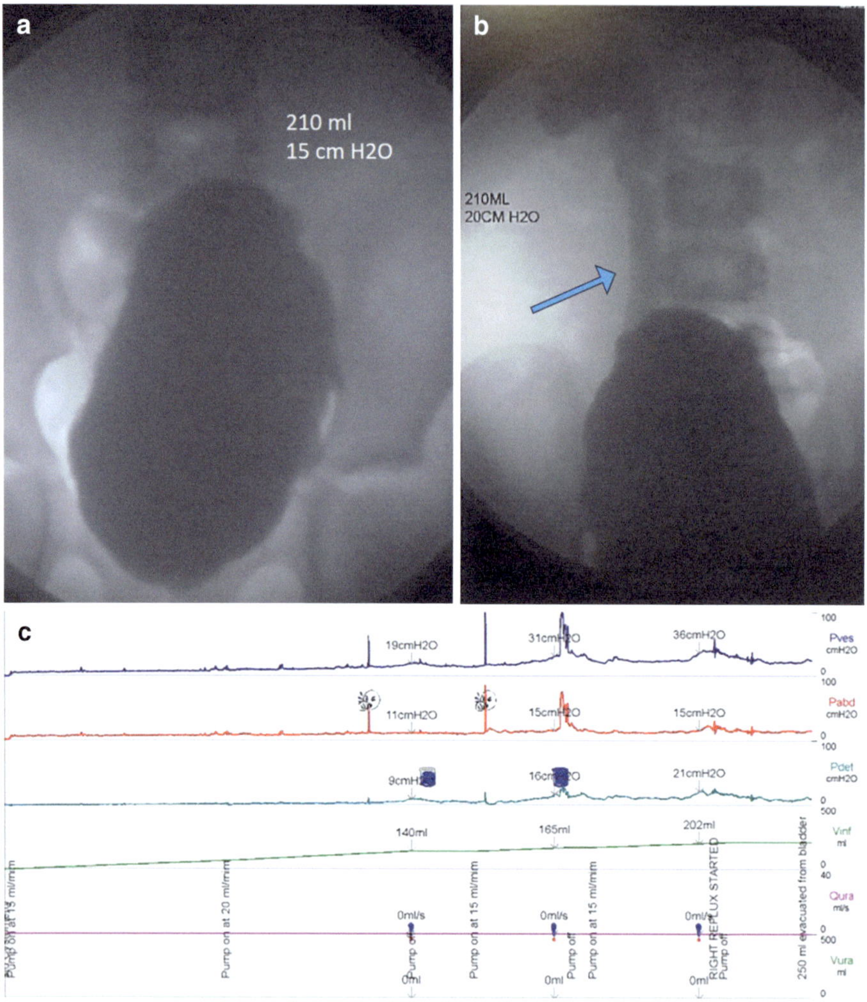

Fig. 17.5 (**a**–**c**) An 8-year-old girl, known case of LSMMC, on CIC and anticholinergics. These are images procured during video-UDS. It shows that at fill volume of 200 ml, there is no reflux when the detrusor pressure is 15 cm H_2O (**a**). Reflux is seen to appear as soon as the detrusor pressure crosses 20 cm H_2O during an episode of IDC (**b**, **c**) at the same volume. So if the detrusor pressure can be maintained under 20 cm H_2O by the use of anticholinergics, reflux can be ameliorated

(d) *Leak*

As one of the main aims of managing an NB patient is to keep him/her dry to achieve social continence, it is important to stop urinary incontinence. The cause of leak has to be identified so that it can be ameliorated.

During the *i*-UDS, we need to identify the point when leak occurs and note any event (straining/detrusor overactivity) and the detrusor/abdominal pressures at that point.

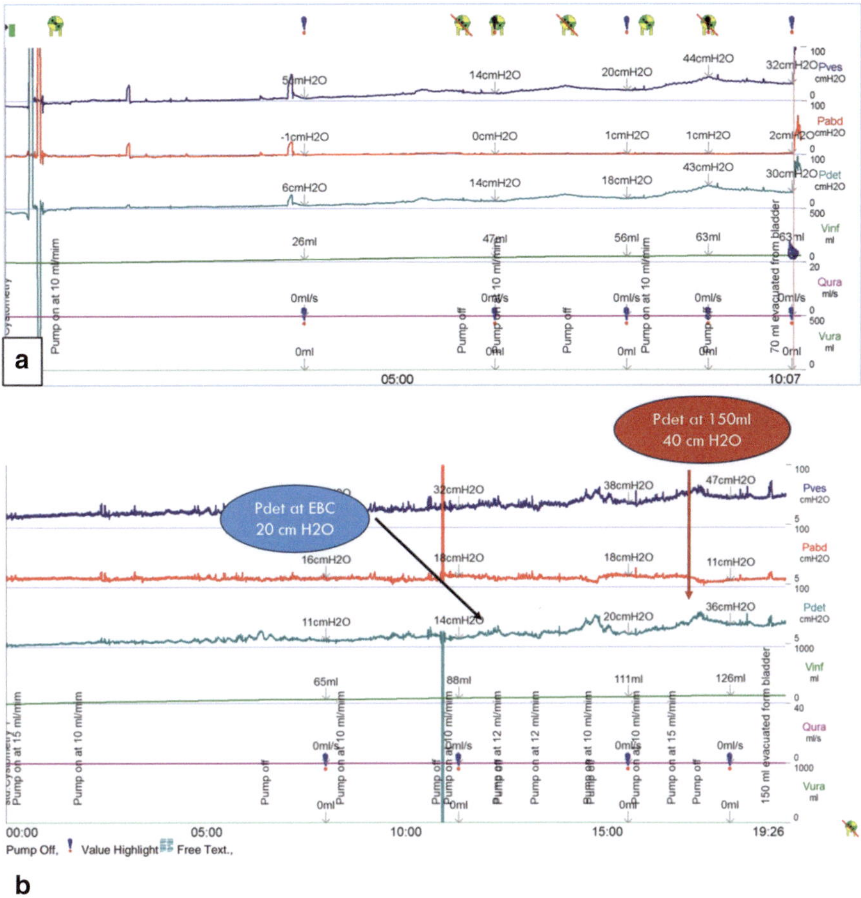

Fig. 17.6 (**a** and **b**) An 8-month-old girl, LSMMC, operated in neonatal period, had history of excessive crying during micturition with passage of small amounts of urine. USG KUB was normal. MCU showed mildly elongated bladder with no VUR. UDS tracing (**a**) shows a normal capacity bladder (60 ml; EBC 40 ml), but the bladder pressures were very high—above 40 cm H_2O at 60 ml. So although the bladder capacity was normal, she was at high risk of upper tact damage and needed anticholinergics to stabilise the bladder pressures. UDS at 2 years of age (**b**) shows that the bladder pressure at EBC (90 ml) is at acceptable range whereas it increases to ~40 cm H_2O pressure at ~120 ml (150% EBC) and places the upper tracts at risk at higher bladder volumes

(i) *DLPP*—Leak can be seen spontaneously in the absence of any detrusor overactivity or rise in abdominal pressure. The detrusor pressure at which this leak occurs is known as detrusor leak point pressure (DLPP). DLPP >40 cm H_2O is classically thought to represent high-risk bladder. If leak is seen at low detrusor pressures of 10–20 cm H_2O, it may signify weak bladder outlet (Fig. 17.8).

(ii) *ALPP*—Leak occurring with rise in abdominal pressure, otherwise known as stress incontinence, usually suggests weak bladder outflow.

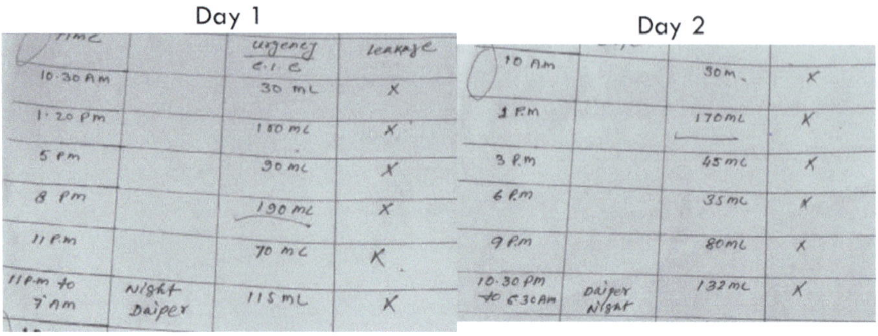

Fig. 17.7 CIC diary of the child in Fig. 17.6 shows CIC volumes to be much higher than the EBC (90 ml at 2 years of age) several times during the day. The bladder pressures would be expected to be dangerously high during these periods

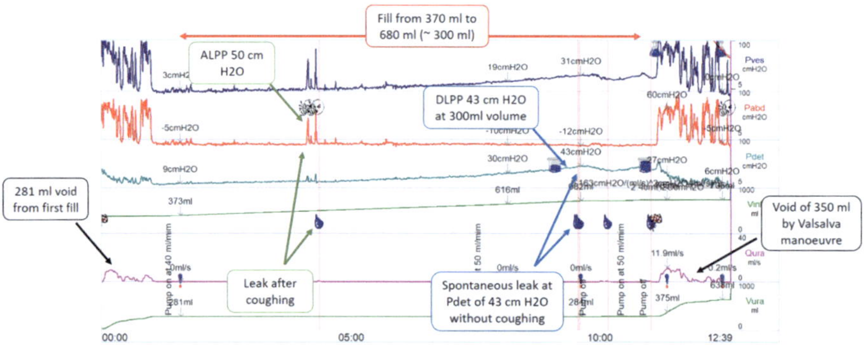

Fig. 17.8 *DLPP and ALPP*. A 16-year-old boy was a follow-up case of lumbar MMC. He was on CIC 4 times a day and had average CIC volumes of 400–500 ml. He started leaking urine 1–2 hours after CIC whenever he performed any activity and needed diapers. He could pass around 250 ml urine by straining. He had history of recurrent episodes of UTI. Investigations revealed thick-walled UB with bilateral HDN and left grade V VUR with poorly functioning kidney. During the UDS, two studies were done in tandem. Early part of the curve shows part of the first void (281 ml urine was voided after 370 ml fill [black arrow]). Rest of the tracing shows filling phase from 370 ml to 670 ml fill (red arrow). Detrusor pressures are seen to increase to 40 cm H_2O at 600 ml fill (i.e., 300 ml capacity) which implies a poorly compliant bladder. He is seen to leak urine after coughing at around 200 ml fill with ALPP around 50 cm H_2O (green arrows) denoting weak bladder outlet. He is also seen to leak urine spontaneously at Pdet of around 40 cm H_2O in the absence of any IDC—DLPP 40 cm H_2O (blue arrows). Voiding command is marked by the 'red chequered flag'. He voids 280 ml of urine by Valsalva manoeuvre (black arrow on right side of image) with a PVR of 150 ml and no detrusor contraction (valsalva voiding). Thus, he has a normal capacity bladder with very high resting pressures (which explains the finding of bilateral HDN and VUR), weak bladder outlet (which is the cause of leaks during activities) and Valsalva voiding. He would benefit from the use of anticholinergics/beta-3 agonists for stabilising bladder pressures (although capacity seems to be normal) along with surgical intervention at the bladder outlet to stop the leakages. He might need CIC for bladder emptying after anticholinergics are added

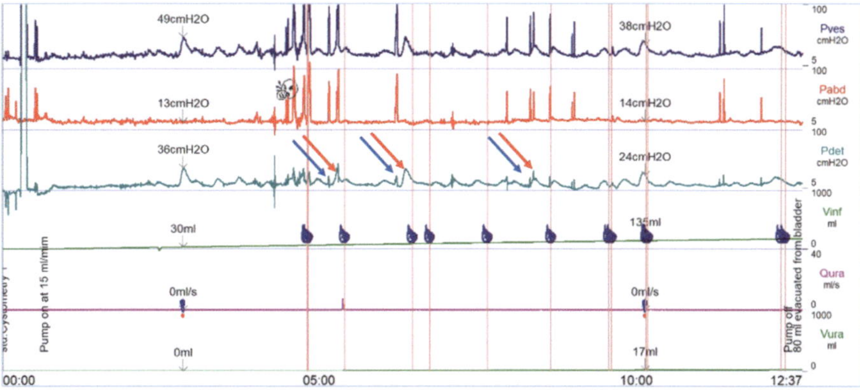

Fig. 17.9 *DO-LPP*. A 5-year-old girl, a case of lumbosacral MMC, operated in neonatal period has history of constant leak of urine with severe perineal excoriations. USG showed normal upper tracts with a thick-walled bladder. UDS showed significant overactivity—spontaneous as well as provoked—and waves of IDC (red arrow) seen immediately following cough artefact (blue arrow). She was seen to leak urine after around 50 ml fill. During the study, it was seen that she was leaking urine only during periods of IDC ('drop' sign). She was not leaking during coughing but leaked immediately after coughing when the IDC was seen. As the study was done in supine position, leaked volume could not be recorded. Compliance was normal. Out of 130 ml filled, 80 ml was evacuated at the end of the study suggesting almost 50 ml leak. She was not able to void on command. She was started on anticholinergics and 3 hourly CIC. At 1-month follow-up, she had no leaks in between CICs and was off diapers, and the excoriations had healed completely

Abdominal leak point pressure (ALPP) is the abdominal pressure at which leak is seen to appear. Patient is asked to cough intermittently, perform Valsalva manoeuvre or, more precisely, blow into an incentive spirometer with graded pressures, and the lowest abdominal pressure at which leak is seen is recorded. ALPP <50 cm H_2O suggests that the patient is going to need bladder neck procedure to keep him/her dry (Fig. 17.8).

(iii) *DO-LPP*—Leak may only be evident when an episode of DO is seen which may be a strong DO or even a weak DO reaching up to 20 cm H_2O. The detrusor pressure during overactivity when leak is seen is known as detrusor overactivity-leak point pressure (DO-LPP). These children can stop leaking by addition of anticholinergics alone (Fig. 17.9).

2. *Whether the child can void on his/her own?*

Voiding parameters can usually be identified in older children who are cooperative. In young children, *i*-UDS can give us only a rough idea of the situation which has to be confirmed by a UDS performed later when the child is older.

If the child is not able to void, CIC is required to empty the bladder.

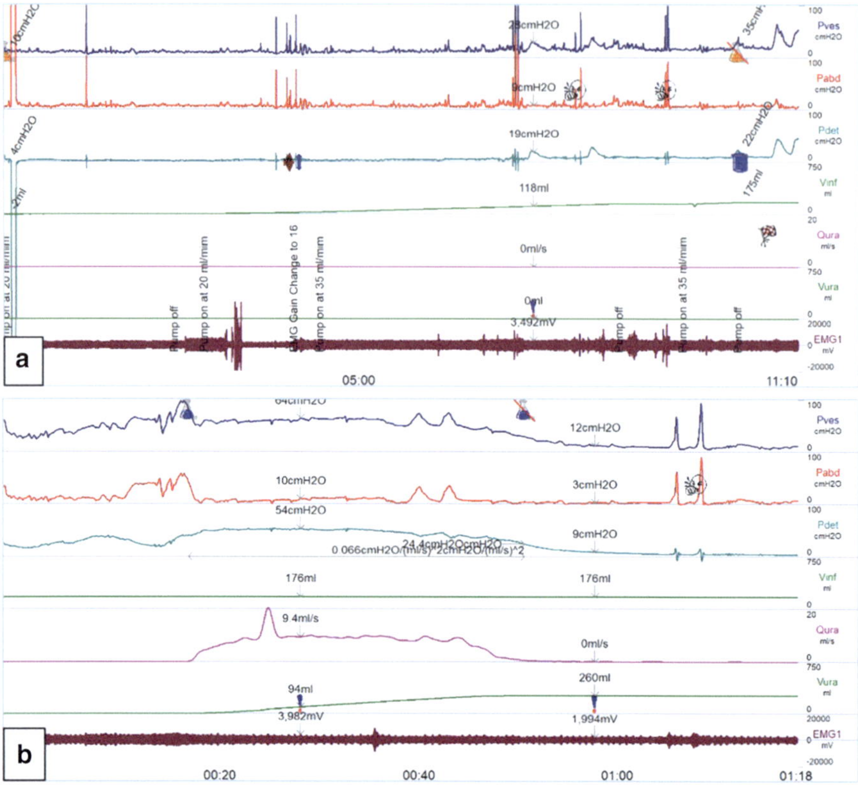

Fig. 17.10 (**a** and **b**) *Voluntary voiding contraction.* A 5-year-old male child underwent LSMMC repair at 1 day of life. He passes urine well with some increased frequency/urgency and constipation. He has no incontinence/enuresis/fecal soiling and no lower limb neurodeficit. USG shows normal upper tracts and bladder. UDS tracings show filling phase (**a**) and voiding phase (**b**) separately. Mild overactivity was noted during filling. He reported urge at 175 ml. He passed 260 ml of urine (implying large capacity bladder) by generating a good intensity, well-sustained voluntary detrusor contraction with no PVR. Voiding detrusor pressures were mildly raised which may be due to presence of catheter in the urethra. Thus, he has a large capacity bladder with mild overactivity and near-normal voiding parameters. The observed abnormalities may be caused due to element of BBD and constipation management should be the first step of therapy

If the child is able to void, it should be further investigated as follows:

(a) *How is the void occurring?*

  (i) *Voluntarily generated detrusor contraction*

    Few children with NB can void volitionally by voluntarily generating voiding detrusor contraction (and do not depend on any IDC/Valsalva for voiding). To assess this, the child is given command to void at variable bladder volumes before the onset of any detrusor overactivity contraction or after cessation of an IDC, and the resultant detrusor contraction and void is noted (Fig. 17.10a and b).

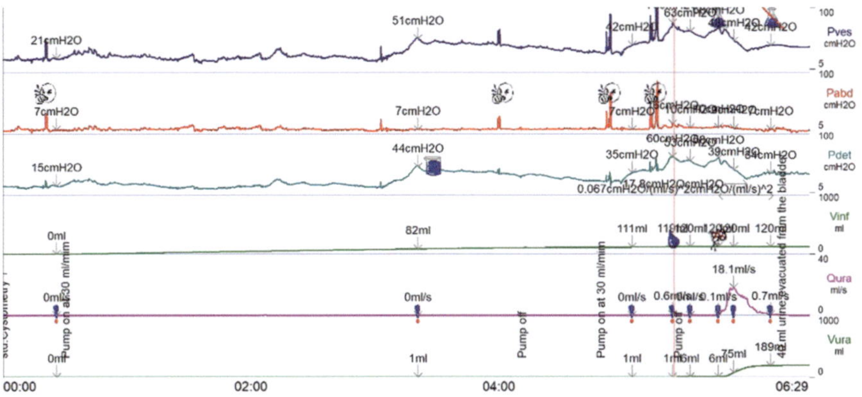

Fig. 17.11 *Spontaneous IDC-induced void.* A 12-year-old female child, NB caused by epidural cyst in region of dorsal spine, presented with recent-onset recurrent UTI. She was detected as having bilateral gross HDUN and thick-walled irregular bladder with no apparent complaints. UDS revealed severe overactivity with poor compliance. She reported urge to void during IDC when Pdet >40 cm H_2O, but she could control the urge to pass urine without any leak. She could pass urine only if she was given command to void during IDC with pressures >50–60 cm H_2O with PVR ranging from 50 to 250 ml. She could not generate any voluntary detrusor contraction if asked to void in the absence of any overactivity. She was started on beta-3 agonists along with CIC/nocturnal catheter drainage after which she improved clinically. Her urinary symptoms had been masked since childhood as she had adapted her lifestyle to her voiding needs

(ii) *IDC mediated*

(a) Spontaneous IDC (Fig. 17.11)

(b) Provoked IDC induced by certain activity or genital stimulation (Figs. 17.12 and 17.13a and b)

These children sense urge to void during an episode of detrusor overactivity and are able to pass urine when the IDC is strong enough. They usually cannot generate a detrusor contraction of their own will. These children have urgency and frequent urge-associated leaks in the early period. As they grow older, they are able to control the leaks to some extent and tend to adjust their daily activities to such an extent that the voiding abnormality may not be perceived by the parents at all. These children typically have thick-walled UB on USG and are predisposed to recurrent episodes of UTIs.

(iii) *Valsalva/Crede's* (Fig. 17.14)

These children have visible straining while passing urine, a poor flow rate and variable PVR. The fact that voiding is possible through Valsalva also implies that urine is able to leak out with increased abdominal pressures. So these patients also have significant degree of outflow incompetence and stress incontinence and may need blader neck procedures to keep them dry. The lower the PVR after Valsalva void, the weaker is the outflow competence. It is important to differen-

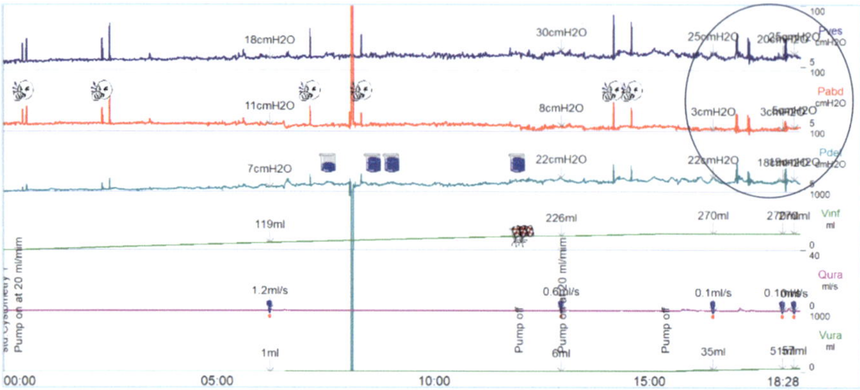

Fig. 17.12 *Provoked/reflex IDC-induced void.* A 10-year-old girl, follow-up case of lumbar lipo-MMC with some foot deformity. USG shows thick-walled bladder with significant PVR with solitary right kidney without any hydronephrosis. She feels the urge to pass urine every 1–2 hours and usually leaks small amounts before reaching the washroom; after reaching the washroom, she cannot pass urine spontaneously. She jumps a few times and then instantly sits on the toilet when she passes some amount of urine. UDS shows a capacity of 270 ml; she felt urge to pass urine at volume of 120–200 ml with mildly reduced compliance and very mild overactivity. She reported significant urge at 220 ml at Pdet >20 cm H_2O, but she could not pass urine spontaneously. When asked to pass urine, she coughed/jumped a few times (artefacts seen in the circled area are due to jumping) after which DO contraction was seen with Pdet rising above 20 cm H_2O when she was able to pass 10–15 ml of urine. She could pass a total amount of 50–60 ml of urine with a PVR of 200 ml. Thus, it was evident that she was able to pass urine only by using provoked overactivity. She was started on mirabegron 25 mg and third hourly CIC and night-time drainage. At 1 month follow-up, she was absolutely dry between CICs and was off diapers with CIC volumes around 300 ml

tiate Valsalva-induced overactivity which causes passage of urine versus Valsalva manoeuvre itself leading to passage of urine because in the first scenario, the detrusor pressures may be high during voiding and the leaks may be controlled by use of anticholinergics only - these patients may not need bladder neck procedures.

(b) *Is the void efficient?*

What is the PVR—Significant PVR suggests inefficient voiding, predisposes to UTIs and needs support of CIC for bladder emptying.

(c) *Is the voiding safe?*

What are the detrusor pressures during voiding—In a child who is able to void voluntarily, high voiding detrusor pressures suggest outflow tract obstruction which is usually due to neurogenic DSD (Fig. 17.15). In such cases, use of alpha-blockers or Botox injection into the bladder neck/sphincter may be attempted.

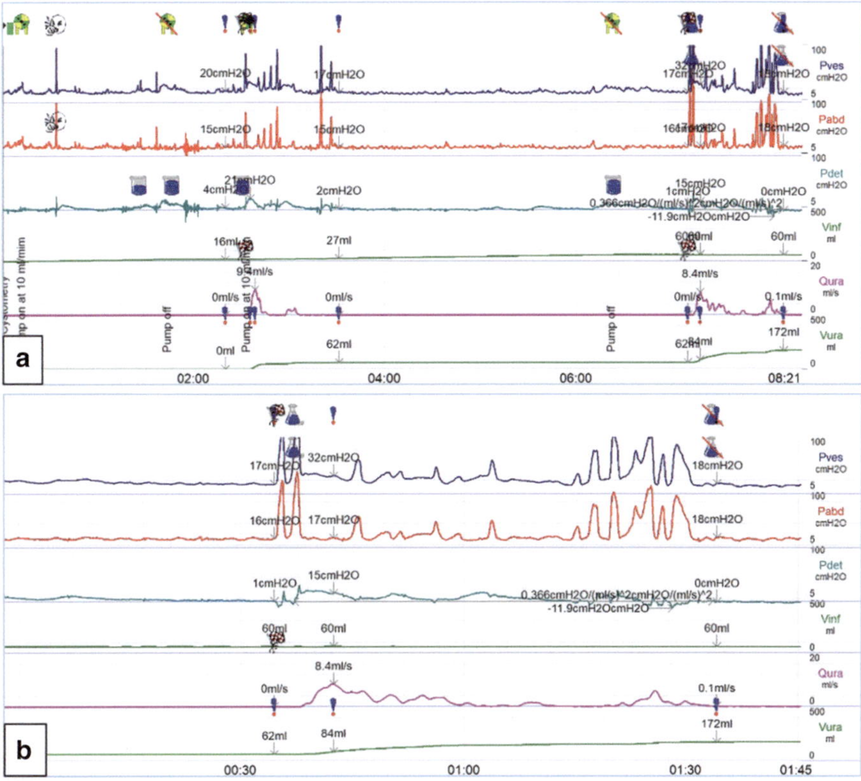

Fig. 17.13 (**a** and **b**) *Provoked IDC-mediated void.* A 7-year-old girl, follow-up case of lumbosacral lipo-MMC, informs urge to pass urine and can hold urine comfortably till she reaches the washroom, has occasional urgency and shows mild straining during passing urine. Does not have any urinary leakage/dribbling and does not need diapers in school or at home. USG showed bilateral upper tract dilatation and thick-walled bladder and was found to have bilateral VUR on MCU. First urodynamic tracing (a) shows two studies done in tandem; IDC is seen intermittently when she reports urgency but does not leak. She passes urine on command (60 ml and 100 ml) by generating voluntary detrusor contraction. The second tracing (b) shows one of the voids in expanded form. It is evident that the voiding detrusor contractions are weak and short-lived and preceded by short strains suggestive of the voiding detrusor contraction being actually provoked IDC. Straining is more pronounced at the end of the void. Flow was weak although there was near-complete emptying of bladder. So she was using provoked IDC along with probably voluntary sphincter relaxations to void to completion. As she was having recurrent episodes of UTI which was presumed to be due to overactivity during the filling phase, she was advised anticholinergics. After starting even low-dose anticholinergics, the child could not void on her own, thus confirming the fact that she was voiding by using provoked IDCs and would need CIC for emptying her bladder. Parents were unhappy with the fact that the child was not passing urine on her own and stopped the medications

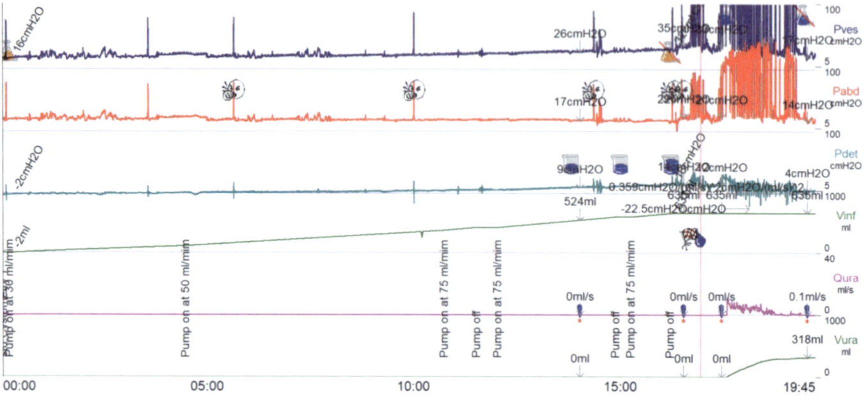

Fig. 17.14 *Valsalva void.* A 16-year-old male child, follow-up case of lumbar lipo-MMC operated at the age of 6 months followed by detethering at the age of 10 years, had h/o increased urinary frequency with urgency. He presently passes good amounts of urine voluntarily by straining and performs night-time catheter drainage. Has had two episodes of UTI in the recent past. USG shows normal upper tracts with thick-walled UB (6 mm). UDS shows a large capacity (630 ml), compliant bladder with no overactivity. He reported urge to void at 530 - 630 ml fill and was given command to void at 630 ml fill. At 630 ml volume, he passed 320 ml solely by Valsalva manoeuvre. There was a PVR of 380 ml after the void. He could not pass urine by Valsalva at volumes <400 ml. So although he had a large bladder capacity, he could efficiently empty only 50% volume leading to increased frequency. Ability to empty by Valsalva implies weak outflow competence which explains the urgency felt at higher bladder volumes. He was advised to perform CIC 2–3 times a day as complete bladder emptying would reduce the urinary frequency and chances of further episodes of UTI

Importance of Assessing the Existence of DSD in Patients with NB

Presence of DSD is considered as an important risk factor which predicts upper tract deterioration. It is seen when *i*-UDS is performed with EMG electrodes in situ. Significantly increased EMG activity is seen during episodes of IDC and/or during voluntary detrusor contraction.

We have found no relevance of assessing existence of DSD in patients who do not void voluntarily. These patients, in any case, need CIC for bladder emptying and presence of DSD adds to the outflow competence and helps the patient remain dry in between CICs. Filling phase parameters can be stabilised by appropriate medical management (Fig. 17.16).

Patients who can void voluntarily need evaluation of voiding detrusor pressures and DSD. If voiding detrusor pressures are high with evidence of DSD, use of alpha-blockers and/or Botox in the sphincters is a valid option (Fig. 17.17).

UDS-Based Practical Working Classification of NB

The following is a practical working classification that we use to manage our children with NB irrespective of the aetiology of NB (Fig. 17.18).

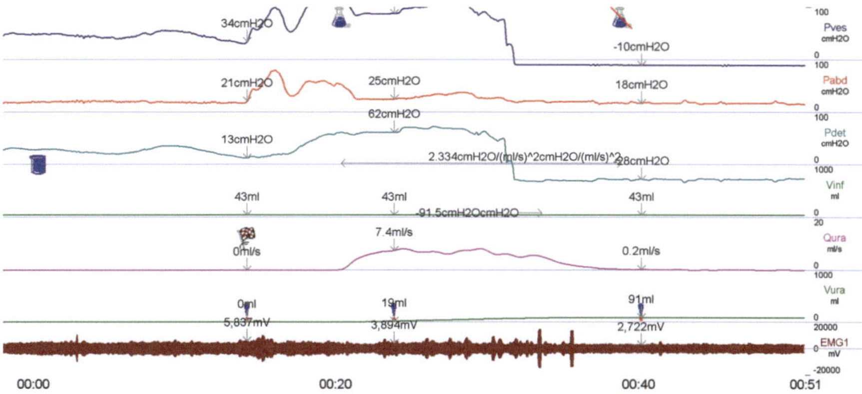

Fig. 17.15 *Voluntary voiding contraction with unsafe voiding pressures*. A 6-year-old girl, follow-up case of LSMMC, had history of urgency and urge incontinence but voided on her own. She showed thick-walled UB on USG with normal upper tracts. During UDS, she showed significant overactivity with urgency during the filling phase with occasional leak. This image shows the voiding phase of the urodynamics in an expanded form. She could generate voiding detrusor contraction on command (voiding command is marked by red chequered flag) and voided till completion. Pdet tracing suddenly drops towards the end of the flow—artefact caused due to slipping out of the catheter. During void, Pdet is seen to be significantly high relative to the flow rates (62 cm H_2O at 7.4 ml/sec) suggesting outflow tract obstruction. EMG activity is also seen to increase to some extent during voiding. So, although she is able to void to completion on her own, she has features of BOO which will be detrimental in the long run and would need alpha-blockers/Botox injection at the bladder neck/sphincter. She was also started on low-dose anticholinergics for the overactivity during filling phase after which symptoms of urgency and urge incontinence improved

How Often Should Repeat Studies be Performed in Patients with NB

In patients with high-risk filling parameters, *i*-UDS should be performed a few months after medical management is instituted to document that bladder pressures have reduced to safe range (Fig. 17.19a–d).

In patients with IDC or reduced detrusor compliance and leaks/ 'self voids' mediated by high detrusor pressures, monitoring the frequency of leaks/ 'self-voids' in between the CICs gives an indirect evidence of persistence of overactivity/poor compliance. Abolishing the leaks by adjusting dose of anticholinergics/beta-3 agonists indicates that detrusor pressure has gone below the value of DLPP or DO-LPP (Fig. 17.20a–c).

In patients with weak bladder outlet, before performing bladder outlet procedure, filling parameters should be documented to be stable (Fig. 17.21a, b).

Once a patient has achieved safe filling bladder pressures, *i*-UDS may have to be repeated if there are fresh changes in clinical or radiological parameters like new onset of leak/UTI/upper tract changes/bladder wall thickening.

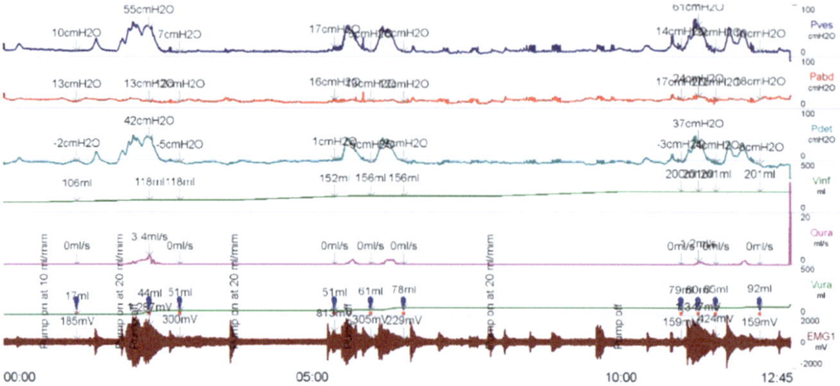

Fig. 17.16 *DSD with no voluntary void.* A 9-year-old boy with cerebral palsy with history of recurrent UTI and bilateral HDUN. This is a small segment of the UDS tracing showing fill from 100 ml to 200 ml. It shows several episodes of IDCs with passage of small volumes of urine and increase in EMG activity during all the episodes of IDCs, suggestive of neurogenic DO with DSD with leaks. The child could not generate a sustained voiding detrusor contraction on command. No complete/effective void was noted during the study. Thus, this child will benefit from anticholinergics to reduce the IDCs and CIC for poor bladder emptying

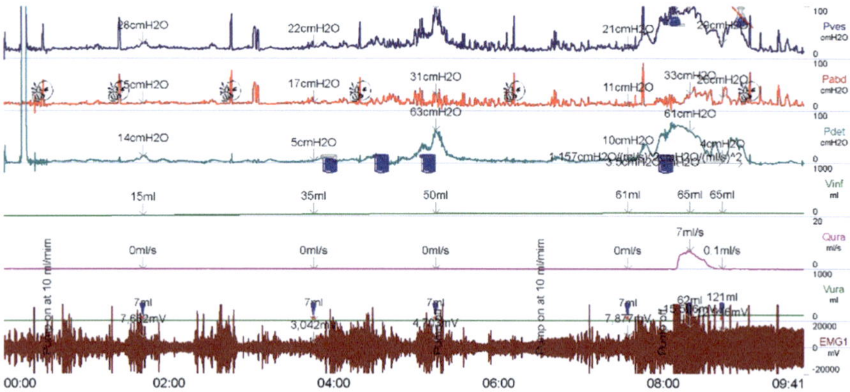

Fig. 17.17 *DSD with voluntary void.* A 7-year-old girl, known case of NB, presented with increased frequency of micturition, urgency, urge incontinence, enuresis and recurrent UTI. USG showed normal upper tracts with a thick-walled bladder. UDS showed a small capacity bladder with normal compliance and detrusor overactivity. There was no overactivity-associated leak. The last contraction seen in the curve was a voluntary sustained detrusor contraction resulting in complete emptying of bladder (although there is no red chequered flag preceding the void). EMG activity shows neurogenic DSD during the voluntary void. Voiding detrusor pressures are very high (60 cm H_2O at 7 ml/sec) suggestive of bladder outflow obstruction probably due to DSD. As this patient has the ability to void voluntarily, she will need alpha-blockers or Botox to reduce obstructive effect of DSD along with careful addition of anticholinergics to control the overactivity

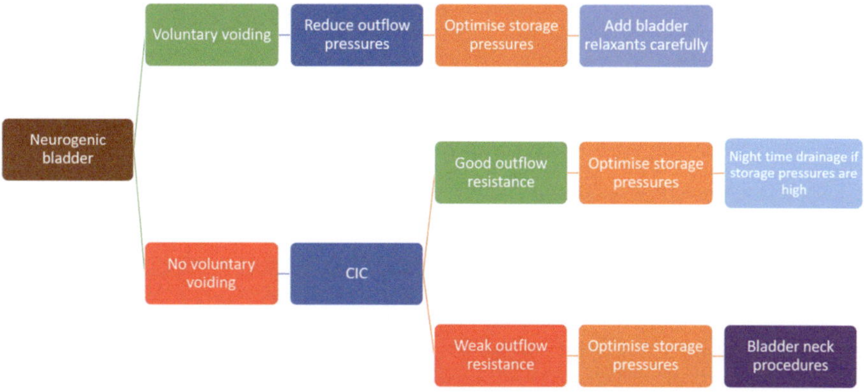

Fig. 17.18 UDS-based practical working classification of NB dysfunction

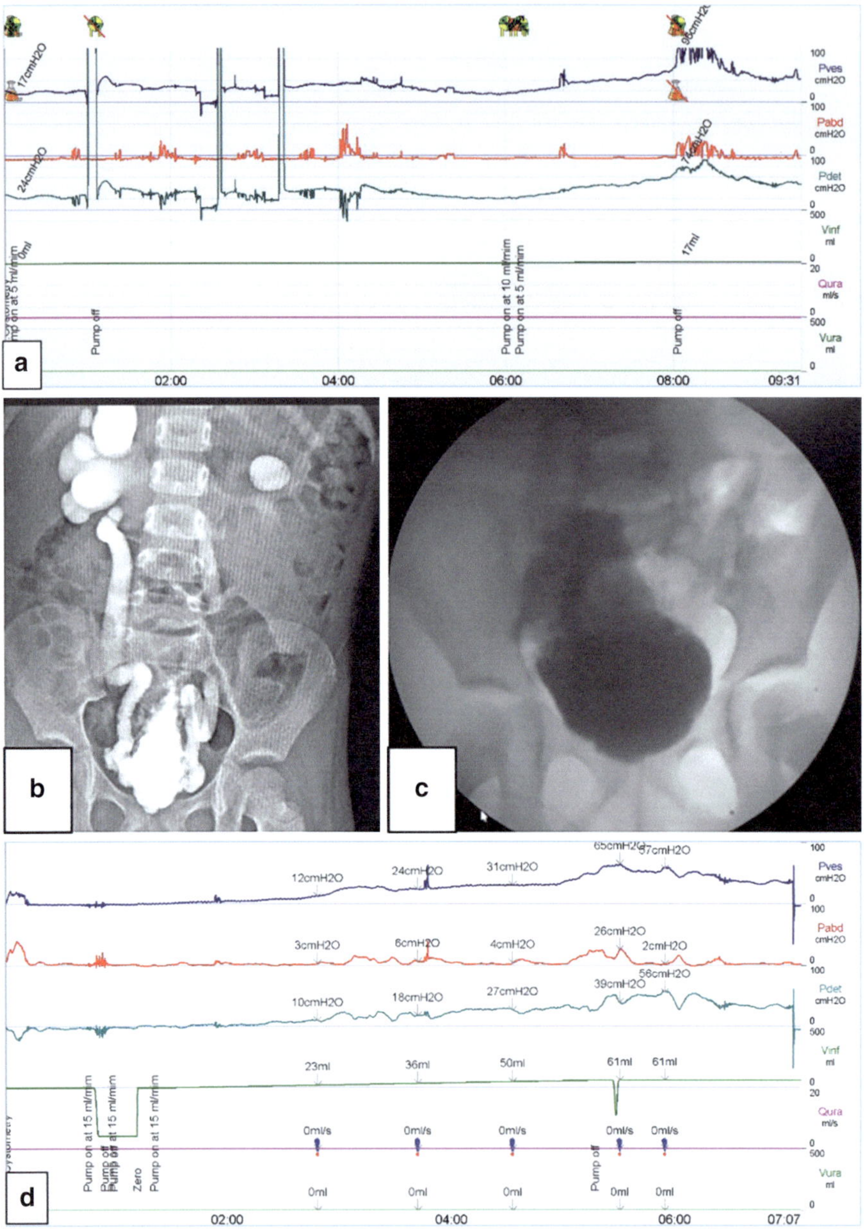

Fig. 17.19 (**a**–**d**) A 4-year-old girl, known case of NB, presented with urosepsis and AKI and was stabilized after catheter drainage (creat 4 mg/dl → 0.4 mg/dl). Initial UDS (**a**) shows very small capacity bladder with severe hypocompliance (70 cm H_2O at 17 ml). MCU at that time showed a small Christmas tree-shaped bladder with bilateral VUR (**b**). She was started on CIC with anticholinergics as parents did not want diversion. After 2 months, she was dry on CIC with CIC volumes being around 100 ml. Repeat study done after 2 months shows significant increase in bladder volumes and improvement in pressures although they are still in the high-risk zone (91 ml at 38 cm H2O) (**d**). MCU was repeated (**c**) to document that the increased storage volumes were due to increase in size of bladder rather than increase in severity of reflux

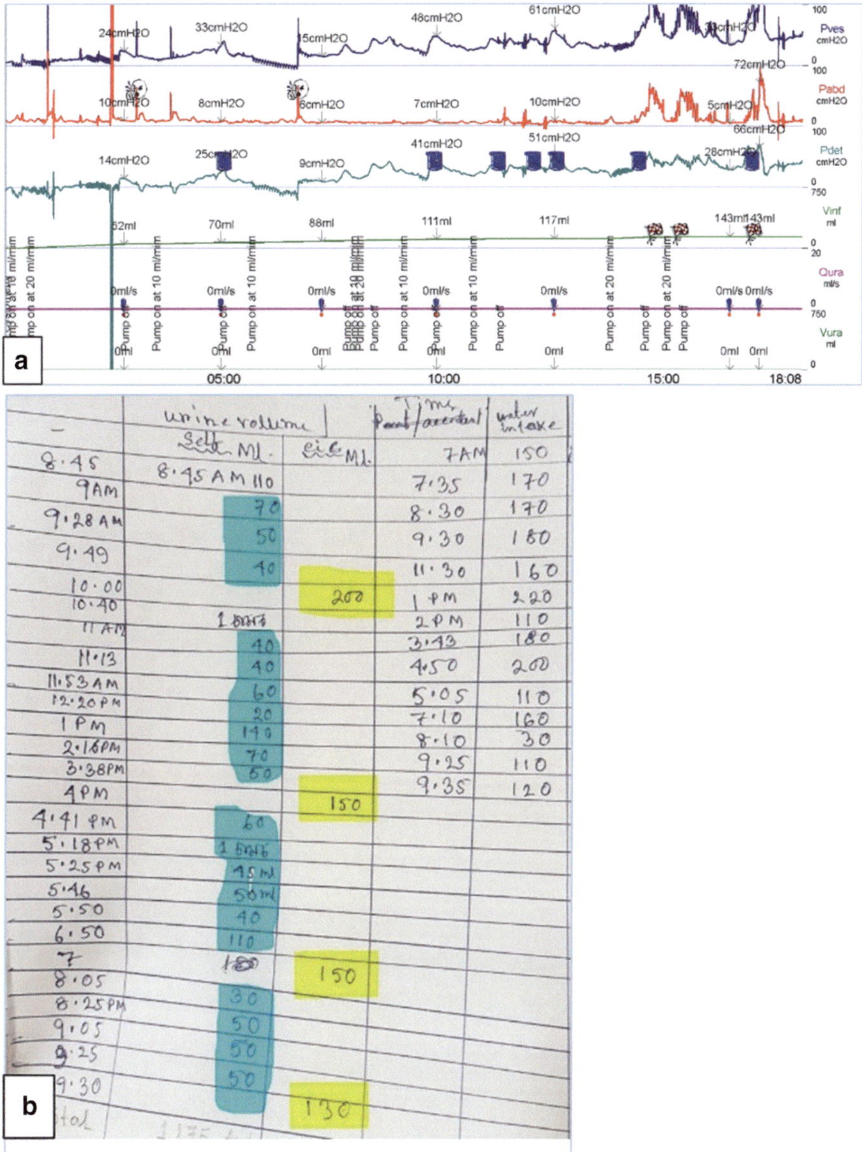

Fig. 17.20 (**a**–**c**) A 7-year-old girl with NB passes urine voluntarily every 30 minutes with urgency but does not leak. CIC is being performed every fourth hourly. USG shows bilateral HDUN with thick-walled UB; MCU showed right Gr V VUR. Initial UDS tracing (**a**) shows a capacity of 140 ml, severe overactivity and hypocompliance. Although she could not void voluntarily during the study, she reported urgency during IDCs only when detrusor pressures reached 30–40 cm H_2O. Her CIC diary (**b**) showed the frequency of self-voids marked in blue and CIC voids marked in yellow. 'Self voids' meant that she had urge to pass urine at those points implying thereby that they actually represented the points where there was significant detrusor overactivity. Doses of anticholinergics were adjusted to reduce frequency of self-voids to zero and she voided only with CIC. The next UDS was repeated after 6 months (**c**) which shows a much stable bladder

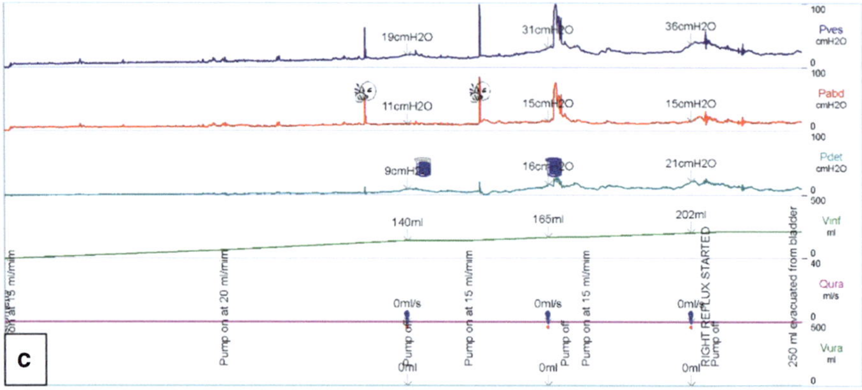

Fig. 17.20 (continued)

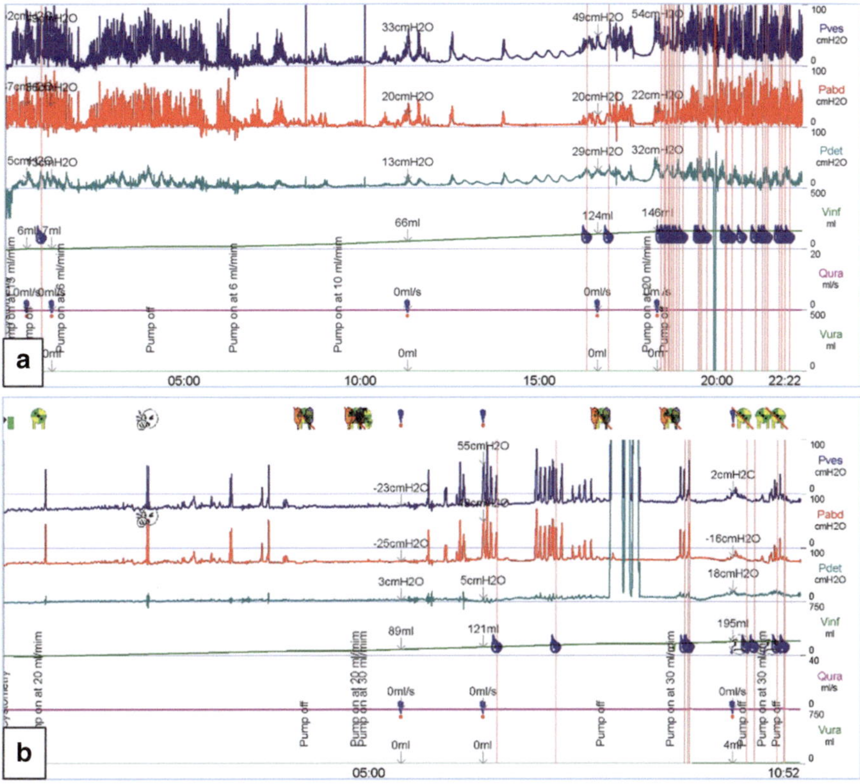

Fig. 17.21 (**a**, **b**) A 3-year-old male child, known case of NB, presented with continuous dribbling of urine and recurrent UTI. USG showed bilateral HDUN with thick-walled UB; MCU showed intermittent left Gr 2–3 VUR. Initial UDS (**a**) showed normal capacity bladder (120 ml) and significant overactivity (spontaneous and provoked). DO-LPP was 30 cm H_2O, ALPP was >40 cm H_2O at 70 ml, but leak of urine was observed when child was crying/straining irrespective of bladder volume (leak was also seen at 6 ml fill). Bladder emptied completely within a minute when child was crying suggestive of weak bladder outlet. He was started on anticholinergics and CIC. At 6 months follow-up, frequency of leaks had reduced significantly; he was leaking only while playing or performing some activities. Repeat UDS (**b**) showed increase in bladder capacity with minimal/no overactivity; ALPP was 50 cm H_2O at 120 ml which confirmed a weak bladder outlet. With the filling parameters stabilized by oral medications, this child was a candidate for bladder neck procedure alone and no augmentation was needed

Declarations

Competing Interests The author(s) has no competing interests to declare that are relevant to the content of this manuscript.

Ethics Approval The author(s) declares that this manuscript does not include primary research with human participants.

The author(s) declares that this manuscript does not include primary studies involving animals.

Role of *i*-UDS Study in Exstrophy Patients

18

Subhasis Saha and Poonam Guha Vaze

The aims of treatment in exstrophy bladder and its variants are:

- Achievement of urinary continence (though the definition varies) allowing the bladder to store urine
- Volitional voiding or emptying the bladder with a catheter
- Preserving the renal function

The three standard methods of repair of exstrophy are:

- CPRE (complete primary repair of exstrophy)
- MSRE (modern staged repair of exstrophy)
- Kelly repair or its variants (soft tissue mobilization without osteotomy)

When the outcome of repair is evaluated, a key concern remains the potential for renal upper tract deterioration. Continence is often achieved at the cost of high intravesical pressure which is transmitted to the upper tract. Volitional initiation and stoppage of micturition is often considered an important parameter of success of this reconstructive effort. But controversy remains whether the voiding is a result of detrusor contraction or contraction of the abdominal musculature.

S. Saha (✉)
Department of Pediatric Surgery, Manipal Hospitals, Kolkata, India

P. G. Vaze
Neotia Bhagirathi Woman and Child Care Centre, Newtown, Kolkata, India

Department of Pediatric Surgery, Nilratan Sircar Medical College and Hospital, Kolkata, India

S. Saha, P. Guha Vaze (eds.), *Comprehensive Atlas of Practical Pediatric Urodynamics*, https://doi.org/10.1007/978-981-95-2709-0_18

All these issues can be assessed to a great extent by urodynamic study and, if possible, video urodynamic study. Video urodynamic study helps to correlate voiding episodes with peristaltic action in the bowel segment or detrusor contractions. A few examples of urodynamic evaluation of the patients are tabulated below. First case is a case of primary bladder closure with no further procedure done. UDS was performed to assess the bladder behavior and decide for bladder neck repair alone versus need for augmentation. The second case is a young female who is continent after bladder neck repair with near normal capacity. The third case had undergone ileal segment bladder augmentation and is continent.

We have seen that a conventional UDS tracks the detrusor activity, and in cases of abdominal voiding, detrusor pressure is not raised. During simultaneous visualization of the contour of the bladder during voiding, we at times see active peristalsis in the colonic augment portion on giving the command for voiding resulting in significant void.

Case 1

A 5-year-old male child underwent bladder closure at the age of 7 months after which he was lost to follow-up. Presently, he had continuous urinary dribbling and leaked intermittently when asleep—passed 80–90 ml urine after waking up. He had recurrent episodes of urinary tract infections. USG showed mild unilateral pelvic fullness. UDS was performed to assess the bladder capacity and behavior (Fig. 18.1).

Fill (Fig. 18.1) was performed at a very slow speed of 5 ml/sec. UDS revealed significant leak of urine shortly after starting filling. Leakage was also noted during coughing with abdominal pressures around 55 cm H_2O (ALPP 55 cm H_2O). Spontaneous dribbling of urine was noted after 12 ml infusion in the absence of

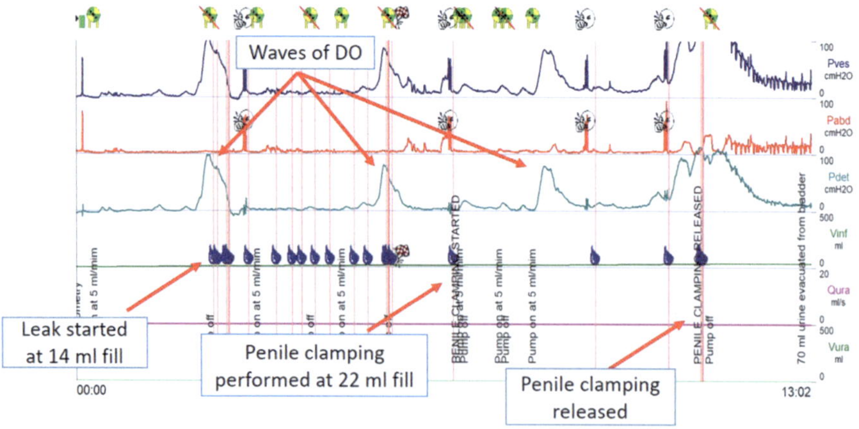

Fig. 18.1 USG showed mild unilateral pelvic fullness. UDS was performed to assess the bladder capacity and behaviour

detrusor overactivity or abdominal straining denoting weak bladder outlet (DLPP 0 cm H_2O at 12 ml volume). Thus, the rest of the study was performed by keeping the penis clamped. Intermittent waves of severe overactivity were noted with pressures reaching 80–100 cm H_2O when patient complained of urge to pass stools. He did not report any bladder sensations. Filling was stopped at 100 ml fill as there was sustained detrusor contraction. He leaked 10–20 ml urine as soon as penile clamping was released. There was 70 ml PVR after the void.

Intermittent severe overactivity and inability to empty the bladder were probably responsible for recurrent UTI in the child. This child would not be a candidate for bladder neck repair alone. He would also require bladder augmentation with Mitrofanoff.

Case 2

An 8-year-old female child had undergone exstrophy repair at neonatal age and bladder neck repair at the age of 5 years. She was now continent. Her voided volumes were around 100–150 ml with no episodes of urine leak during the day. She had history of enuresis.

UDS was performed to assess bladder function (Fig. 18.2). She could not be catheterized when awake, so the study was done under sedation in the operation theater under fluoroscopic screening. She could be catheterised under anaesthesia. Detrusor was found to be stable with no evidence of overactivity. Compliance was normal/mildly reduced. Filling was stopped at 200 ml as the bladder appeared to be tense on video-fluoroscopic screening. The bladder outline was lobulated, with a suspected diverticulum noted on the posterior aspect. A lobulated filling defect was noted in the region of the bladder neck probably attributable to previous bladder neck repair. No VUR was noted. No leak was noted on suprapubic pressures.

Thus, the study revealed a decent capacity stable bladder (200 ml; EBC, 270 ml). As the study was done under sedation, findings like reduced functional capacity/ urgency, leak point pressures, and overactivity may have been masked.

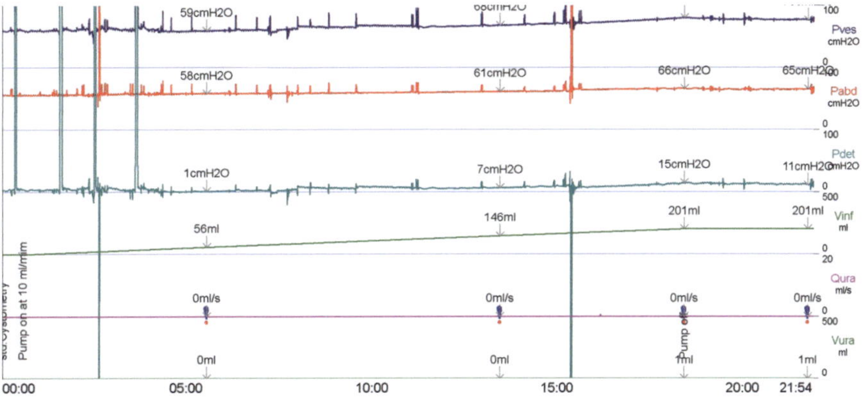

Fig. 18.2 UDS was performed to assess bladder function

Case 3

A 9-year-old girl underwent primary bladder closure at 2 years followed by Young-Dee's bladder neck repair with colocystoplasty at 5.5 years. She developed bladder stone and at the age of 8 years-underwent open cystolithotomy and Mitrofanoff stoma creation for bladder washes. Presently, she passed urine voluntarily via naturalis during the day with occasional dribbling/leakage when running/dancing. She had occasional enuresis.

Voiding diary showed small volume voids of 80–100 ml 5–6 times per day with morning void of 150 ml. She could pass 54 ml urine in a bell-shaped curve with the flow rate proportional to the voided volume during uroflowmetry without any PVR (Fig. 18.3).

During UDS (Fig. 18.4), bladder capacity was found to be 200 ml although she reported urge to pass from 50 ml fill onward (sensory urgency of unknown cause).

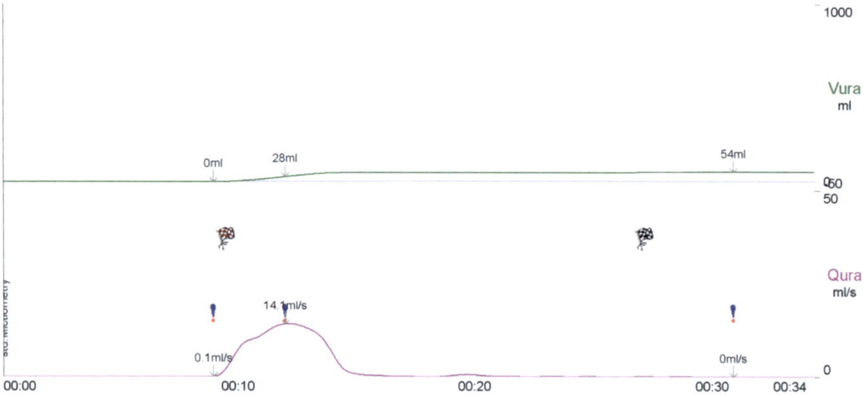

Fig. 18.3 Uroflowmetry tracing

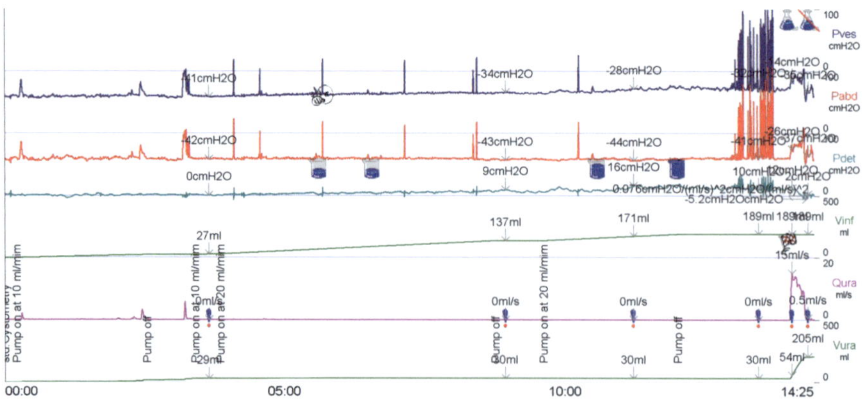

Fig. 18.4 During UDS, bladder capacity was found to be 200 ml, although she reported urge to pass from 50 ml fill onwards (Sensory urgency)

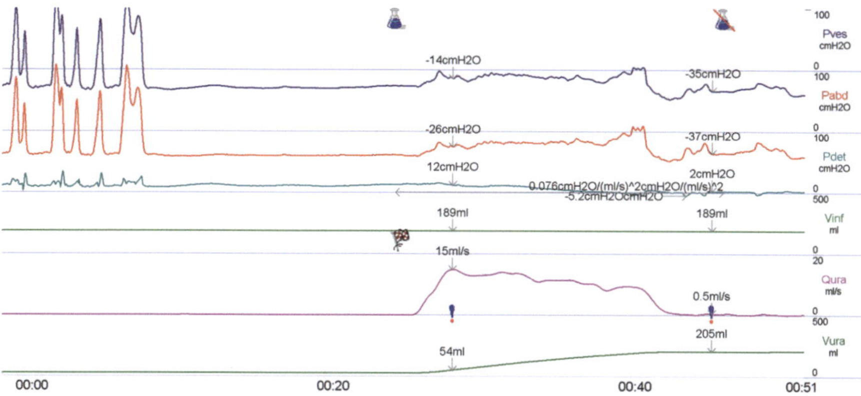

Fig. 18.5 Voiding phase of the UDS tracing in an expanded form

Compliance was seen to be normal/very mildly reduced (10 cm H_2O at 200 ml). Intermittent waves of very mild DO were noted with pressures reaching 10–16 cm H_2O when she reported urgency. No leak was observed during the study—ALPP >100 cm H_2O—suggesting good competence of outflow tract.

Bladder was lobulated in shape and irregular in outline. The upper half of the bladder appeared like the colonic augment and lower part resembled native bladder. Periodic peristalsis was seen in the upper half of the bladder which coincided with the overactivity recorded on UDS and caused urgency. No VUR was seen.

She could pass urine on command. Void was primarily by Valsalva maneuver with good flow rates and complete emptying of bladder (Fig. 18.5).

So this child was having a decent capacity bladder with features of urgency due to periodic colonic peristalsis.

In a nutshell, we can decipher the following from the *i*-UDS study of an exstrophy child:

- Bladder volume (cystometric volume and functional bladder capacity)
- Presence of detrusor contractions or Valsalva and we know whether they are effective
- Any loss of compliance or presence of overactivity during filling or excessive bladder pressure during voiding
- Degree of leakage

Accordingly, we may plan the following procedures as necessary for these children:

- Bladder neck reconstruction (YDL/sling)
- Surgical augmentation/Botox
- Mitrofanoff stoma

There are only a few published articles in international literature who have looked at urodynamic findings and correlated them with the type of repair of exstrophy bladder.

Unaugmented exstrophy bladders often have the potential of damaging the upper tracts secondary to dilating VUR as well as functional obstruction at the VUJ or bladder outlet. Small capacity and high pressure in the bladder add to the problem. Kondabolu et al. [4] have suggested a novel ileocecal doughnut augmentation in children with exstrophy bladder. They have done cystometry on 91% of the 33 cases. The mean cystometric capacity was 300 ml which represented 95% of the expected bladder capacity for that age. The end filling pressure was less than 20 cm in 80% of these patients.

When a child achieves dry state with preserved upper tracts on serial USG, cystometry may not be done.

On the other hand, Weaver and colleagues [5] have managed many exstrophy patients without augmentation, and they have done UDS to prove that effective detrusor contraction is possible resulting in volitional voiding. They are of the opinion that a greater emphasis should be laid on performing routine UDS assessment in complete bladder exstrophy patients to understand the physiology of bladder emptying better as more and more patients are opting not to have their bladder augmented.

Declarations

Competing Interests The author(s) has no competing interests to declare that are relevant to the content of this manuscript.

Ethics Approval The author(s) declares that this manuscript does not include primary research with human participants.

The author(s) declares that this manuscript does not include primary studies involving animals.

Further Reading

1. Bhatnagar V. Bladder exstrophy: an overview of the surgical management. J Ind Ass Ped Surg. 2011;16(3):81–7.
2. Di Carlo HN, Maruf M, Jayman J, et al. The inadequate bladder template: its effect on outcomes in classic bladder exstrophy. J Ped Urol. 2018;14:427e1–7.
3. Fay T, Deshpande AV, Blanc T, et al. Pediatric urodynamic studies: emerging technologies and new frontiers. Ther Adv Urol. 2025;17:1–14.
4. Kondabolu GC, Barla RK, Arunachalam P, et al. Ileocecal doughnut augmentation in children with exstrophy-epispadias complex – a study of 100 cases. J Ped Urol. 2024;20:644e1–8.
5. Weaver JK, Eftekharzdeh S, Lee T, et al. Early urodynamic findings after complete primary repair of exstrophy. J Ped Urol. 2023;19:565e1–5.

Atlas of Disease-Wise Curves

19

Poonam Guha Vaze

Children present with bladder dysfunction due to several causes which include PUV, neurogenic bladder and functional bladder dysfunctions. Bladder dysfunction is also commonly seen in setup of neurodevelopmental disorders like cerebral palsy, Down syndrome and cases of anorectal malformation. This chapter presents a brief outline of the basics of abnormal bladder function in each of the aforementioned disease states followed by few representative case scenarios with their UDS findings and their subsequent management. Neurogenic bladder has been dealt with in a separate chapter.

1. PUV—Post-fulguration follow-up
   - 1.1 PUV with DO but normal outflow parameters
   - 1.2 PUV with DO and BOO
   - 1.3 PUV with hypocompliant bladder
   - 1.4 PUV with weak bladder outlet
   - 1.5 PUV with presumed myogenic failure—residual BOO
   - 1.6 PUV with presumed myogenic failure—blader neck dysfunction
2. Functional bladder disorders
   - 2.1 Sensory urgency
   - 2.2 Genital/abdominal pain
   - 2.3 DO presenting as primary enuresis

Supplementary Information The online version contains supplementary material available at https://doi.org/10.1007/978-981-95-2709-0_19.

P. G. Vaze (✉)
Neotia Bhagirathi Woman and Child Care Centre, Newtown, Kolkata, India

Department of Pediatric Surgery, Nilratan Sircar Medical College and Hospital, Kolkata, India

S. Saha, P. Guha Vaze (eds.), *Comprehensive Atlas of Practical Pediatric Urodynamics*, https://doi.org/10.1007/978-981-95-2709-0_19

- 2.4 DO presenting as recurrent UTI
- 2.5 NNNB—inefficient voiding
- 2.6 NNNB—bladder neck dysfunction

3. Neurodevelopmental disorders
   - 3.1 Down syndrome
     - 3.1.1. Down syndrome with bladder neck dysfunction
     - 3.1.2. Down with variable voiding pattern
     - 3.1.3. Down with VUR
     - 3.1.4. Down with weak bladder outlet
   - 3.2 Cerebral palsy
     - 3.2.1. CP with urinary retention
     - 3.2.2. CP with recurrent UTI—DO
     - 3.2.3. CP with recurrent UTI—BOO
4. Anorectal malformation
   - 4.1 ARM with neurogenic DSD
   - 4.2 ARM with underactive bladder
   - 4.3 ARM with hypocompliant bladder
   - 4.4 ARM with weak bladder outlet

PUV: Post-Fulguration Follow-Up

i-UDS has a definite role in the management of patients after PUV fulguration. Bladder dysfunction is seen in long term in the majority of patients of PUV. The pattern of bladder behaviour varies depending on the severity of primary disease, surgical procedure performed (diversion vs fulguration), age at diagnosis, time elapsed following definitive procedure and presence of any residual outflow tract obstruction (residual valves, strictures, bladder neck hypertrophy/dysfunction).

PUV bladder is classically known to change from small capacity, overactive/hyper-contractile bladder early after fulguration to large capacity bladder with poor emptying and myogenic failure in adolescence. Several studies have documented that myogenic failure can develop in children well before adolescence also.

Few studies have documented that residual HDUN after valve fulguration is often attributable to some form of bladder dysfunction and can be reversed by appropriate evaluation and management of bladder dysfunctions. Few of the so-called 'myogenic failures' can also be reversed by relieving residual outflow obstruction.

We have highlighted the UDS findings in six different case scenarios following PUV fulguration and the management strategies employed.

Case 1: PUV with DO but Normal Outflow Parameters

A 10-year-old male child, FUC of PUV, underwent fulguration of valves at the age of 1.6 years. He had been well after the surgery and was lost to follow-up. He presented at 10 years of age with history of urgency, urge incontinence, wetness of pants during the day and enuresis (several episodes every night). He was passing urine in good uninterrupted stream. He had unremarkable stool habits.

USG showed normal upper tracts and thick-walled UB (2.9 mm) with insignificant PVR; rectal diameter was noted to be 32 mm. Voiding diary showed that he voided 14–15 times per day with usual voided volumes—50–100 ml; maximum voided volumes were 130–140 ml suggesting small capacity bladder/detrusor overactivity.

His serum creatinine was 1 mg/dl.

The working diagnosis was either detrusor overactivity or a poorly compliant bladder probably due to residual BOO.

Uroflowmetry (Fig. 19.1a) showed good flow pattern with supranormal flow rates (160 ml @ 16 ml/sec). There was no PVR after the void.

UDS and MCU were performed to assess the bladder behaviour and urethral/bladder neck appearance as he had no post-operative evaluations/check cystoscopy.

UDS (Fig. 19.1 b) showed a small capacity bladder (130 ml) with severe DO at 70 ml fill with pressures reaching 40 cm H2O when he reported urgency (blue beaker). The compliance was normal. During voiding (Fig 19.1c), Qmax was 13 ml/sec with PdetQmax being 29 cm H2O suggesting normal voiding pressures and flow rates. There was no PVR after the void.

MCU (Fig. 19.1d) showed a small capacity, smooth-walled, rounded bladder with normal appearance of bladder neck/urethra during voiding.

Thus, the uroflow/UDS/MCU showed that he had normal outflow parameters with significant overactivity which was responsible for his symptoms. Rectal diameter of 32 mm suggests rectal loading and probable BBD, and he was started on constipation management and mirabegron.

Case 2: PUV with DO—Residual BOO

A 9-month-old child with PUV had undergone cystoscopy and fulguration at the age of 2 days. He was passing urine well in good stream. He had intermittent episodes of increased frequency. Preoperative USG KUB had shown bilateral HDUN with thick-walled bladder. USG at 9 months showed right small kidney with mild HDN, normal left kidney and thickened bladder mucosa. A uroflowmetry (Fig. 19.2a) could be recorded which showed good flow rates with bell-shaped curve. MCU (Fig. 19.2b) showed significant resolution of preoperative changes. A persistent radiolucent filling defect was seen in the posterior urethra (yellow arrow) with good calibre of distal urethra. The present investigations did not provide any evidence of residual BOO. The child was on oxybutynin 2.5 mg twice a day. As there were episodes of increased frequency in spite of being on oxybutynin along with the persistent radioloscent defect in the urethra, a UDS was performed to rule out any residual BOO and to assess the bladder behaviour - whether any change in dose of oxybutinin was warranted.

UDS (Fig. 19.2c) showed a large capacity bladder (100 ml; EBC 60 ml) with severe overactivity in the filling phase with pressures reaching 50–100 cm

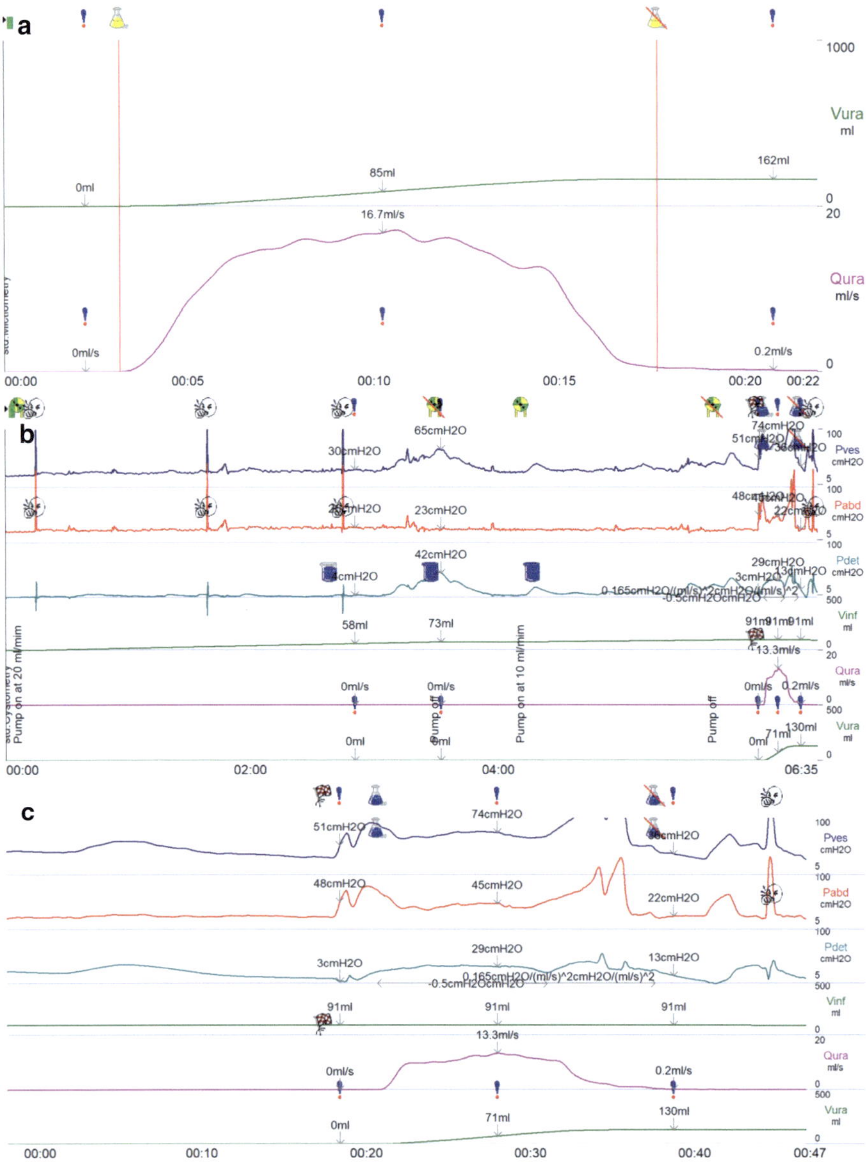

Fig. 19.1 (**a**) Uroflowmetry curve. (**b**) UDS tracing. (**c**) Voiding phase of the UDS tracing in an expanded form. (**d**) MCU images

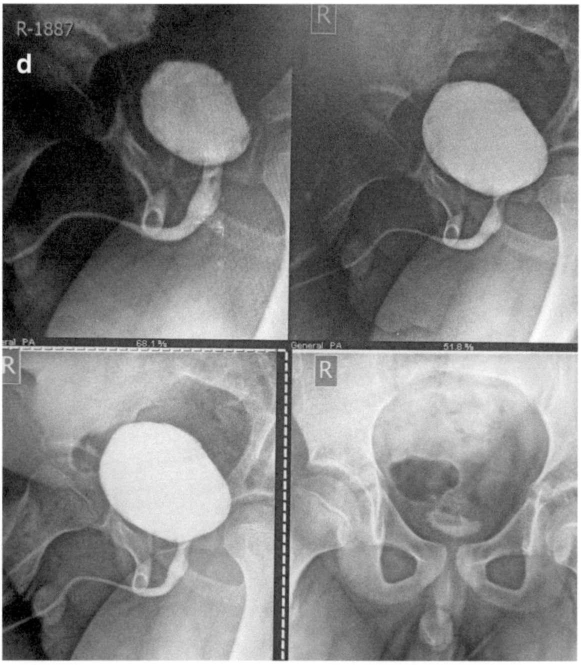

Fig. 19.1 (continued)

H2O. Compliance was normal. During voiding (Fig 19.2d), flow rates were appropriate for age, but the detrusor pressures were very high (100 cm H2O). Although high voiding detrusor pressures have been classically considered as normal in infants due to physiological dys-synergic voiding, flow rates and detrusor pressures in this child were rather uniform throughout the flow which did not suggest raised pressures due to sphincteric contraction. Also, the child was on oxybutynin, which would be expected to lower the detrusor pressures to some extent. High voiding detrusor pressures in spite of the child being on oxybutynin, with low/normal flow rates, suggested BOO.

The child underwent a check cystoscopy which revealed residual valves which were incised (video).

This case highlights certain very pertinent facts:

1. MCU appearance in post-operative cases of PUV can be deceptive and the whole clinical picture needs to be considered.
2. Uroflowmetry curves in children can be bell shaped in the presence of BOO.
3. Informative UDS curves including voiding phase assessment can the achieved in infants and can guide further management.

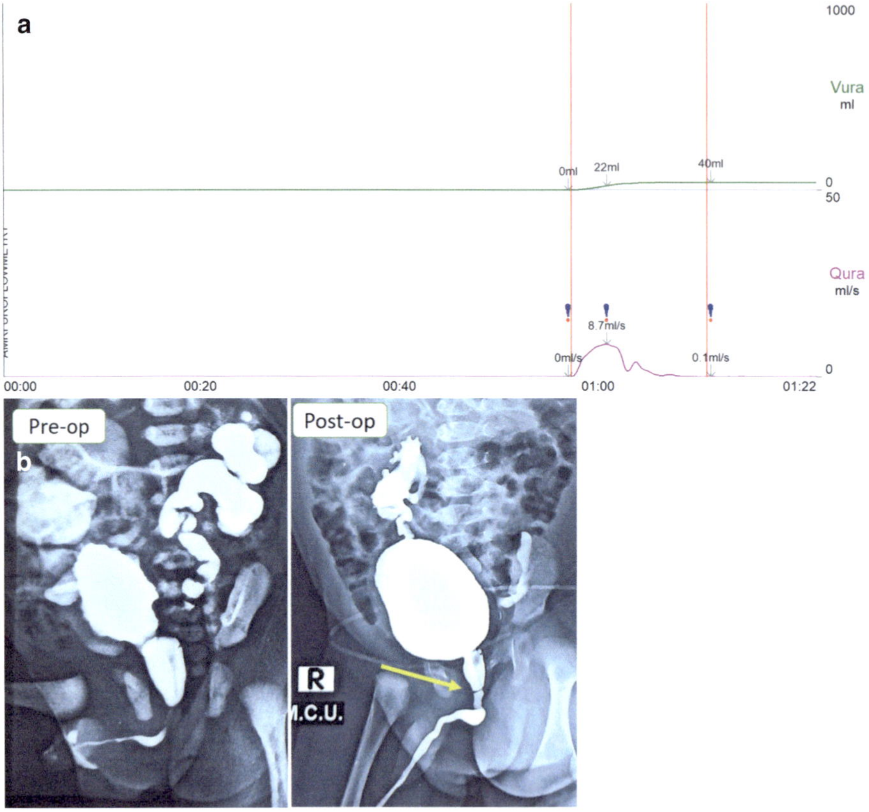

Fig. 19.2 (**a**) Uroflowmetry curve. (**b**) Preoperative and post-operative MCU images. (**c**) UDS tracing showing severe overactivity during the filling phase. (**d**) Voiding phase of the UDS tracing (in an expanded form) to show high-pressure voiding

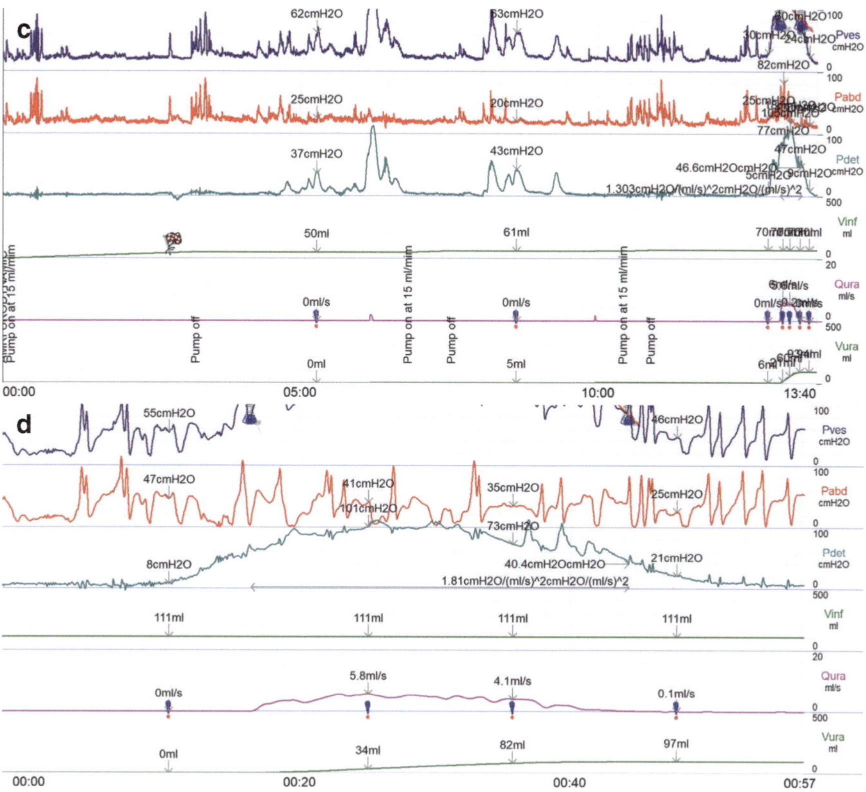

Fig. 19.2 (continued)

Case 3: PUV with Hypocompliant Bladder

A 4-year-old male child was a follow-up case of PUV. He had undergone fulguration of valves at the age of 1 ½ years, residual valve fulguration and circumcision at 2.5 years of age and check cystoscopy and bladder neck incision at the age of 2.9 years which did not reveal any valves. He leaked urine frequently, did not inform before passing urine and passed urine in variable amounts when asked to do so; pants were wet almost continuously. He had recurrent episodes of UTI, two in the current year. He was on oxybutynin 2.5 mg twice a day.

His serum creatinine was 0.9 mg/dl which increased to 1.5 mg/dl during episodes of febrile UTI. USG showed bilateral gross HDN (right and left APD of 24 and 26 mm, respectively); ureters were dilated; UB wall was thickened and trabeculated.

Preop MCU (Fig. 19.3a) had shown a small bladder with very prominent bladder neck impression and evidence of PUV. Post-op MCU (Fig. 19.3d) showed a small irregular bladder with poor visualisation of urethra.

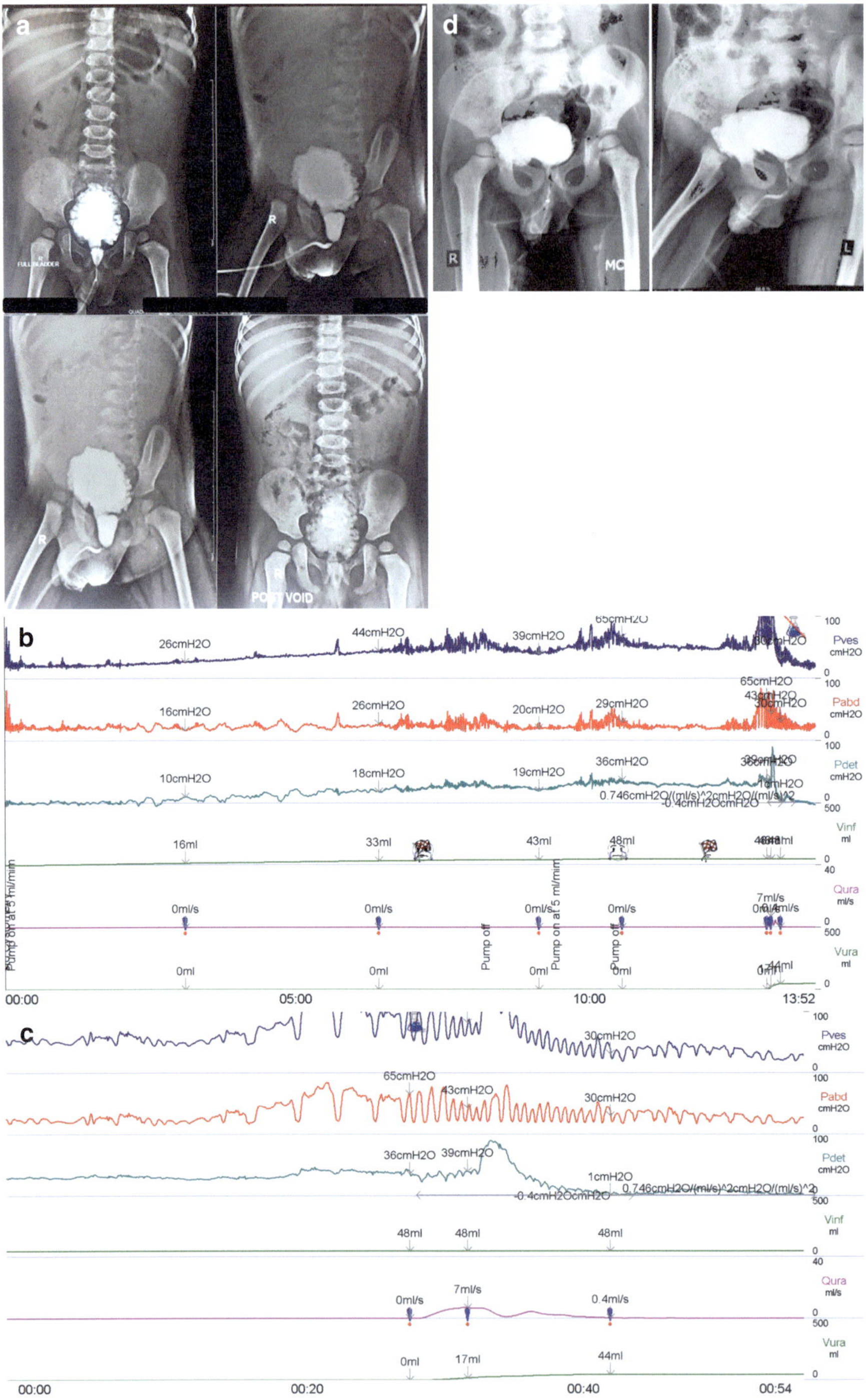

Fig. 19.3 (**a**) Preoperative MCU showed a small bladder with very prominent bladder neck impression and evidence of PUV. (**b**) UDS tracing. (**c**) Voiding phase of the UDS tracing shown in an expanded form (**d**) Post operative MCU

Voiding diary could not be maintained as the child leaked almost continuously.

During uroflowmetry, he passed only 5–10 ml urine on two occasions. UDS was performed after stopping oxybutynin for 1 week to assess baseline bladder behaviour in the absence of medications. Urine leak was seen to increase after stopping oxybutynin.

UDS (Fig. 19.3b) showed a small capacity, very poorly compliant bladder with pressures reaching 36 cm H2O at 48 ml. There was a suspicion of tonic overactivity also. The child became irritable at 33 ml ('cry' sign) when he was given command to void (red chequered flag). Filling was continued till 48 ml when he became irritable again and pressures reached 36 cm H2O and he voided on command. No leak was observed during the study.

During voiding (Fig. 19.3c), detrusor pressures were seen to be normal (39 cm H2O) and flow rates were appropriate. PVR was insignificant. Thus, UDS showed high-pressure, very poorly compliant bladder with no evidence of BOO.

He was offered the option of diversion/augmentation in view of HDUN, rising creatinine and recurrent UTI with poorly compliant bladder. As the family did not agree for any further operative interventions, he was started on anticholinergics to reduce the detrusor pressures, but the PVR was seen to increase. So he was started on CIC with night-time catheter drainage.

Case 4: PUV with Weak Bladder Outlet

A 2-year-old male child was antenatally detected as having left-sided hydronephrosis and postnatally worked up and diagnosed as having PUV. He underwent fulguration at the age of 9 months. Presently, he passed urine in good stream on cue and *dribbled often* during crying/playing or before micturition.

USG KUB showed normal bladder with left-sided mild HDN.

Uroflowmetry (Fig. 19.4a) could be performed as he passed 100 ml urine in a good stream generating Qmax of 18 ml/sec which was supranormal for his age.

UDS was performed to identify the reason for urinary dribbling. UDS (Fig. 19.4b) showed a normal capacity bladder with normal compliance. Intermittent tonic overactivity was seen with pressures reaching 10–20 cm H2O when he was seen to leak a few drops of urine ('drop'/'leak' sign on UDS tracing) implying DO-LPP of 10 - 20 cm H2O. After 100 ml fill, suprapubic compresses were given to check for 'cough impulse'. He was seen to leak significant amounts of urine with abdominal compresses (marked on the tracing by black arrows) at abdominal pressures of 20 cm H2O (ALPP 20 cm H2O) denoting a very weak bladder outlet. Voiding phase has been highlighted by a black oval in the full tracing and shown in an expanded form separately (Fig. 19.4c). During voiding, he voided 80 ml of urine with normal detrusor pressures and flow rate.

The findings of supranormal Qmax on free-flow uroflowmetry, ALPP of 20 cm H2O and normal voiding detrusor pressures suggest a weak bladder outflow. He also had a significant element of detrusor overactivity. Weak bladder outlet with detrusor overactivity could be implicated as the cause of urinary leak based on the urodynamic findings. Review of his operative records showed that the baby had undergone BNI at the time of PUV fulguration.

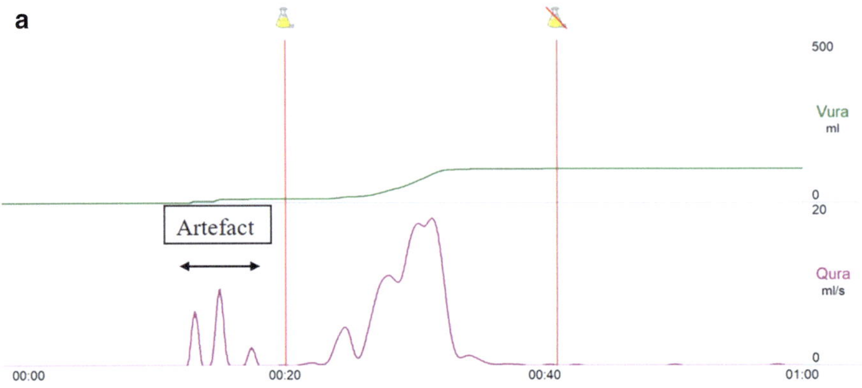

Parameter	Value
Voiding time	20.9s
Flow time	20s
Time to maximum flow	11.2s
Maximum flow rate	18.1ml/s
Volume at maximum flow	85ml
Mean flow rate	4.4ml/s
Total voided volume	92ml
Residual volume	10ml

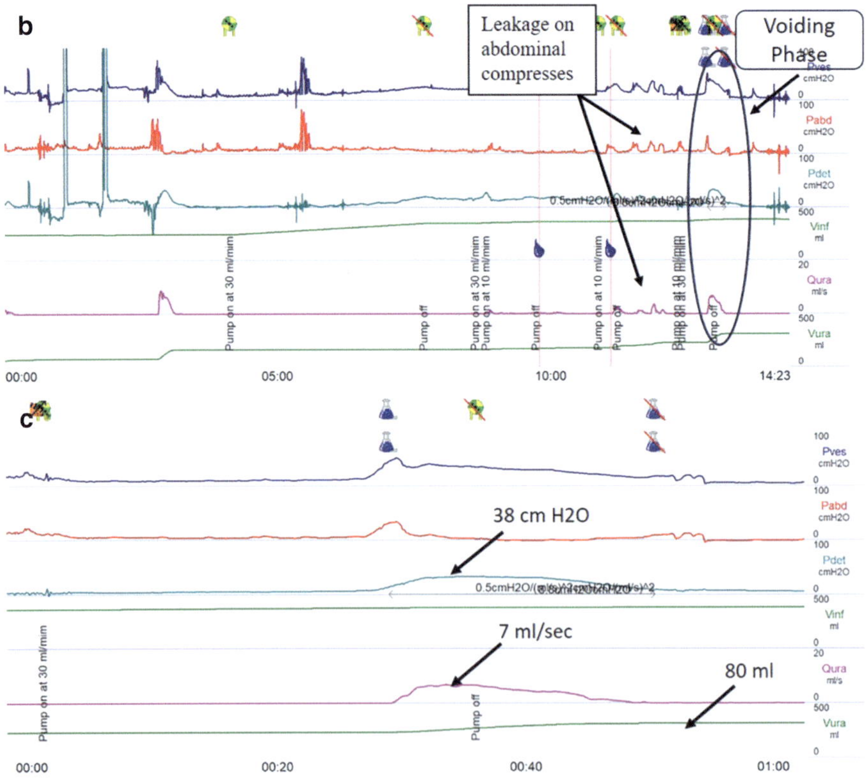

Fig. 19.4 (**a**) Uroflowmetry curve. (**b**) UDS curve. (**c**) Voiding phase of the UDS curve in an expanded form

Case 5: Presumed Myogenic Failure—Residual Valves

A 15-year-old male child, follow-up case of PUV, had undergone fulguration at the age of 10 days and check cystoscopy at the age of 4 years. He had had 3–4 episodes of UTI in the last 11 years. He passed urine normally in good stream. He had no urgency, increased frequency, incontinence, wetness of pants or enuresis.

USG KUB showed that he had bilateral gross HDUN. UB wall was mildly trabeculated and thickened. There was no PVR. Voiding diary showed 5–7 voids per day, usual volumes of 300 ml, maximum daytime volume of 400 ml and morning void of 450–500 ml.

Uroflowmetry (Fig. 19.5a) showed a weak flow with a plateau-shaped curve.

Bilateral HDUN with weak flow in a long-term follow-up case of PUV may indicate myogenic failure. But this child had normal capacity bladder (myogenic failure should have large capacity bladder), and the finding of thick-walled UB along with few episodes of UTIs suggested that he might be having an element of detrusor overactivity as well. So an invasive UDS was performed.

UDS (Fig. 19.5b) showed a normal capacity bladder with some overactivity after 250 ml fill. During voiding (Fig. 19.5c), flow rate was poor with high detrusor pressures reaching up to 50–60 cm H2O during periods of void with flow rates of 5–7 ml/sec (which was poor for the age) suggesting obstructed pressure flow relation. There was no straining during the void (no rise in abdominal pressure) which also points against myogenic failure. So the plateau curve on uroflowmetry was probably because of BOO and not myogenic failure. During voiding, the detrusor contraction was seen to be waxing-waning in nature which is usually seen in underactive detrusors. This child was probably having early decompensation due to longstanding outflow tract obstruction. To verify the findings, MCU was performed which showed a linear filling defect in the posterior urethra (Fig. 19.5d).

The child underwent cystoscopy which showed residual valves which had probably been missed at the check cystoscopy - these were incised. At 6 months follow up, bilateral HDUN had improved considerably and the flow rates (Fig. 19.5e) improved considerably.

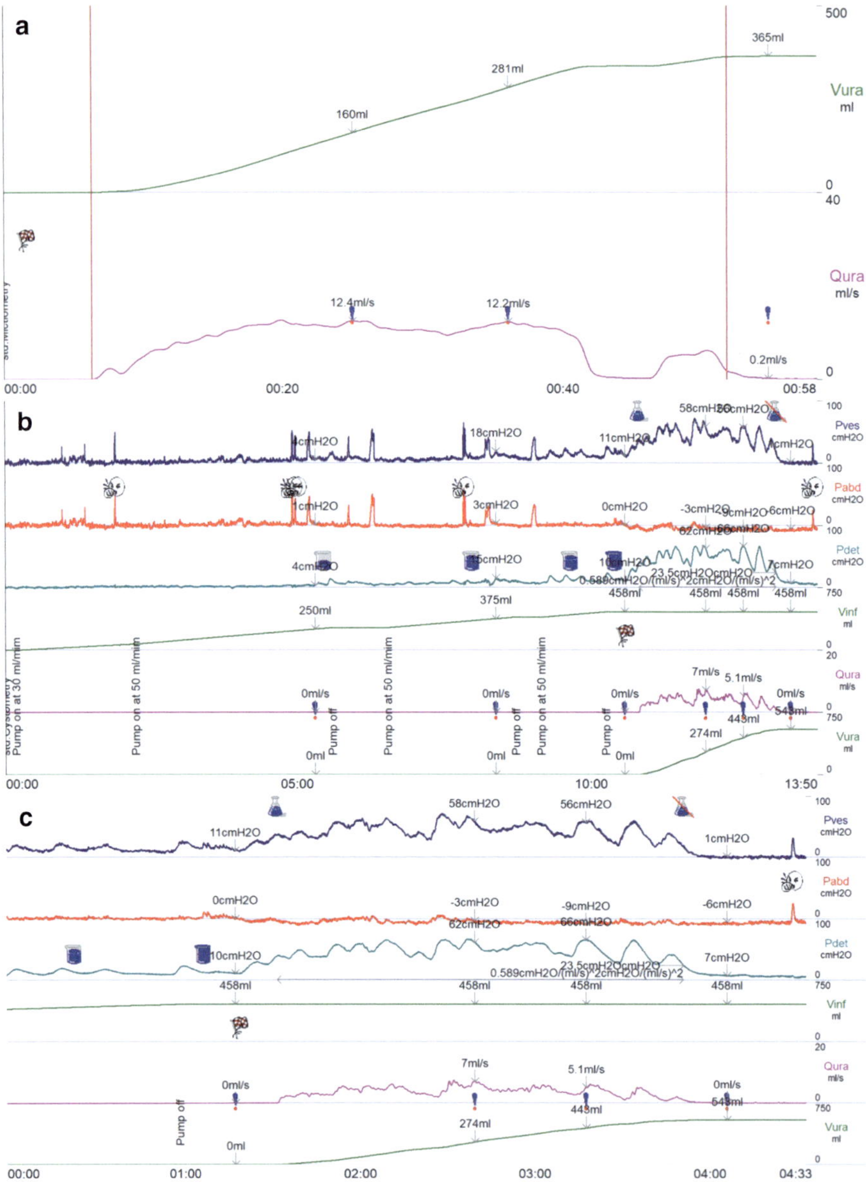

Fig. 19.5 (**a**) Uroflowmetry curve (at baseline). (**b**) UDS tracing. (**c**) Voiding phase of UDS in an expanded form. (**d**) MCU images. (**e**) Uroflowmetry tracing at 6 months follow up after the cystoscopy, the flow rates improved considerably

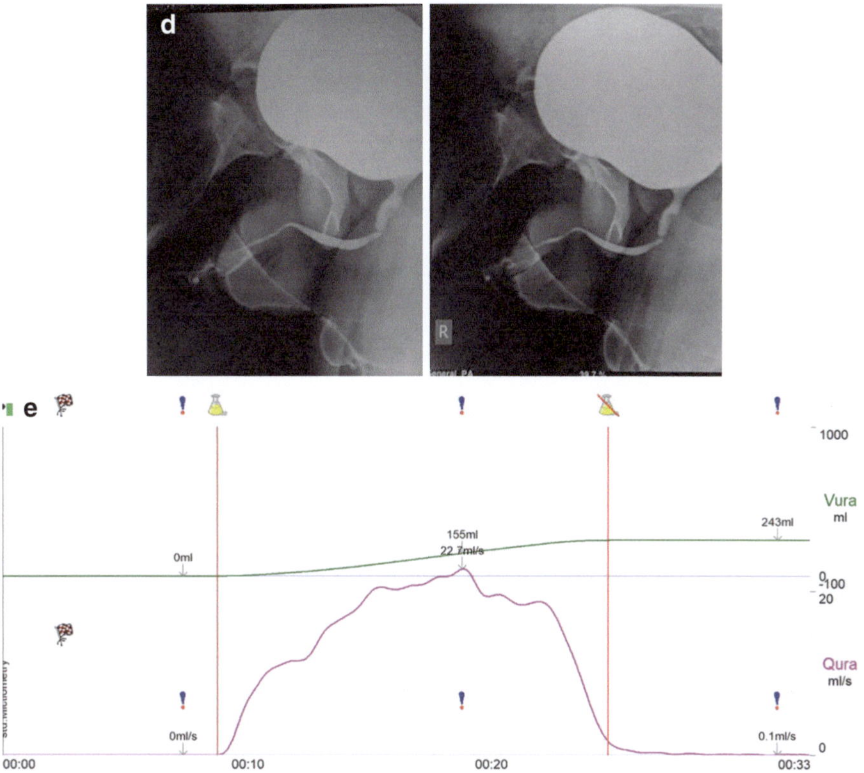

Fig. 19.5 (continued)

Case 6: Presumed Myogenic Failure—Bladder Neck Dysfunction

A 14-year-old boy, follow-up case of PUV, had undergone cystoscopy and fulguration at the age of 2 1/2 years and 6 months and check cystoscopy at the age of 5.5 years. He had been well after that with no history of UTIs and he passed urine normally.

USG showed bilateral HDUN and right APD being 44 mm and left being 24 mm; bladder wall was 3.7 mm thick and there was a PVR of 110 ml.

Voiding diary showed that he voided 8–9 times per day, usual voided volume was 200–300 ml, max daytime volume was 350 ml and urgency was present during voids >300 ml.

Uroflowmetry (Fig. 19.6a) showed an interrupted void with poor flow rates. He voided 160 ml in the primary flow and 25 ml in subsequent spurts. There was a PVR of 25 ml after the void.

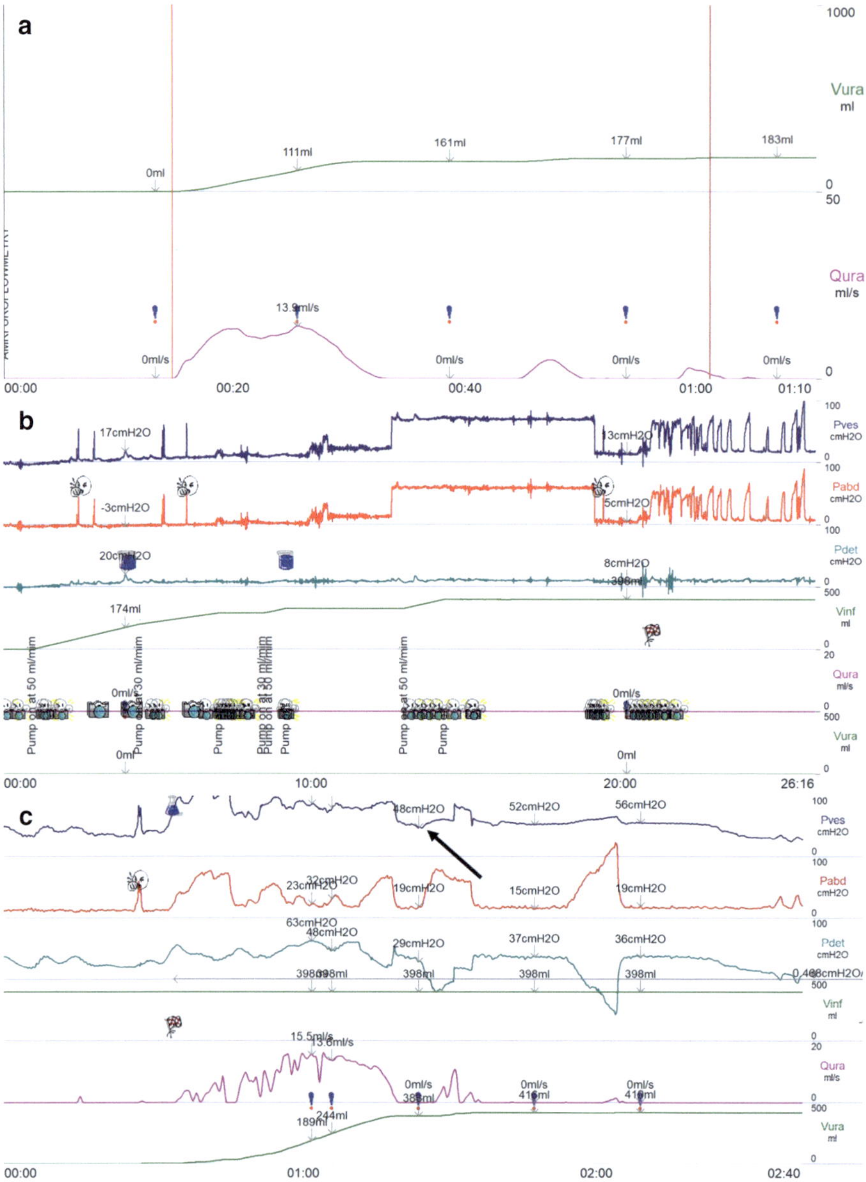

Fig. 19.6 (**a**) Uroflowmetry curve. (**b**) Filling phase of the video-UDS curve. (**c**) Voiding phase of the UDS curve in expanded form. The urethral catheter malfunctioned at the end of the primary void (black arrow) after which the vesical readings are absent. (**d**) Fluoroscopic images of voiding showing poor opening of bladder neck (black arrow). (**e**) Uroflowmetry curve at 2 months follow-up

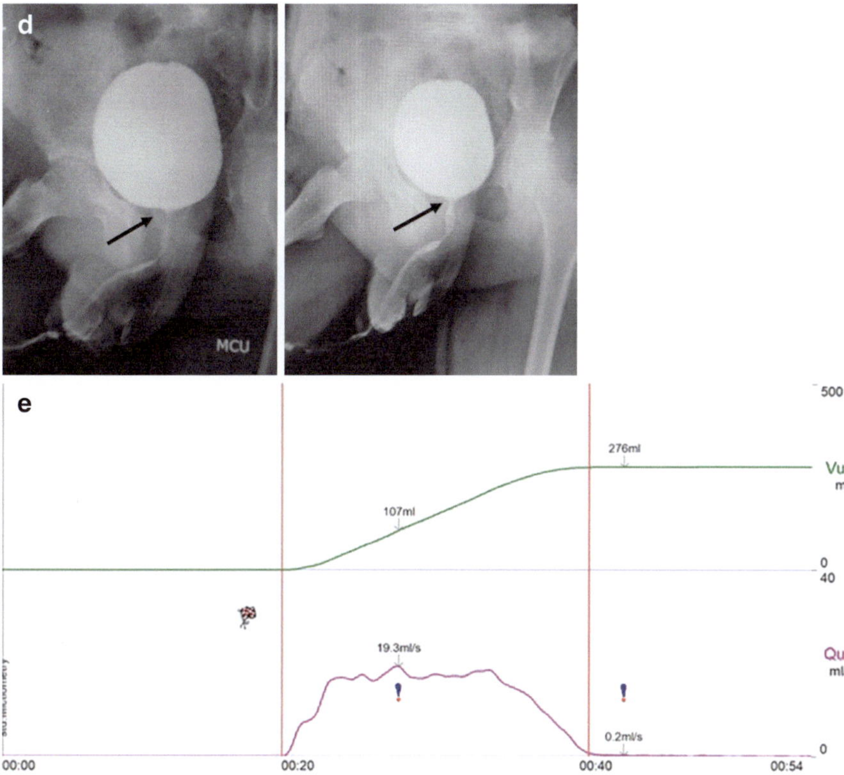

Fig. 19.6 (continued)

Bilateral HDUN with poor flow rates and significant PVR in a long-term follow-up patient of PUV suggested myogenic failure. But the bladder size as per the voiding diary appeared normal. He had urgency at volumes >300 ml, which did not fit with the diagnosis of myogenic failure or suggested probable detrusor overactivity.

He underwent video-UDS. UDS (Fig. 19.6b) showed normal capacity bladder with mildly reduced compliance (20 cm H2O at 500 ml) and mild overactivity after 100 ml filling. DO of intensity around 20 cm H2O was noted at 175 ml volume associated with urgency. This corroborated with his usual voided volumes of around 200 ml. He complained of urge to void from 175 ml fill onwards which he was able to control. He could tolerate fill up to 500 ml when he had significant urge to pass urine. Bladder was seen to be smooth walled and rounded in shape on fluoroscopic images.

During voiding (Fig. 19.6c), PdetQmax was seen to be around 60 cm H2O at Qmax of 15 ml suggesting normal contractility (BCI 135) and an equivocal pressure flow relation (BOOI 30). He passed 380 ml of urine in the primary void and 25 ml in the subsequent voids with a PVR of 75 ml. Some straining was also noted during the void.

In this patient, voiding detrusor pressures are normal suggesting good contractile strength of the bladder which points against myogenic failure. At the same time,

PVR was probably caused due to inadequate duration of detrusor contraction suggesting some element of detrusor underactivity which also explains the straining seen during voiding and poor flow rates seen on free-flow uroflowmetry. Thus, this UDS shows evidence of probable long-standing outflow obstruction with early decompensation.

Voiding fluoroscopic images (Fig. 19.6d) showed normal appearance of urethra but poor opening of bladder neck. Corroborating this finding with UDS finding, it was inferred that he had bladder neck dysfunction and was started on alpha-blockers. At 2 months follow-up, his flow rates had improved significantly (Fig. 19.6e) and upper tract dilatation and PVR on USG had reduced considerably (right APD 44 mm → 18.4 mm; left APD 24 mm → 18 mm; PVR 100 ml → 15 ml).

Functional Bladder Problems

Most of the functional bladder problems can be diagnosed and managed appropriately based on findings on non-invasive investigations, i.e., proper history, voiding diary, USG and uroflowmetry with or with EMG (single channel or double channel). Role of *i*-UDS in functional bladder problems is controversial and limited to therapy-resistant cases with refractory symptoms.

The nomenclature used for identifying functional bladder problems have been laid down by ICCS, the details of which is outside the purview of this book.

We have listed a few cases of functional bladder problems where the diagnosis was obscure and the UDS findings guided the further management.

Case 1: Sensory Urgency

A 7-year-old male child presented with increased frequency of micturition and urgency since the last 5 months. He passed urine every 10–15 minutes. There was no history of incontinence, straining or interrupted stream. There were no nocturnal symptoms or enuresis. He had history of constipation and had been started on stool softeners since the last 3 months with partial improvement in urinary symptoms.

USG KUB showed normal study.

Uroflowmetry (Fig. 19.7a) showed an obstructed flow with Qmax of 9 ml sec for a flow of 300 ml; uroflowmetry was repeated with EMG (Fig. 19.7b) 11 ml/sec for a flow of 200 ml; EMG activity was silent during void but increased at the end of the void. There was no PVR after the void.

He was suspected of having bladder outflow obstruction in view of poor flow rates in absence of EMG activity and features suggestive of overactive bladder and MCUG was performed.

MCU (Fig. 19.7c) showed smooth-walled, rounded bladder with normal appearance of urethra and bladder neck—ruling out BOO. He underwent UDS to rule out underactive detrusor.

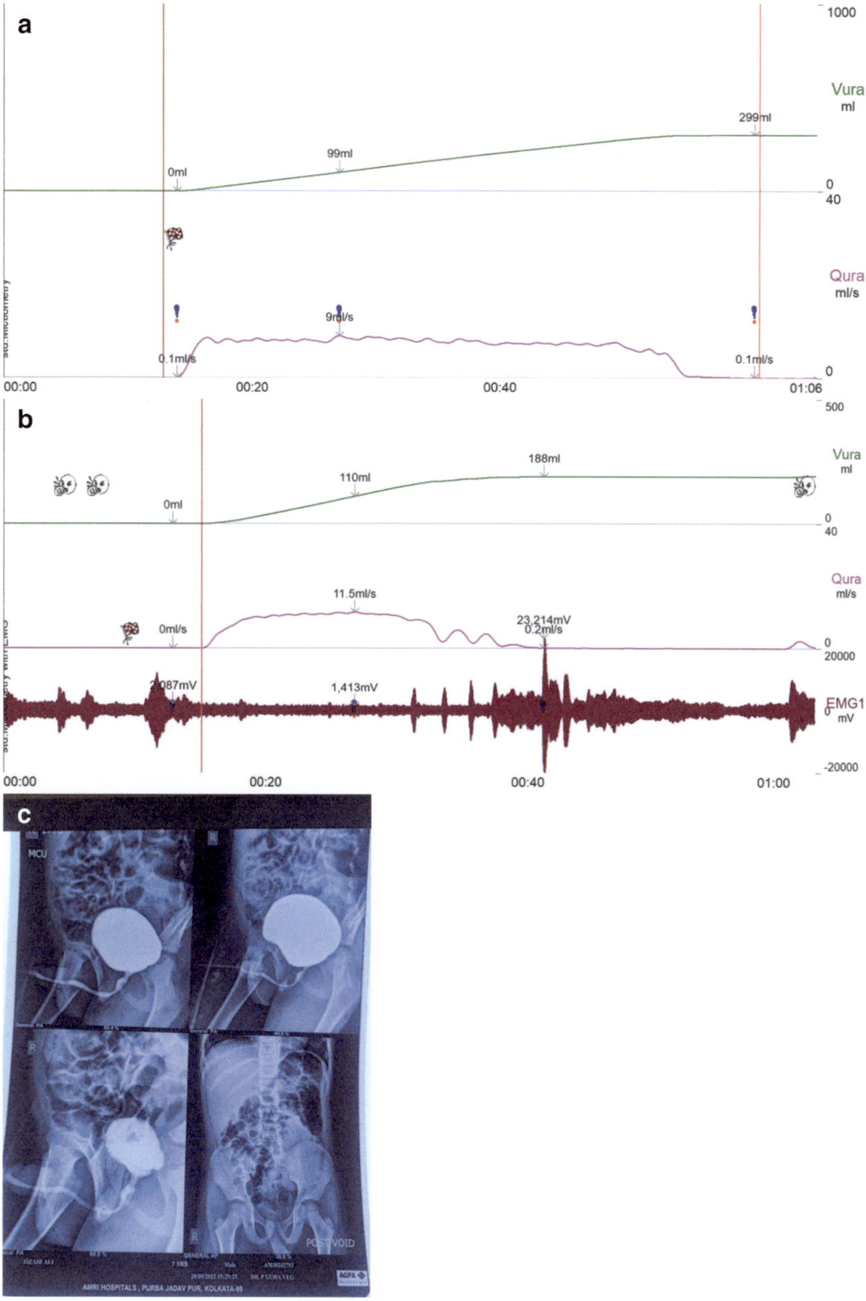

Fig. 19.7 (**a**) Uroflowmetry curve. (**b**) Uroflowmetry with EMG. (**c**) MCU images. (**d**) UDS tracing. (**e**) Voiding portion of the UDS curve shown in expanded form

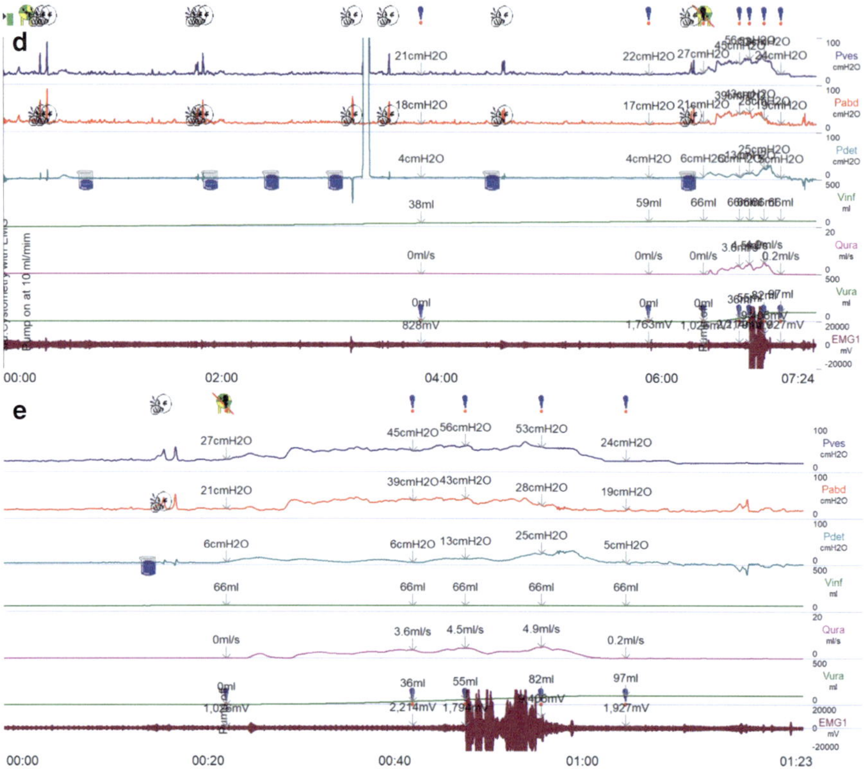

Fig. 19.7 (continued)

UDS (Fig. 19.7d, e) showed a small capacity but stable bladder with no overactivity and normal compliance. He complained of urge to void from beginning of fill in the absence of any overactivity or detrusor pressure rise ('sensory urgency') but allowed the fill to continue if he was distracted. During voiding, the observed flow rates were poor and the detrusor pressures were also low suggestive of low-pressure-low-flow state, i.e., underactive detrusor. Significant straining was noted during voiding which corroborates with detrusor underactivity. EMG activity was seen to increase transiently during voiding which may be artefactual due to straining.

Thus, the child had daytime-only increased urinary frequency without any history of incontinence suggestive of pollakiuria. He showed a poor/obstructive pattern on uroflowmetry and features of 'sensory urgency' with detrusor underactivity on UDS. We have seen similar UDS findings in children with pollakiuria or in children who have rectal loading, and the symptoms improve once aggressive management of constipation is instituted.

Case 2: Genital/Suprapubic Pain

A 12-year-old girl presented with history of two documented episodes of UTI in the last 1 year and distressing pain in the genitals and suprapubic region on and off since the last 3 months. Lower abdominal pain was colicky, starting before micturition, continuing during micturition and lasting for 5–10 minutes after micturition. There was history of occasional straining, hesitancy and sense of incomplete evacuation. She had history of primary enuresis till the age of 10 years.

USG KUB showed bilateral mild pelvic fullness, bladder wall thickness of 4 mm and a PVR of 19 ml. Voiding diary showed 5–7 voids per day, 350–400 ml, maximum daytime volume 500 ml and urgency at volumes >350 ml. Voiding diary showed that she had difficulty in initiating urinary stream and complained of pain during passing urine at each void.

Uroflowmetry (Fig. 19.8a) showed good forceful stream with increased EMG activity showing DV. This was corroborated on MCU (Fig. 19.8b) which showed spin top urethra. Sphincteric/perineal muscle spasm could explain the occurrence of genital pain, but the present evidence did not provide explanation for suprapubic pain. So she underwent UDS.

UDS (Fig. 19.8c) showed a normal capacity bladder (500 ml) with normal compliance. Intermittent mild overactivity was seen with pressures reaching 10 cm H2O. She

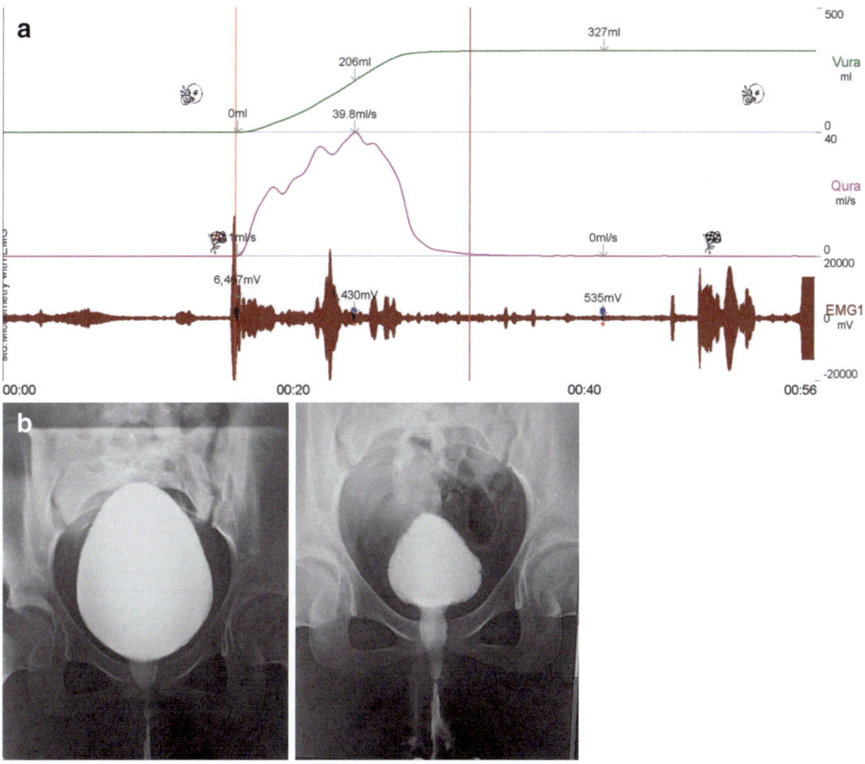

Fig. 19.8 (**a**) Uroflow curve. (**b**) MCU images. (**c**) UDS tracing. (**d**) Voiding phase of the UDS curve in an expanded form

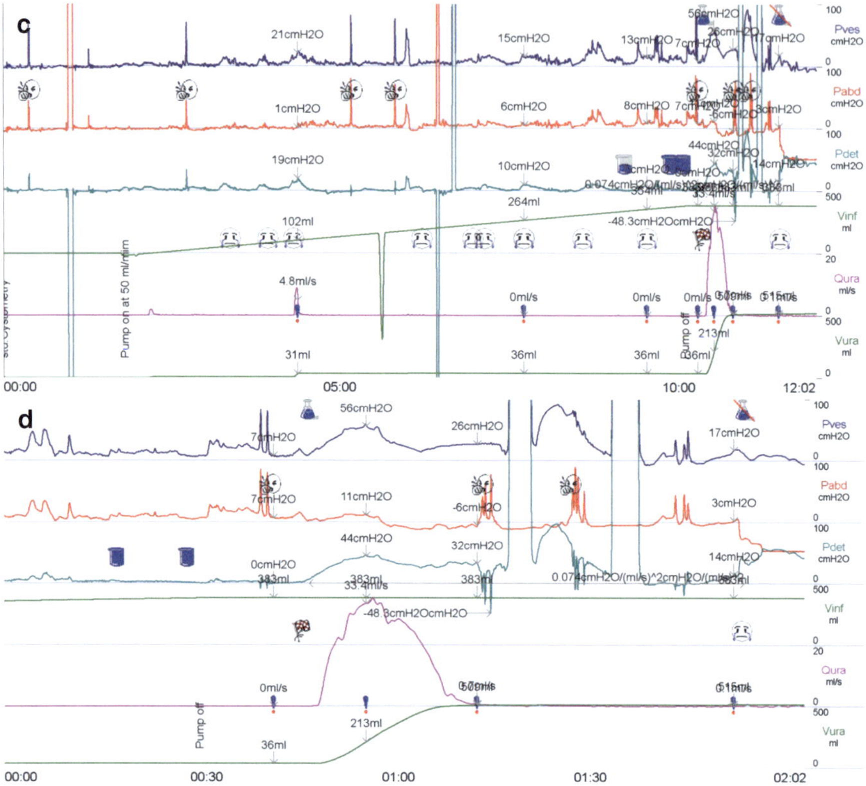

Fig. 19.8 (continued)

complained of suprapubic pain during each episode of DO (marked by 'cry' sign). During voiding (Fig 19.8d), flow rate was good, but there was evidence of raised voiding detrusor pressures. Significant after contraction was also noted. She complained of suprapubic pain during the strong voiding detrusor contraction and the after contraction as well. Thus the cause of suprapubic pain was detrusor overactivity contractions during filling and strong after-contraction after voiding.

She was started on aggressive management of constipation, pelvic floor relaxation exercises and mirabegron. At 2 weeks follow-up, her pain episodes had improved significantly.

Case 3: Primary Detrusor Overactivity Presenting as Enuresis

An 11-years old male child presented with complaints of primary enuresis 2–3 times per night. Parents and the child denied any daytime symptoms. He passed urine in good stream with no history of hesitancy, straining or sense of incomplete evacuation. Passed stools daily.

USG KUB showed normal upper tracts and bladder with insignificant PVR.

The parents couldn't maintain a voiding diary.

During uroflowmetry (Fig. 19.9a) he passed 160 ml of urine when he had severe urge. Flow rates were very good, generating a tower-shaped curve. This was suggestive of detrusor overactivity.

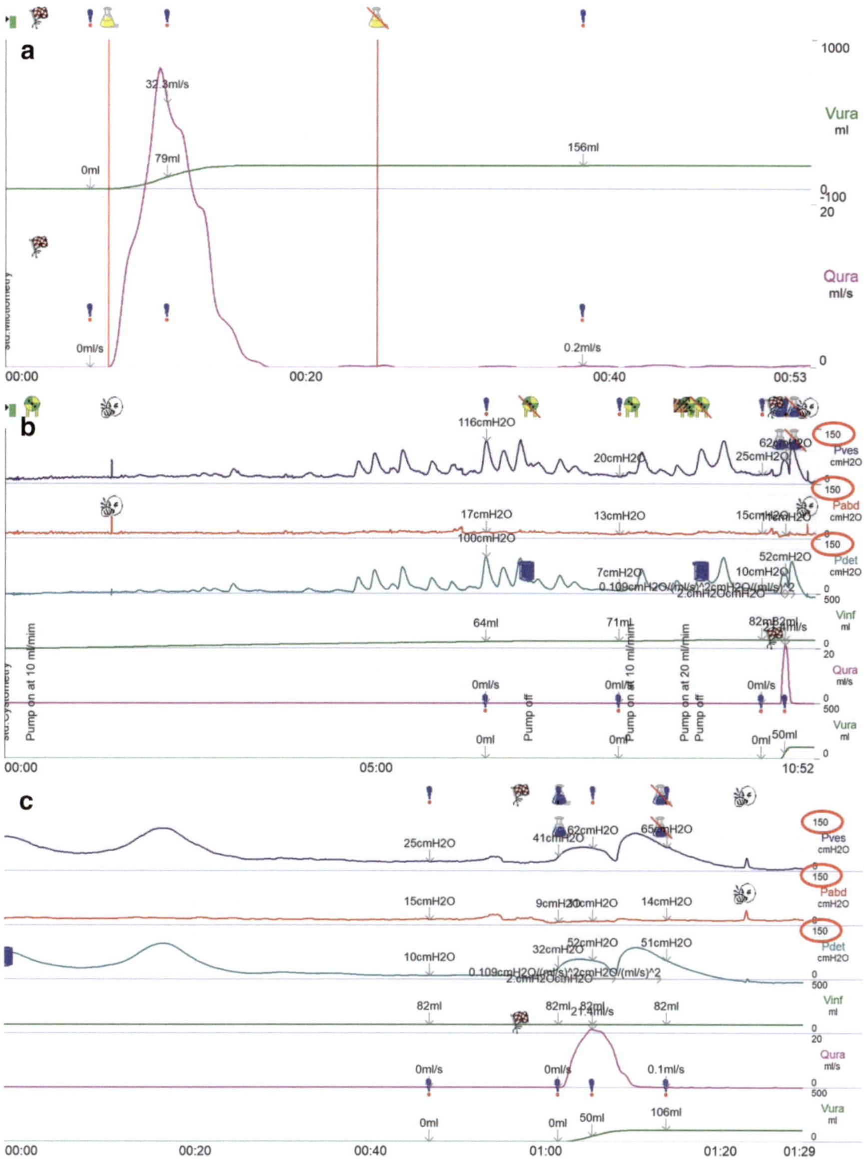

Fig. 19.9 (**a**) Uroflowmetry showing tower-shaped curve. (**b**) UDS tracing showing severe overactivity with small capacity bladder—filling stopped at 80 ml. Note that the pressure limits are set at 150 cm H2O (highlighted by red oval) rather than the usual 100 cm H2O, as the detrusor pressures during the episodes of DO cross 100 cm H2O and would have otherwise moved out of the range covered in the print. (**c**) UDS tracing—voiding phase in an expanded form. Note that the pressure limit is set at 150 cm H2O (highlighted by red oval) rather than the usual 100 cm H2O. (**d**) MCU images

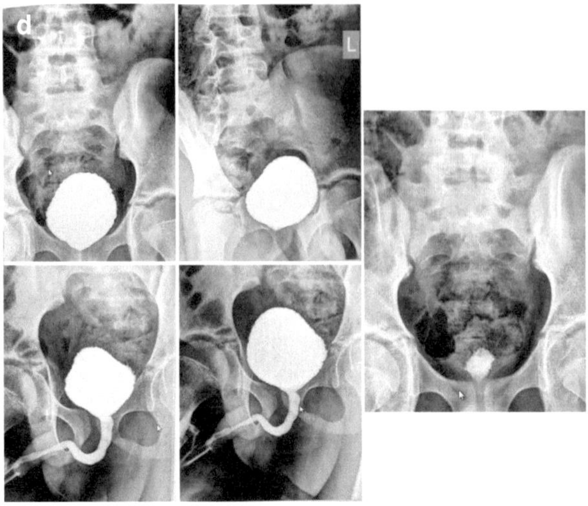

Fig. 19.9 (continued)

When the parents were asked again, they gave history suggestive of daytime urgency and occasional urge incontinence (frequent episodes of daytime wetting till 7 years of age).

The available information was suggestive of probable detrusor overactivity, but as the child had complaints since beginning, UDS + MCU was planned to look for any other anatomical abnormalities.

UDS (Fig. 19.9b) revealed a small capacity bladder with normal compliance and severe detrusor overactivity without any urgency. During voiding (Fig 19.9c), Pdet Qmax was 50 cm H2O which seemed higher than pdetQmax usually seen in cases with no outflow obstruction, but the Qmax was also high (22 ml/sec); BOOI = 8 → unobstructed outflow; BCI = 160 → supranormal detrusor contraction. Thus, the raised detrusor pressure during voiding was not because of high outflow resistance, but it was primary due to the detrusor overactivity and forceful detrusor contraction generating supranormal flow rates. There was no PVR after the void.

MCU findings (Fig. 19.9d) corroborated with UDS findings—small bladder with crenated outline, widely open bladder neck and well-distended urethra during voiding because of strong detrusor contraction with no evidence of outflow tract obstruction.

He was diagnosed as having primary detrusor overactivity and started on mirabegron with relief of symptoms.

Case 4: Primary Detrusor Overactivity Presenting as Recurrent UTI

A 2.6-year-old girl presented with episodes of recurrent febrile UTI in the last 6 months. She had no voiding complaints, passed urine every 1–2 hours and informed before passing urine. Although she was very young, but still she had no history of enuresis in the last 8 months. USG showed a normal study.

MCU (Fig. 19.10a) done elsewhere showed normal bladder and urethra with no reflux.

She had some history of constipation which was considered to be the cause of UTIs and she was started on stool softeners and uroprophylaxis. She had an episode of breakthrough UTI in the next 2 months when she was started on rectal washes for constipation. She had complete compliance with the medicines and rectal washes but had yet another episode of UTI in the next month when she was taken up for UDS.

Uroflowmetry (Fig. 19.10b) showed good flow rates with no PVR. The flow rates were high for the age and voided volume raising the suspicion of detrusor overactivity.

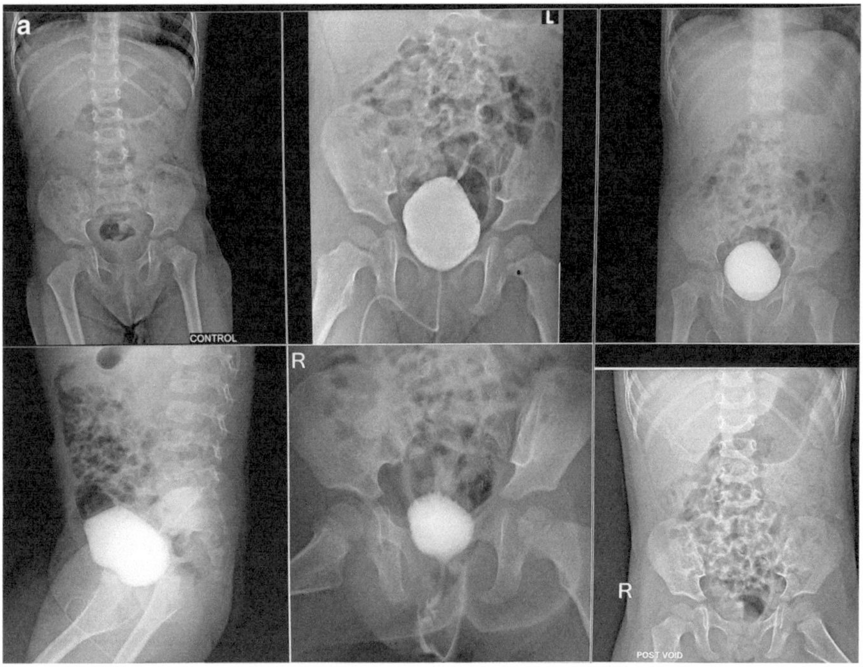

Fig. 19.10 (**a**) MCU image. (**b**) Uroflowmetry image. This tracing shows a time span of 18 seconds instead of the standard 1 min. Thus, the flow curve is stretched and appears to be bell shaped instead of tower shaped. (**c**) UDS tracing

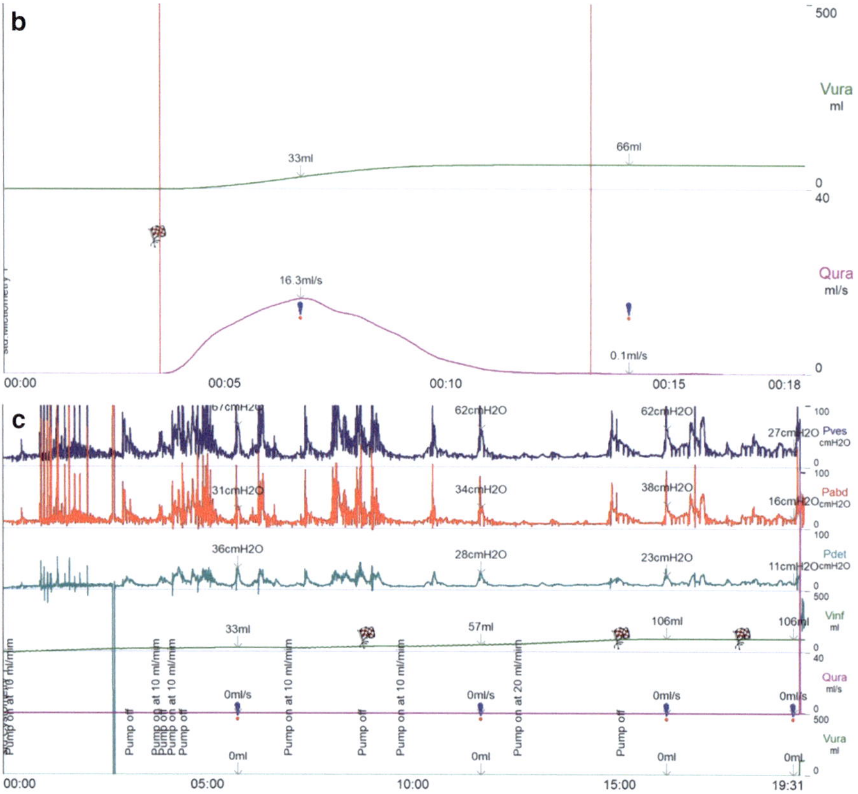

Fig. 19.10 (continued)

UDS (Fig. 19.10c) showed a normal capacity bladder with significant overactivity throughout the study (pressures reaching 25–35 cm H2O). Voiding phase could not be evaluated as the child did not void with the catheter in the urethra.

She was started on anticholinergics and did not have any further UTIs in the next 6 months.

So this child had detrusor overactivity which was suggested by uroflowmetry and was evident only on urodynamic evaluation, although there were no clinical or radiological manifestations other than recurrent UTI. She was started on Oxybutinin and continued on bowel management. She did not have any UTIs in the next 1 year of follow up.

Case 5: Non-neurogenic Neurogenic Bladder—DO with Inefficient Voiding

A 6-year-old girl presented with history of repeated episodes of UTI since the last 1 year. There was history of holding manoeuvres, Vincent's curtsy, urgency and urge incontinence since the last 1.5 years. She had continuous wetness of pants during the day and primary enuresis. She had habitual constipation since childhood.

Voiding diary showed that she voided 10 times per day, usual volumes of 60–90 ml, maximum daytime volume of 180 ml and several episodes of leakages.

USG KUB showed bilateral mild ureteric dilatation with thickened and trabeculated UB wall and a PVR of 55 ml.

She had undergone an MCU elsewhere which showed an irregular bladder wall with spin top appearance of bladder (Fig. 19.11a).

She was started on bowel management, urotherapy, abdominal breathing exercises and alpha-blockers. Biofeedback could not be done as the child was not cooperative. UDS was planned when there was no change in symptoms after 2 months of conservative therapy. She passed small volumes of urine during uroflowmetry, so the findings were unreliable. UDS (Fig. 19.11b) showed a small capacity bladder (complained of urge at 100 ml), normal compliance, significant overactivity (after 50 ml fill, with pressures reaching 25–50 cm H2O), urgency during periods of severe overactivity and leak of small amounts of urine during strong detrusor contractions. During attempted voiding (Fig. 19.11c), strong, but ill-sustained, detrusor contractions were seen with small spurts of void. After each small void, she passed another spurt of urine on coaxing. She voided a total of 150 ml of urine in small spurts of 20–40 ml each time and could empty the bladder.

Thus, this child had a severely overactive bladder during filling with detrusor underactivity during voiding (voiding detrusor contraction of insufficient duration) resulting in significant PVR and recurrent UTIs. She underwent cystoscopy with Botox injection at external sphincter, but her symptoms continued. So she was diagnosed as having NNNB and advised anticholinergics along with CIC.

Fig. 19.11 (**a**) MCU images. (**b**) UDS tracing. (**c**) Voiding phase of the UDS tracing in an expanded form

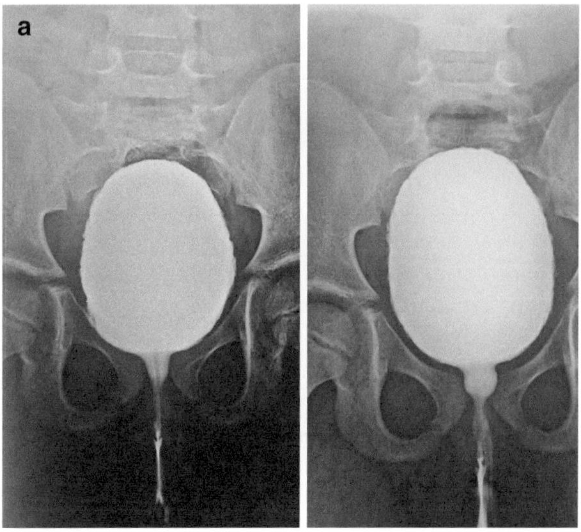

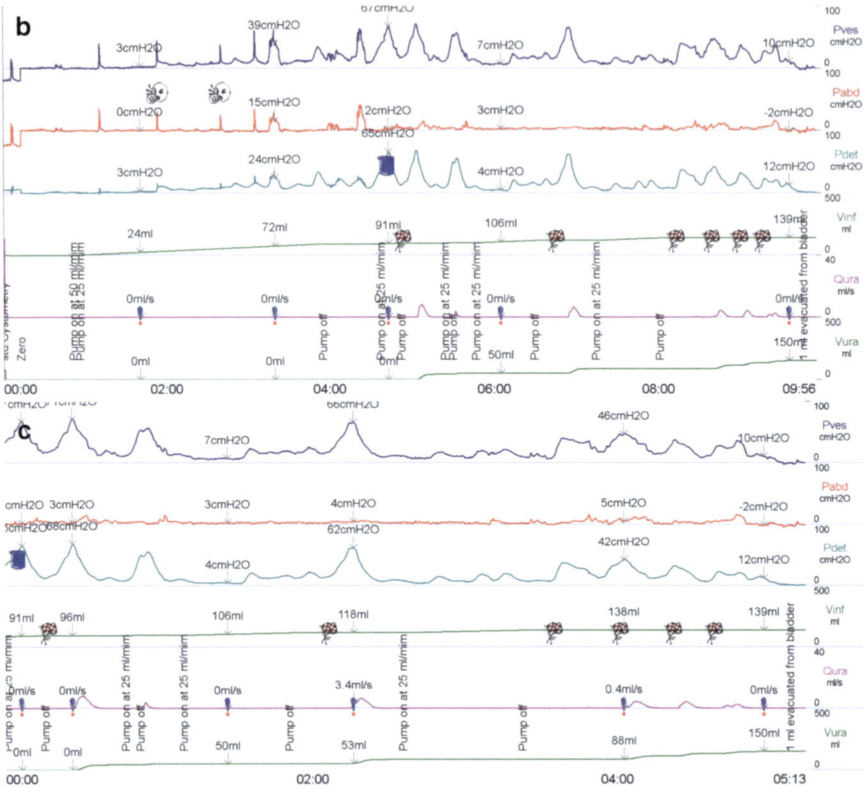

Fig. 19.11 (continued)

Case 6: Non-neurogenic Neurogenic Bladder—DO with Bladder Neck Dysfunction

A 3.6-year-old female child was a follow-up case of right grade V VUR with hydroureteronephrosis with non-functioning right kidney and recurrent/persistent UTI She had undergone right nephrectomy with end ureterostomy of distal stump of right ureter at the age of 6 months. Presently, she passed urine primarily through the ureterostomy, intermittently passed small amounts of urine per urethrally and occasionally reported urge to pass urine. She passed stools normally.

USG showed normal bladder with normal left kidney.

Video-UDS was performed to decide whether right ureterostomy could be closed off. Child did not pass urine for uroflowmetry.

During UDS (Fig. 19.12a), contrast was seen to leak through the ureterostomy after 20 ml fill, after which it was kept occluded by digital compression. The bladder was seen to be stable with no overactivity till 100 ml fill; baseline detrusor pressures increased up to 10 cm H2O at 100 ml denoting mildly reduced compliance. At 120 ml and 160 ml fill, waves of strong detrusor contraction were seen

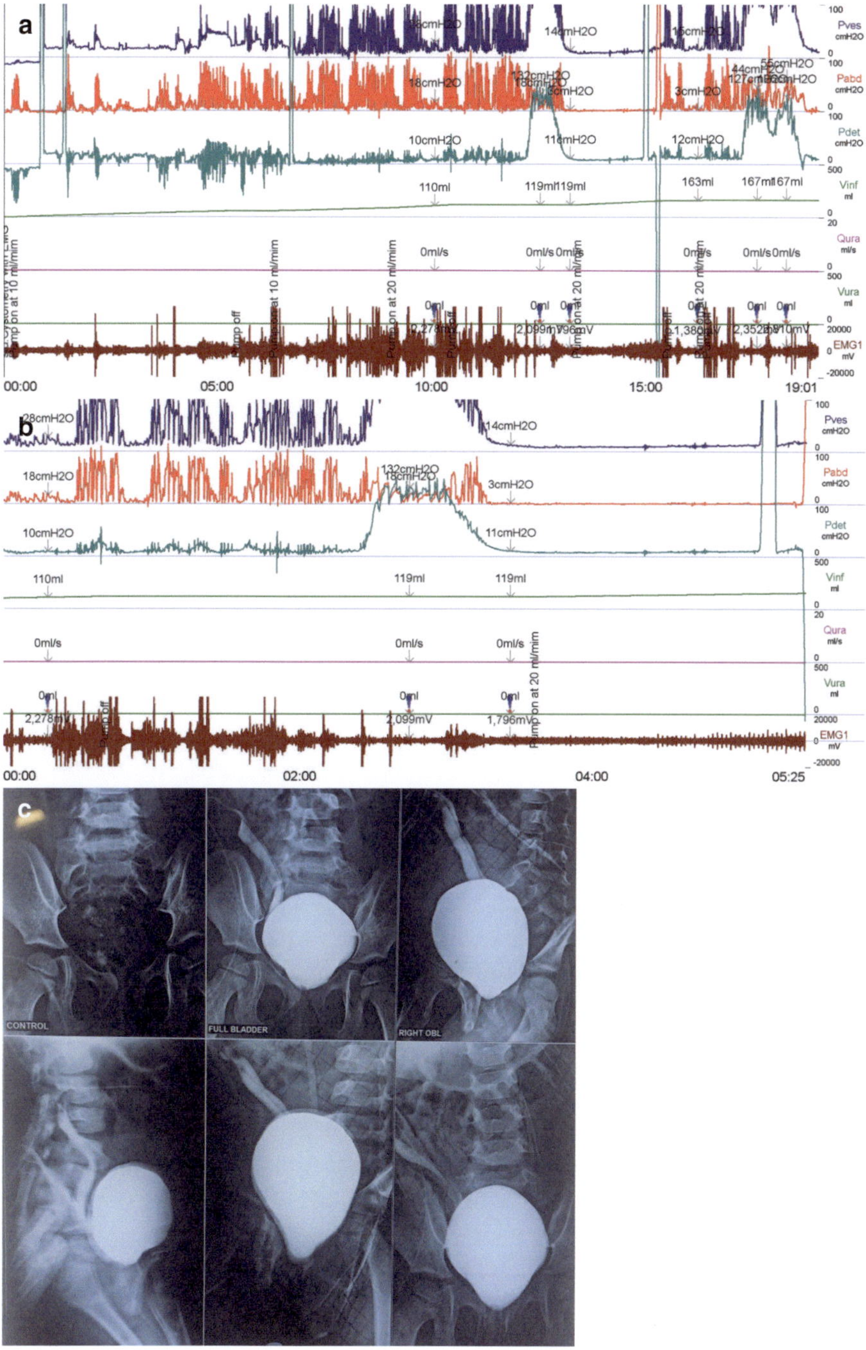

Fig. 19.12 (**a**) UDS tracing. (**b**) Suspected voiding contraction in an expanded form. (**c**) MCU images obtained during video-UDS. (**d**) UDS tracing. 'Leak'/'drop' mark demonstrates the point where leak/reflux was noted through the ureterostomy after which it was kept occluded. (**e**) Voiding contraction in an expanded form

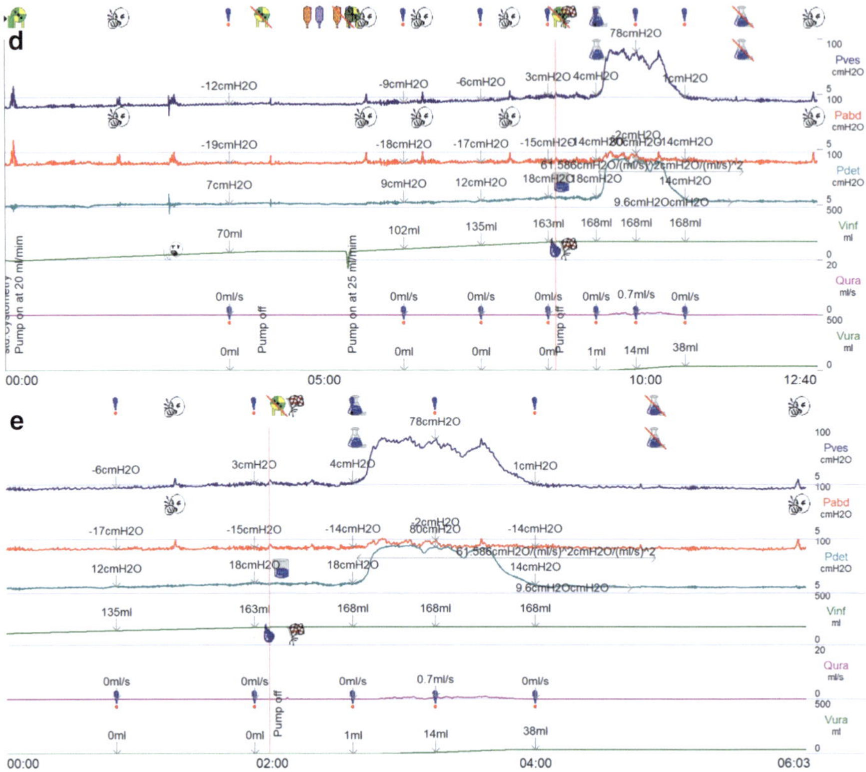

Fig. 19.12 (continued)

(Fig. 19.12b) with pressures reaching 100–130 cm H2O with passage of very small amount of urine. Voided volume is not recorded as the study was performed in supine position. On fluoroscopic screening (Fig. 19.12c), right gross VUR was recorded from 20 ml fill onwards. During the strong detrusor contractions, small amount of urine was seen to be passed perurethrally, but bladder neck was not seen to open appropriately and urethra could not be demonstrated.

These contractions were presumed to be voiding detrusor contractions, but the child did not void—either due to voluntary withholding or due to bladder neck dysfunction, which could not be confirmed due to young age of child. Under usual circumstances also, as the child passed urine primarily through the stoma and occasionally per urethrally, probability of bladder dysfunction was more likely. Ureterostomy was retained and she was started on alpha-blockers.

She underwent cystoscopy which revealed a tortuous urethra with abnormal appearance of bladder neck. Botox injection was given at the bladder neck after which per-urethral urine output increased to some extent.

At 5 years of age, she was passing urine intermittently per urethrally. She could feel the urge to pass urine, passed small amounts of urine perurethrally by straining and felt the urge to defecate while passing urine. Repeat UDS (Fig. 19.12d) was performed at the age of 5 years. Bladder capacity was seen to be 220 ml (filled up till 160 ml, voided 40 ml with PVR 180 ml). Detrusor pressures reached 18 cm H2O at 165 ml suggesting reduced compliance, and reflux/leak through ureterostomy was noted at 18 cm H2O pressures at 165 ml volume after which it was kept occluded. Child felt uncomfortable at 165 ml fill and voided urine. During voiding (Fig 19.12 d), strong voiding detrusor contraction was noted with pressures reaching 80 cm H2O and passage of 40 ml of urine in a poor stream with a PVR of 180 ml. Thus, she had an obstructed outflow with high pressure-poor flow during void with significant PVR which corroborated the previous UDS findings. MRI spine was normal. She was diagnosed as having NNNB and advised CIC through the ureterostomy.

Bladder Dysfunction Associated with Neurodevelopmental Problems

Down Syndrome

Bladder dysfunction/incontinence is seen frequently in individuals with Down syndrome. Involvement of LUT can range from innocuous incontinence/enuresis to florid NNNB. In individuals with Down syndrome, features of pelvic floor spasticity with NNNB have been reported more frequently in boys than in girls. Coexistence of anatomical abnormalities like PUV or neural tube defects have also been reported. Functional BOO in cases of Down syndrome more often require operative interventions as compliance with behavioural and other conservative therapies is an issue.

Case 1: Down with Bladder Neck Dysfunction

A 3.9-year-old male boy, diagnosed as trisomy 21, presented with difficulty in passing urine, severe straining and crying with poor urinary stream. He had three episodes of febrile UTI. USG showed right moderate HDN with left small kidney; bladder wall was normal, but there was a PVR of 110 ml. An MCU had been done elsewhere which showed a smooth-walled, rounded bladder, but urethra was not visualised.

Child strained significantly during uroflowmetry (Fig. 19.13a) and produced a weak interrupted stream with 40 ml PVR. USG and uroflow findings suggested either an underactive bladder or significant element of dysfunctional voiding.

UDS (Fig. 19.13b) revealed a bladder capacity of 180 ml (EBC 150 ml) with mild to moderate overactivity during one of the studies, no overactivity during the second study and mildly reduced compliance (10 cm H2O at 180 ml). Child strained significantly during voiding with very high detrusor pressures and poor flow rates (2.8 ml/sec at 128 cm H2O) suggestive of BOO. There was some increase in EMG activity during voiding, but that can be attributed to artefact caused by straining. He underwent cystoscopy which revealed a very prominent bladder neck, no evidence of PUV and very prominent sphincteric impression. He was started on alpha-blockers and the dose was titrated based on response and tolerability. He improved symptomatically. At 2 years follow-up, he had no voiding complaints, USG changes had improved and uroflowmetry pattern (Fig. 19.13c) was significantly better.

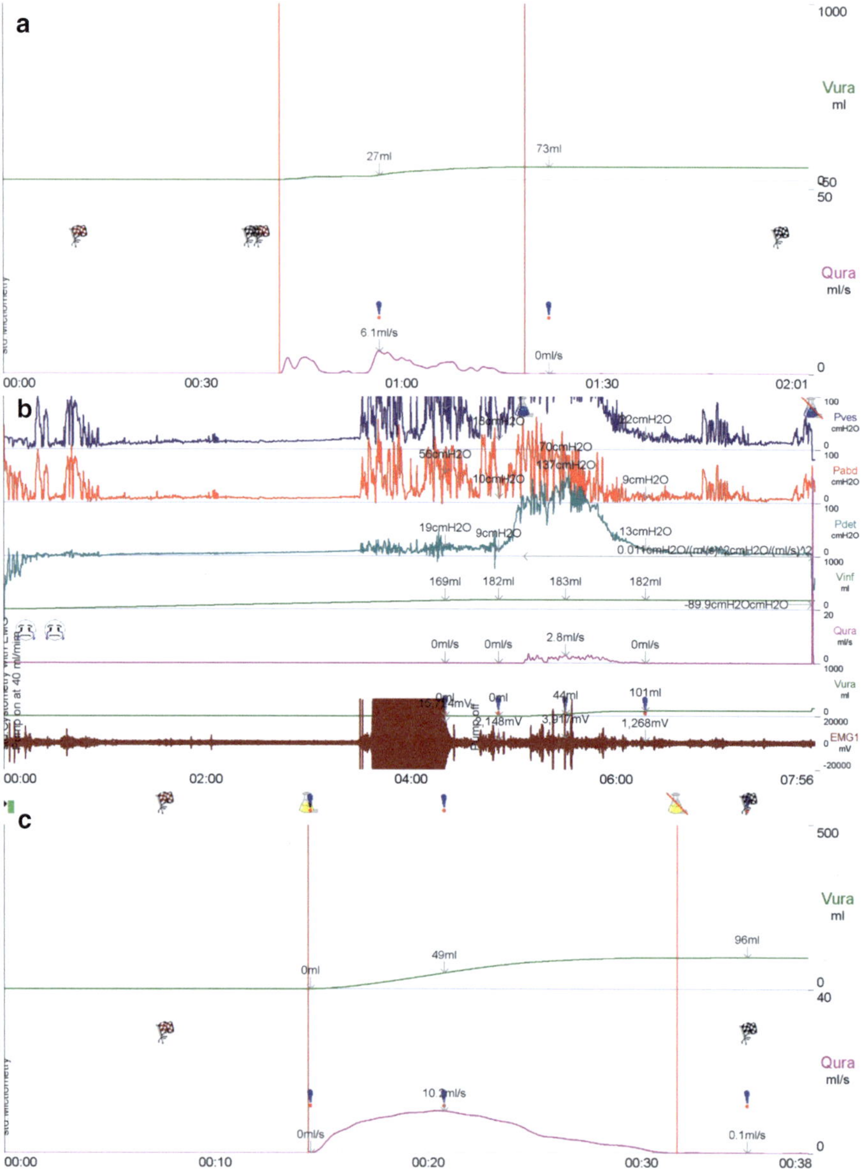

Fig. 19.13 (**a**) Uroflowmetry image. (**b**) UDS tracing. (**c**) Follow-up uroflowmetry image

Case 2: Down with Variable Voiding Pattern

A 2-year-old male child, known case of trisomy 21, presented with variable urinary stream, straining while passing urine and dribbling of urine with two episodes of UTI in the last 2 months. He had variable urinary frequency ranging from once every 15 minutes to once in 7 hours. There was history suggestive of voiding

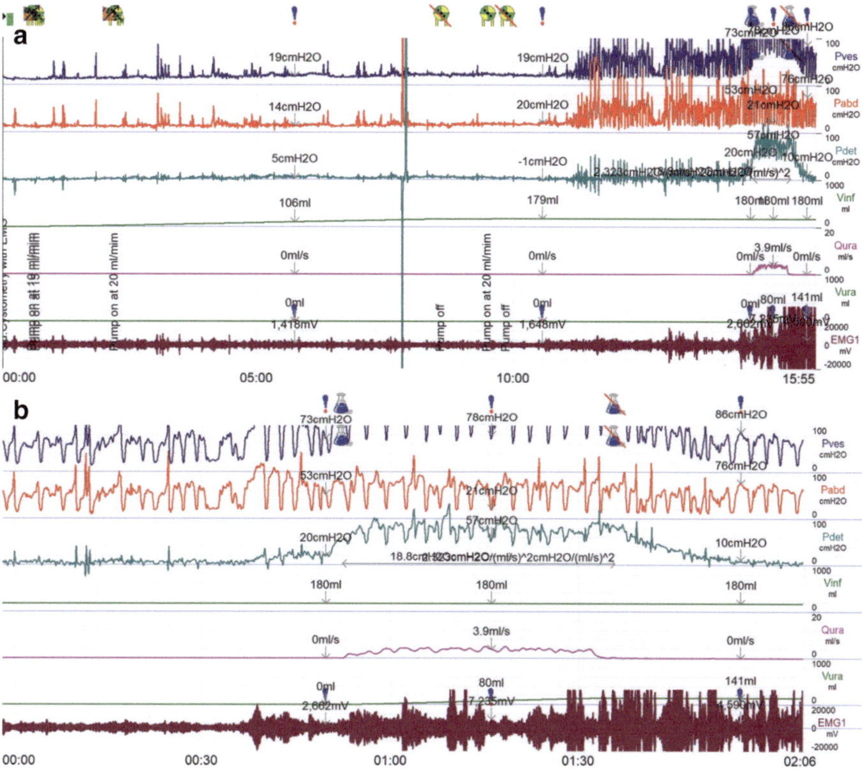

Fig. 19.14 (**a**) UDS tracing. (**b**) Voiding phase of the UDS tracing in an expanded form

postponement and he did not void on cues. USG showed thick-walled trabeculated bladder with mild left lower ureteric dilatation. MCU showed elongated irregular bladder with left grade V VUR and normal appearance of urethra. Due to the variability of urinary pattern, anatomical outflow obstruction seemed unlikely.

UDS (Fig. 19.14a) showed large capacity bladder (180 ml; EBC 90 ml) with mild overactivity towards end of fill (which may be considered physiological). During voiding (Fig. 19.14b), the flow rate was poor (around 4 ml/sec) with relatively high detrusor pressures and increased EMG activity during voiding suggesting probably dysfunctional element.

Because of the variability in voiding behaviour, he was thought to have a central component to his bladder dysfunction. He was started on clonidine and improved significantly.

Case 3: Down with VUR

A 1.3-year-old girl, known case of trisomy 21, had no voiding symptoms. She had an episode of UTI at the age of 1 year. USG KUB revealed bilateral HDUN with thick-walled UB and significant PVR. MCU (Fig. 19.15a) revealed mildly elongated bladder with bilateral grade IV–V VUR and poor visualisation of urethra.

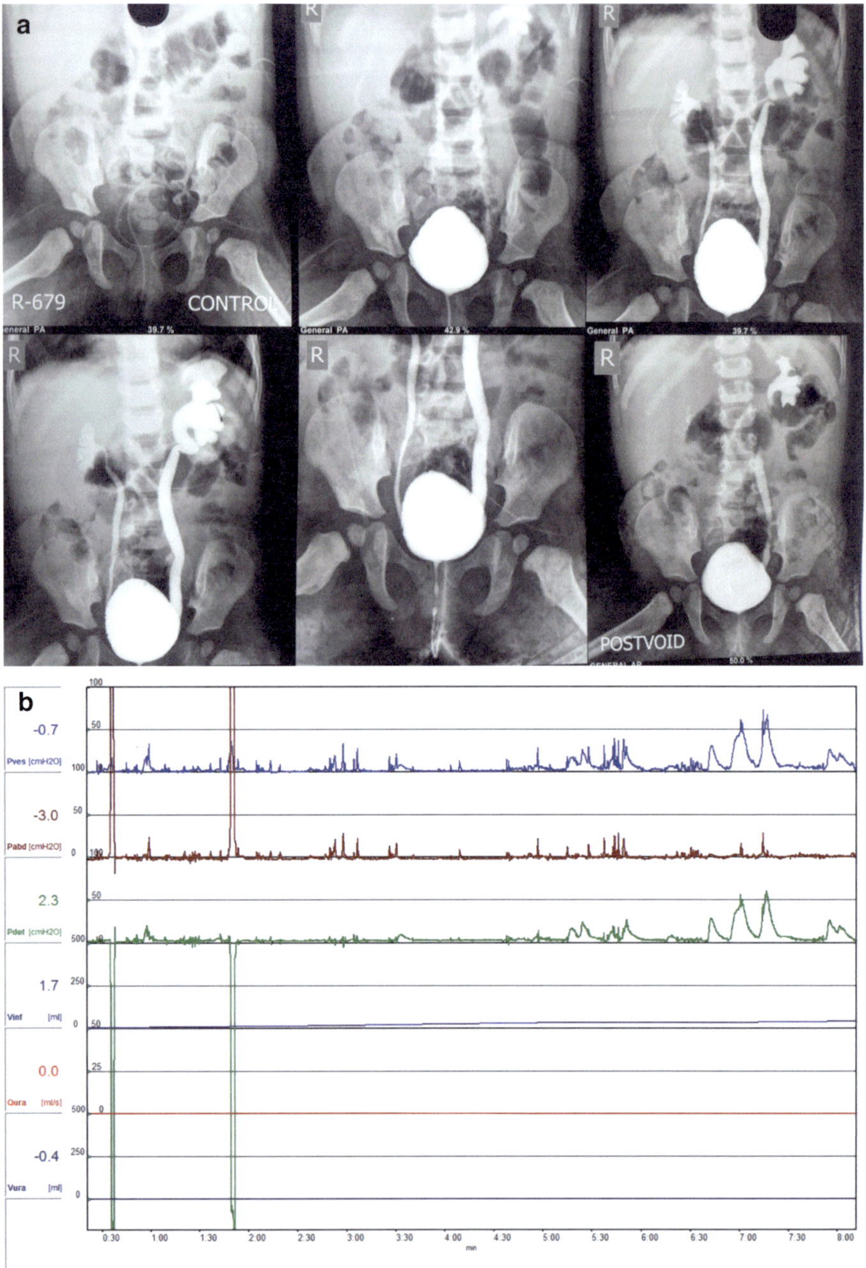

Fig. 19.15 (**a**) MCU images. (**b**) Filling phase of the UDS tracing showing waves of detrusor overactivity. (**c**) Voiding phase of the UDS tracing showing very high voiding pressure and poor flow rates. The rectal catheter slipped out midway during the void (black arrow), thus falsely elevating the detrusor tracing beyond that point. The Pdet reading is reliable before that point

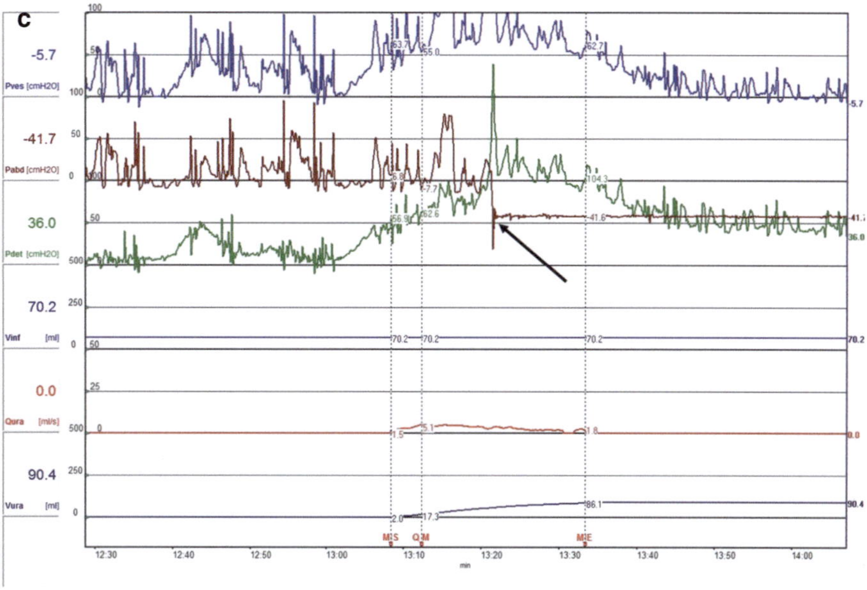

Fig. 19.15 (continued)

UDS (Fig. 19.15b) was performed to rule out secondary VUR. It revealed normal capacity bladder with normal compliance but significant overactivity. During voiding (Fig. 19.15c), voiding detrusor pressures were markedly raised (60–80 cm H2O) with poor flow rates. There was a PVR of 15 ml after the void. Thus, the diagnosis was detrusor overactivity and probable dysfunctional voiding causing BOO with secondary VUR.

She was started on alpha-blockers but continued to have UTIs. So she was started on anticholinergics and CIC following which she did not have any further UTI.

Case 4: Down with Poor Outflow Competence

A 6-year-old male child, known case of trisomy 21, presented with history of dribbling of urine since the age of 3 years, more during the day, increased dribbling with activity/straining. There was no history of urgency/urge incontinence. He passed urine voluntarily in the toilet. There was no history of constipation. USG showed normal bladder and upper tracts with variable PVR—70 ml on one occasion and 4 ml on another. Uroflowmetry (Fig. 19.16a) revealed a poor flow suggesting BOO or underactive bladder.

MCU revealed normal bladder and no VUR with intermittent opening of bladder neck with contrast entering the posterior urethra seen during the filling phase which was more prominent on full bladder. During voiding, urine stream was visibly poor with poor delineation of urethra.

UDS was performed to differentiate between BOO and underactive detrusor and to ascertain the cause of dribbling. UDS (Fig. 19.16b) showed a normal capacity

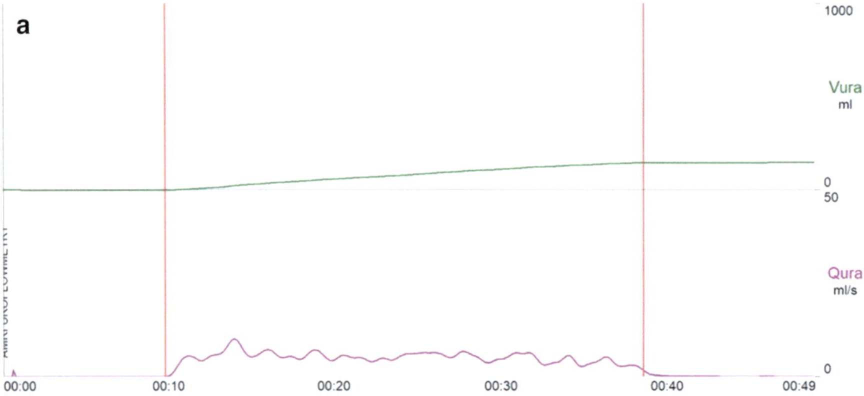

Parameter	Value
Voiding time	28.8s
Flow time	28.8s
Time to maximum flow	4.2s
Maximum flow rate	10.1ml/s
Volume at maximum flow	23ml
Mean flow rate	5.1ml/s
Total voided volume	146ml
Residual volume	30ml

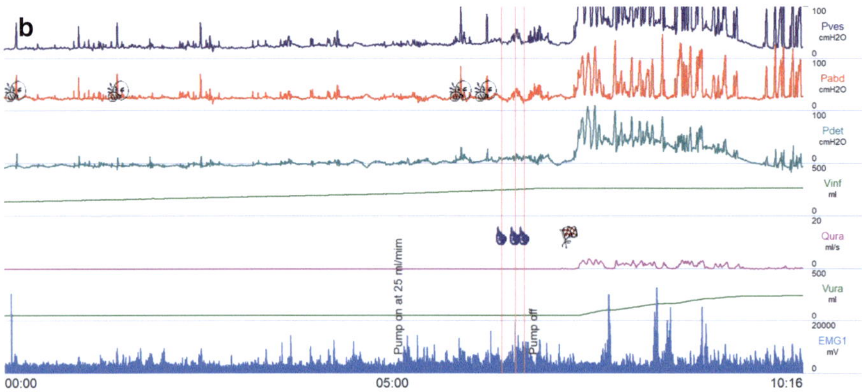

Fig. 19.16 (**a**) Uroflowmetry curve. (**b**) UDS tracing

bladder with normal compliance and mild overactivity. Mild dribbling was noted towards the end of fill in the absence of any detrusor overactivity or straining suggesting probable intermittent bladder neck opening as evident on MCU. During voiding, flow rates were poor, detrusor contraction was weak and there was no significant increase in EMG activity suggesting detrusor underactivity as the cause of weak flow.

He was started on timed voiding with a trial of imipramine.

Cerebral Palsy

Bladder dysfunction is common in children with cerebral palsy (CP) which may or may not manifest as LUT symptoms. Symptoms of bladder dysfunction include increased frequency, urgency, intermittent daytime incontinence and enuresis; voiding abnormalities can manifest as hesitancy, poor stream and increased PVR. Bladder dysfunction is a result of upper motor neuron lesion with neurogenic DO which is responsible for the storage symptoms. Patients with upper motor neuron dysfunction are expected to have synergic sphincters. But patients with CP usually show features of DSD. This can be explained by pelvic floor hypertonia due to spasticity. This phenomenon, also known as pseudo-DSD, is responsible for abnormalities in voiding phase in patients with CP.

Case 1: CP with Urinary Retention

A 15-year-old male child, known case of spastic CP, passed urine on his own or on cues and was in diapers continuously. He had an episode of urinary retention at the age of 15 years when he required catheterisation. Afetr the episode, he continued to have intermittent episodes of restlessness/discomfort due to inability to pass urine because of which his mother was taught to perform CIC. He also had history of significant constipation for which he was started on bowel washes. USG showed thick-walled UB (6.5 mm) with normal upper tracts.

MCU (Fig. 19.17a) showed elongated irregular bladder with poor distension of membranous urethra during voiding and suggestion of high-pressure voiding.

UDS (Fig. 19.17b) showed an extremely small capacity bladder with spontaneous voids after every 20–30 ml fill. The patient signalled urge to void but could not postpone/hold micturition, suggesting that the voids were due to waves of detrusor overactivity. During voiding, detrusor pressures were in the range of 100–130 cm H2O with flow rates of 4.5 ml/sec suggesting BOO. EMG activity was seen to increase during the voids indicating pseudo-DSD. There was complete emptying of bladder during the voids.

He was suggested anticholinergics along with CIC, but as the parents were not comfortable with the added burden of CIC, they opted for a trial of Botox at the sphincter.

Case 2: CP with Recurrent UTI—DO

A 7-year-old female child, known case of spastic CP, presented with recurrent episodes of febrile UTI (once in every 2 - 3 months)since the age of 11 months and two to three episodes in the last 1 year. She passed urine in good stream every 40 minutes to 1 hour and occasionally signalled before passing urine. She also had history of constipation for which she was on bowel washes. Voiding diary was maintained by diaper weight method—weighing the diapers after each void- 12–14 times per

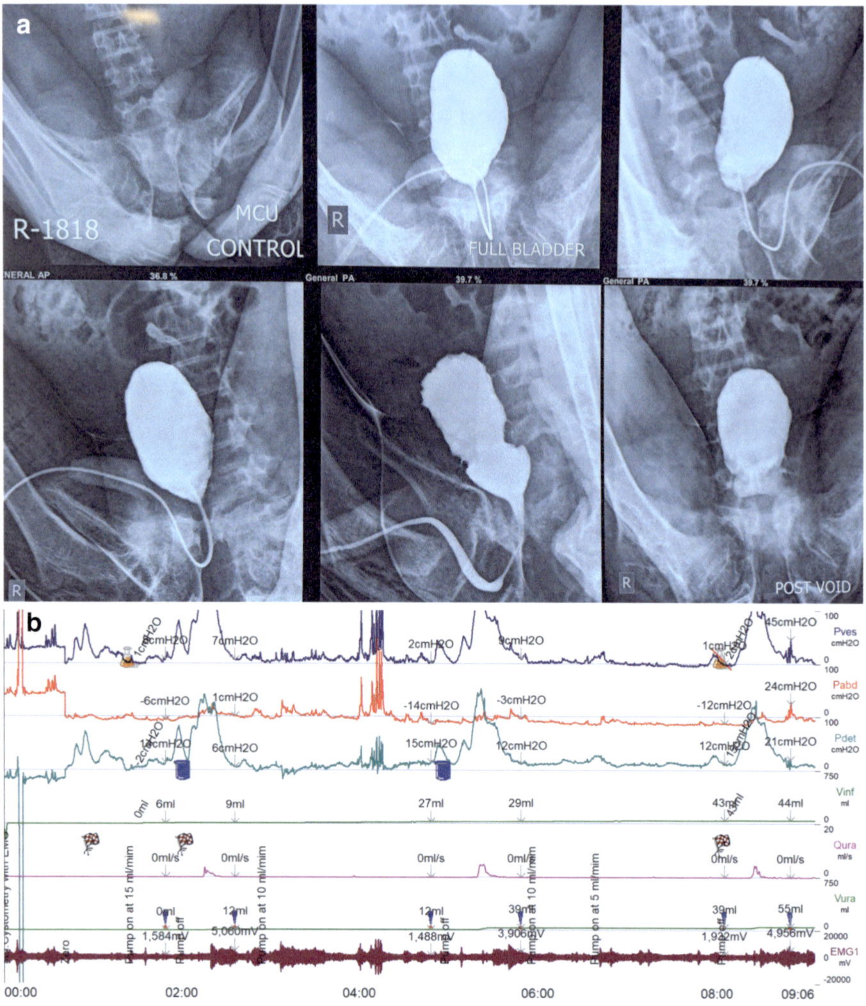

Fig. 19.17 (**a**) MCU showed elongated irregular bladder with poor distension of membranous urethra during voiding and suggestion of high-pressure voiding. (**b**) UDS showed a extremely small capacity bladder with spontaneous voids after every 20–30 ml fill

day, usual volumes of 120–150 ml, few volumes of 50–90 ml and 3 times per night (EBC 400 ml). USG showed mild bladder wall thickening with normal upper tracts. MCU revealed smooth-walled, rounded bladder with no VUR (Fig. 19.18a).

UDS was performed to check for any overactivity or obstructed voiding pattern. Positioning the children of CP for UDS may be tricky as they very often have contractures of limbs and poor trunk control (Fig. 19.18b).

UDS revealed voiding at variable bladder volumes ranging from 40 ml to 200 ml (Fig. 19.18c). The child showed some signalling before passing urine. During voiding, flow rates were appropriate and detrusor pressures were normal. There was no

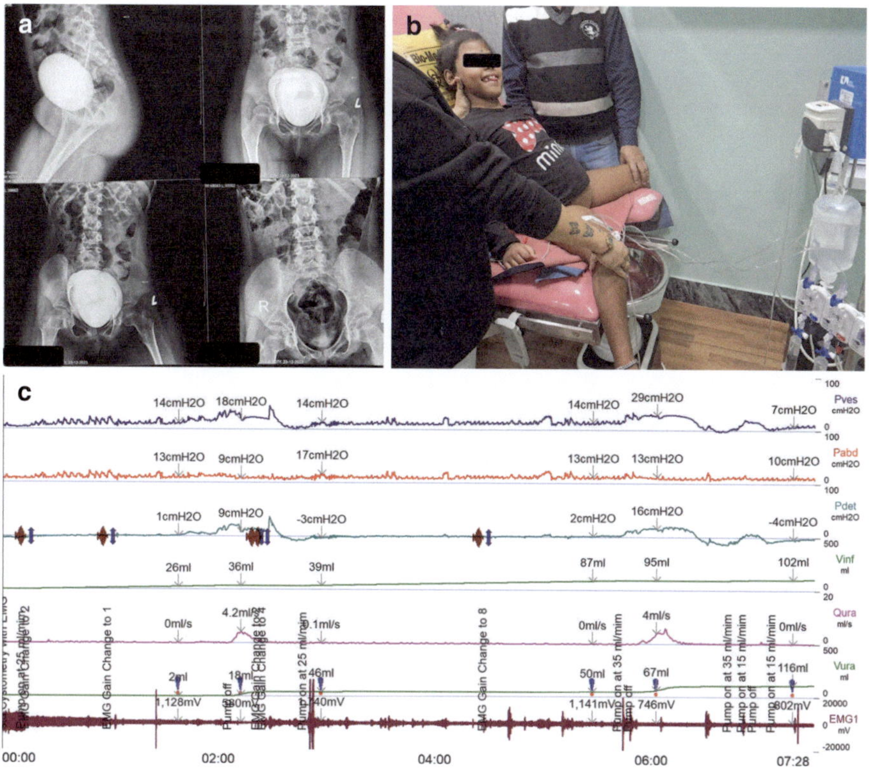

Fig. 19.18 (**a**) MCU images. (**b**) Positioning of the child with back rest of the bed elevated and parents supporting the child from either side. Voided volume and flow rate can be assessed as the urine falls into the uroflowmetry jar. (**c**) UDS revealed voiding at variable bladder volumes ranging from 40 ml to 200 ml.

abnormal EMG activity during voiding and PVR was 18 ml after the last void. Spontaneous voids at small bladder volumes may indicate voids due to detrusor overactivity for which she was started on mirabegron and PVR was checked by serial USGs. At 1 year follow-up, voiding frequency and voided volumes had improved to some extent, but there were no further episodes of UTI. It was presumed that the unrecognised DO was responsible for the UTIs.

Case 3: CP with Recurrent UTI—BOO

A 1.10-year-old female child had history of birth asphyxia. She had developmental delay and could not stand with support. She presented with history of recurrent episodes of UTI. She had no apparent urinary complaints, passed urine every hourly in occasionally interrupted stream and had no history of straining while passing urine.

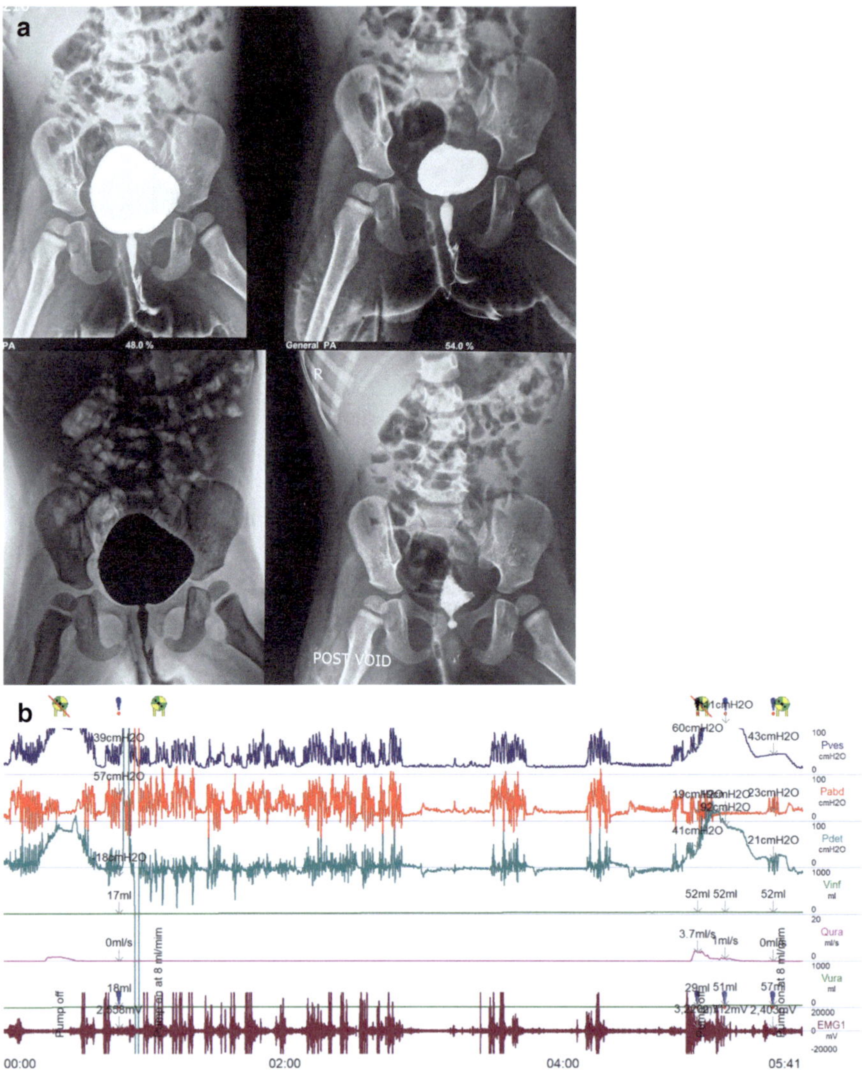

Fig. 19.19 (**a**) MCU images. (**b**) A portion of the UDS tracing in an expanded form expanded to show filling between 17 ml and 52 ml. Child is seen to void at 17 ml fill and then at 52 ml fill. Increased EMG activity is noted during the second void. (**c**) Further portion of UDS tracing showing filling from 52 ml to 75 ml with two voids at 52 ml (same as the second void in Fig. CP 3a) and 75 ml. Increased EMG activity is noted during both the voids

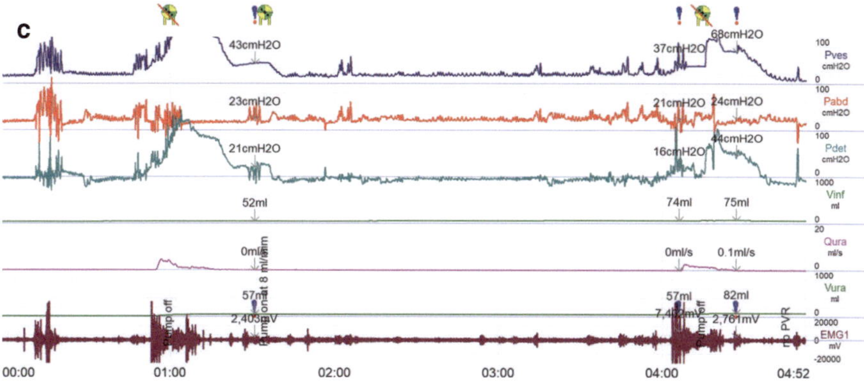

Fig. 19.19 (continued)

USG KUB showed left HDUN with bladder wall thickness of 2.2 mm. MCU showed rounded bladder with no VUR but evidence of dysfunctional voiding (Fig. 19.19a).

UDS (Fig. 19.19b, c) showed a small capacity bladder with voids at volumes of 20, 30 and 40 ml—probably due to detrusor overactivity. Voiding pressures were high (50–100 cm H2O) with relatively poor flow rates suggestive of BOO; EMG activity was seen to increase during two out of three voids suggestive of (? pseudo) DSD. There was complete emptying of bladder.

Detrusor overactivity with DSD was thought to be responsible for UTIs and she was started on anticholinergics with alpha-blockers.

Bladder Dysfunction Associated with Anorectal Malformation

A significant proportion of the children with anorectal malformation (ARM) have bladder dysfunction suggestive of neurogenic bladder. It may be as a result of inherent spinal abnormality or may be iatrogenic due to the corrective surgery. The higher the defect, the higher is the propensity of bladder dysfunction.

In patients with high type of ARM, even in the absence of any urinary symptoms, patients may show significant urodynamic abnormalities.

Case 1: ARM with Neurogenic DSD

A 3.10-year-old male child, follow-up case of ARM, underwent colostomy in neonatal period; PSARP was done at 3 years of age. He was passing urine relatively well and in good stream before PSARP, used to inform before passing urine and passed urine in equal amounts per urethrally and through the distal stoma. He had intermittent episodes of increased frequency and frequent episodes of UTI/hematuria. After PSARP, the child did not pass urine in stream. He had history of continuous dribbling, leaked larger amounts of urine on crying/shouting/straining and leaked continuously while asleep.

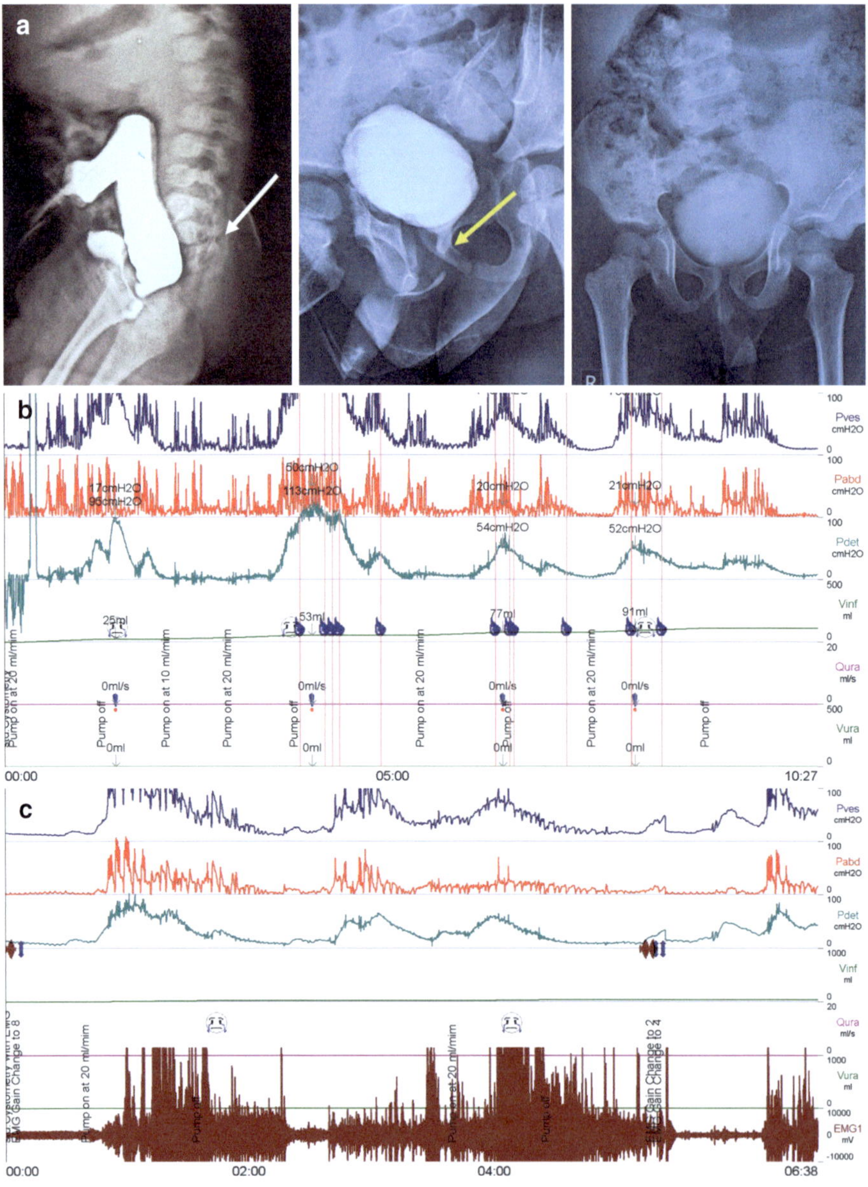

Fig. 19.20 (**a**) Distal cologram and MCU images. White arrow highlights sacral agenesis on the image of distal cologram. Yellow arrow highlights abrupt cutoff of the urethra at distal end of posterior urethra. (**b**) UDS showed a small capacity bladder (filling was stopped at 100 ml due to severe overactivity and urine leak), severe detrusor overactivity and overactivity associated leakage of urine. (**c**) When study was performed with EMG in situ, EMG activity was seen to increase significantly during episodes of detrusor overactivity suggesting neurogenic DSD

USG showed normal bladder with left HDN. Image of distal cologram (Fig. 19.20a) was suggestive of partial sacral agenesis (white arrow). MCU (Fig. 19.20a) performed elsewhere showed normal appearance of bladder with poor urethral delineation. Abrupt cutoff of urethra was seen at level of membranous urethra – probable DSD (yellow arrow) with significant PVR.

The child could not pass urine for uroflowmetry. UDS (Fig. 19.20b) showed a small capacity bladder (filling was stopped at 100 ml due to severe overactivity and urine leak), severe detrusor overactivity and overactivity-associated leakage of urine. When study was performed with EMG in situ (Fig. 19.20c), EMG activity was seen to increase significantly during episodes of detrusor overactivity suggesting neurogenic DSD. The child could not void on command which may be due to neurogenic cause or inability to obey command due to young age of the child also.

This child had a pre-existing neurogenic element (partial sacral agenesis) with probable bladder dysfunction even before the PSARP, but the voiding symptoms became prominent after the surgery. This can be explained by an added element of iatrogenic injury to neural innervation during posterior sagittal dissection or loss of the venting effect of distal stoma after disconnection of the fistulous communication.

Case 2: ARM with Detrusor Underactivity

A 4.10-year-old male child, follow-up case of high type of ARM, underwent staged repair with abdomino-perineal pull through at the age of 3 years. He had history of recurrent episodes of UTI before the abdomino-perineal pull through which improved after the surgery. Presently, he passed urine voluntarily in relatively poor stream and had straining while passing urine. Occasional dribbling was noted when he was engrossed in activities and he had no enuresis. USG showed mildly thick-walled bladder with normal upper tracts.

Voiding diary was incomplete, but it suggested that he passed 50–100 ml of urine each time at frequent intervals of 30 min to 1 hour.

Uroflowmetry showed a poor stream with possibility of detrusor underactivity or dysfunctional voiding (Fig. 19.21a).

UDS (Fig. 19.21a) showed normal capacity, stable bladder with normal compliance. During voiding (Fig. 19.21b), he had weak detrusor contraction with poor flow rates and significant straining indicating detrusor underactivity as the cause of poor flow rates. There was variable PVR after the voids.

Because of the finding of bladder dysfunction, he underwent MRI spine which revealed a low-lying tethered cord with cystic lesion at cauda equina.

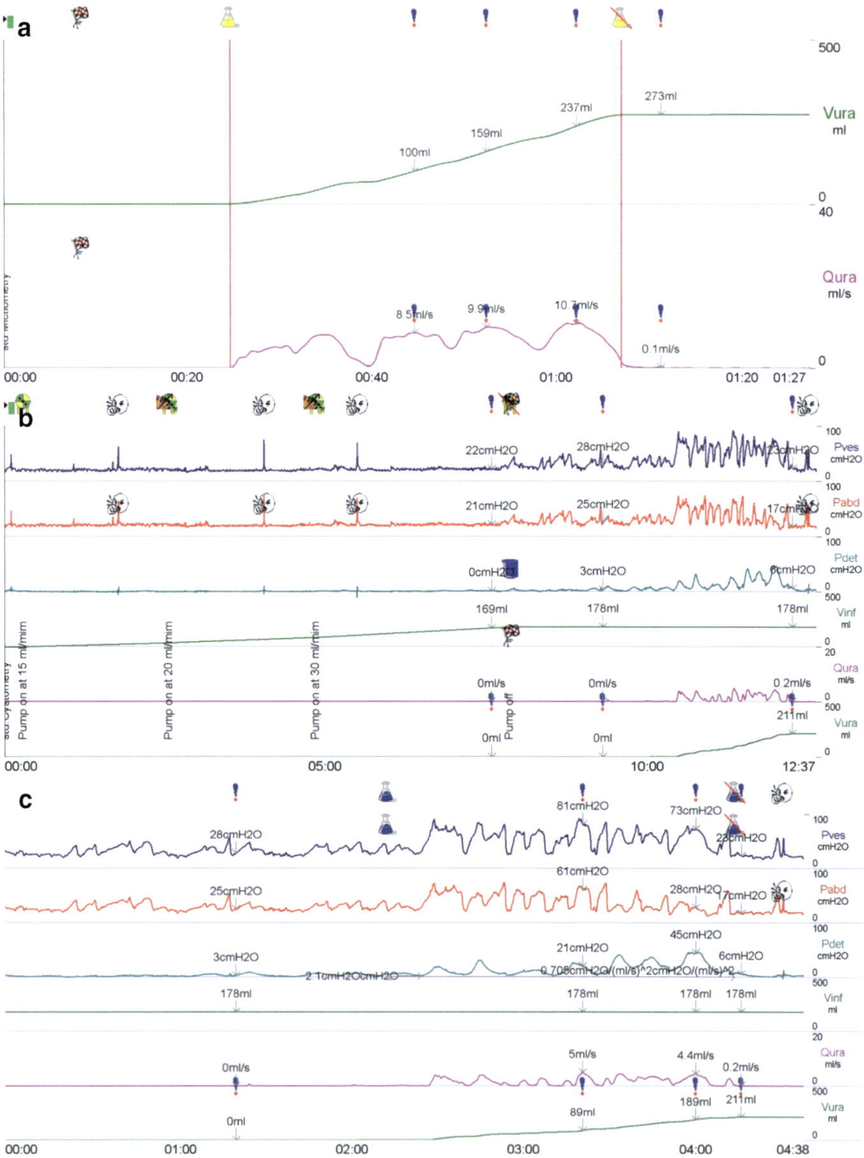

Fig. 19.21 (**a**) Uroflowmetry curve. (**b**) UDS tracing. (**c**) Voiding portion of the UDS tracing in an expanded form

Case 3: ARM with Poorly Compliant Bladder

A 7.7-year-old male child, follow-up case of ARM, underwent PSARP at the age of 2.5 years after which he developed urinary retention and had to be started on CIC. He had been on regular CIC every 2–3 hourly since then. He could feel urge to pass urine intermittently and could pass some urine voluntarily. He leaked urine if he had to hold urine for some time.

He was on rectal washes for fecal soiling.

As per the voiding diary, he passed urine voluntarily every 1 ½ to 2 hours (40–110 ml); post void CIC volumes were 90–200 ml. USG KUB revealed thick-walled bladder with normal upper tracts.

During uroflowmetry (Fig. 19.22a), he passed 50 ml urine in a poor stream with 150 ml PVR suggesting either underactive detrusor or BOO.

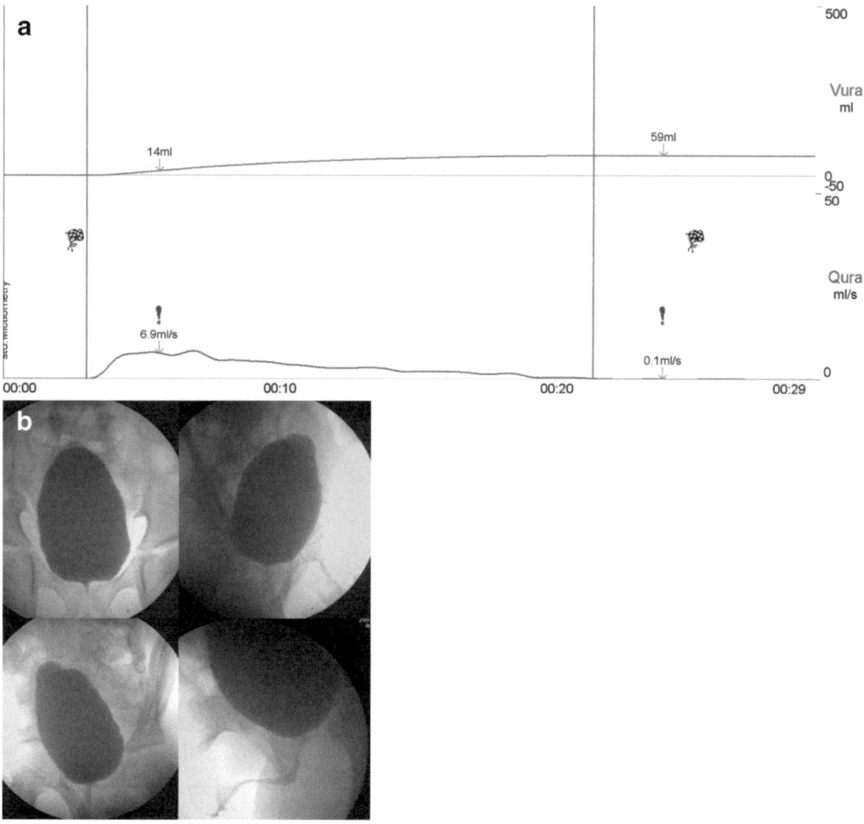

Fig. 19.22 (**a**) During uroflowmetry, passed 50 ml urine in a poor stream with 150 ml PVR suggesting either underactive detrusor or BOO. (**b**) MCU showed elongated bladder with irregular outline and no VUR. (**c**) UDS tracing. (**d**) Voiding phase of the UDS tracing in an expanded form

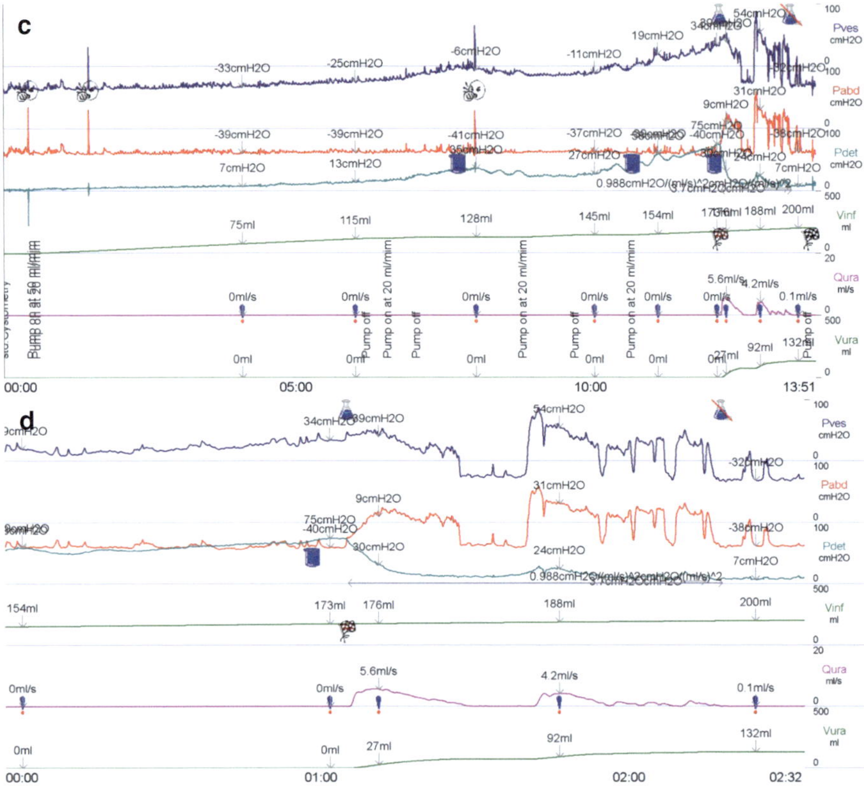

Fig. 19.22 (continued)

MCU (Fig. 19.22b) showed elongated bladder with irregular outline and no VUR. Poor opening of bladder neck was seen during voiding with visualised urethra being normal. MCU appearance of the bladder was suggestive of neurogenic bladder.

UDS (Fig. 19.22c) revealed a normal capacity bladder with severely reduced compliance (27 cm H2O at 140 ml) and significant overactivity (tonic rise in pressures up to 36 cm H2O at 128 ml and 70 cm H2O at 170 ml). He complained of urge to void during episodes of significant overactivity, but there was no leak (this shows that DO-LPP > 70 cm H2O and DLPP >27 cm H2O). On command to void (Fig. 19.22d), no voiding detrusor contraction was noted. On the contrary, detrusor pressures were seen to decrease rapidly as around 90 ml of urine was emptied from the bladder. This void was probably initiated by sphincteric/bladder neck relaxation on the face of high prevoid detrusor pressures. Around 50 ml of urine was passed as a second bout by Valsalva and a weak detrusor contraction. There was a PVR of 90 ml after the void.

Thus, this patient had severely reduced compliance with significant overactivity and voiding by use of raised prevoid detrusor pressures. He was started on anticholinergics and continued on CIC. MRI spine was advised.

Case 4: ARM with Weak Outflow Resistance

An 8-year-old male child, FUC of ARM with staged repair done (all stages completed by age of 1 year). He had history of increased crying in initial months of life, was diagnosed as having bilateral hydroureteronephrosis with thick-walled bladder and underwent cystoscopy at the age of 1 year which did not reveal any PUV.

He had history of continuous urinary dribbling/dampness of undergarments since 1 month of age; he could pass small amounts of urine by straining when asked to.

USG KUB showed bilateral pelvic fullness with left ureter grossly dilated. Bladder wall thickness was normal with a PVR of 8 cc.

As per the voiding diary (Fig. 19.23a), he had a frequency of 9–13 times/day, daytime volumes of 50–90 ml, morning void of 150 ml and maximum daytime volume of 135 ml. There was continuous wetness of pants requiring several changes of pants per day.

MCU (Fig. 19.23b) showed elongated bladder with smooth walls, capacity of 150 ml and no VUR. Urethra was normal but the bladder neck impression was very prominent. Leak was noted on two occasions—small amount just after coughing on full bladder.

During uroflowmetry (Fig. 19.23b), he passed a small amount on urine with a weak stream.

Overall voiding history and voiding diary suggested small capacity bladder with urinary leak, but the cause of urinary leak was uncertain.

UDS (Fig. 19.23d) showed significant leak of urine from beginning of fill ('leak'/drop sign). The leak was seen in the absence of any DO or straining—probably due to intermittent opening of bladder neck. He leaked 17 ml urine till 100 ml fill when penile clamping was performed and the filling was continued. He tolerated a fill of 150 ml when he complained of urge to void and penile clamping was released. No overactivity was noted during the study; detrusor pressures were 20 cm H2O at 150 ml suggesting reduced compliance. He voided (Fig. 19.23e) on command with an appropriate flow rate but very weak/imperceptible detrusor contraction suggesting reduced outflow resistance. There was complete emptying of bladder at the end of the void.

As per the UDS, poor compliance explained the upper tract changes and reduced outflow resistance explained the dribbling of urine. So he was started on a low dose of anticholinergics with imipramine following which there was significant improvement in voiding frequency and voided volumes (Fig. 19.23f) as well as his uroflowmetry (Fig. 19.23g).

a Time	Voided Volume
8am	150 ml
9.30 am	60 ml
10.30 am	80 ml
12.20 pm	50 ml
1.45 pm	60 ml
3.20 pm	55 ml
3.45 pm	75 ml
5.45 pm	50 ml
7.00 pm	10 ml
8.00 pm	34 ml
8.35 pm	20 ml
9.00 pm	12 ml
9.45 pm	105 m
10.30 pm	90 ml

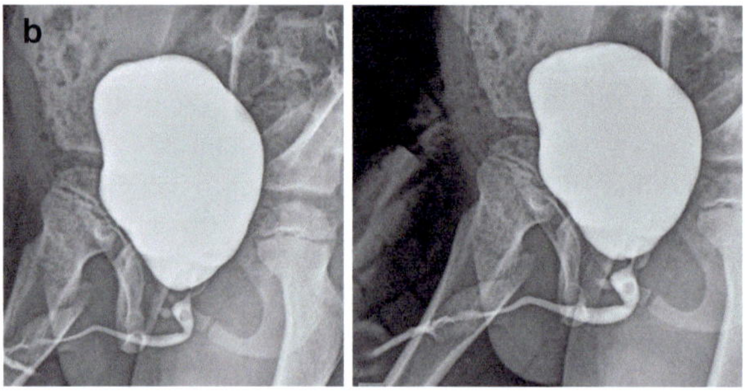

Fig. 19.23 (**a**) Voiding diary. (**b**) MCU images. (**c**) Uroflowmetry curve. (**d**) UDS tracing. Points where penile clamping was started and released have been highlighted. (**e**) Voiding phase of the UDS in expanded form. (**f**) Voiding diary at 6 months follow-up. (**g**) Uroflowmetry at follow-up

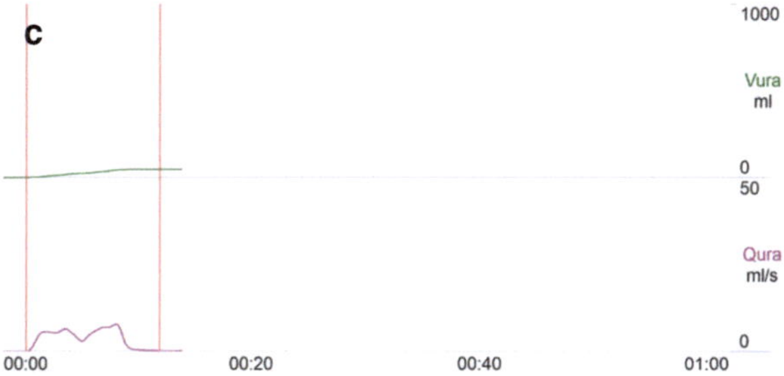

Parameter	Value
Voiding time	11.9s
Flow time	11.9s
Time to maximum flow	8s
Maximum flow rate	7.9ml/s
Volume at maximum flow	42ml
Mean flow rate	3.9ml/s
Total voided volume	47ml

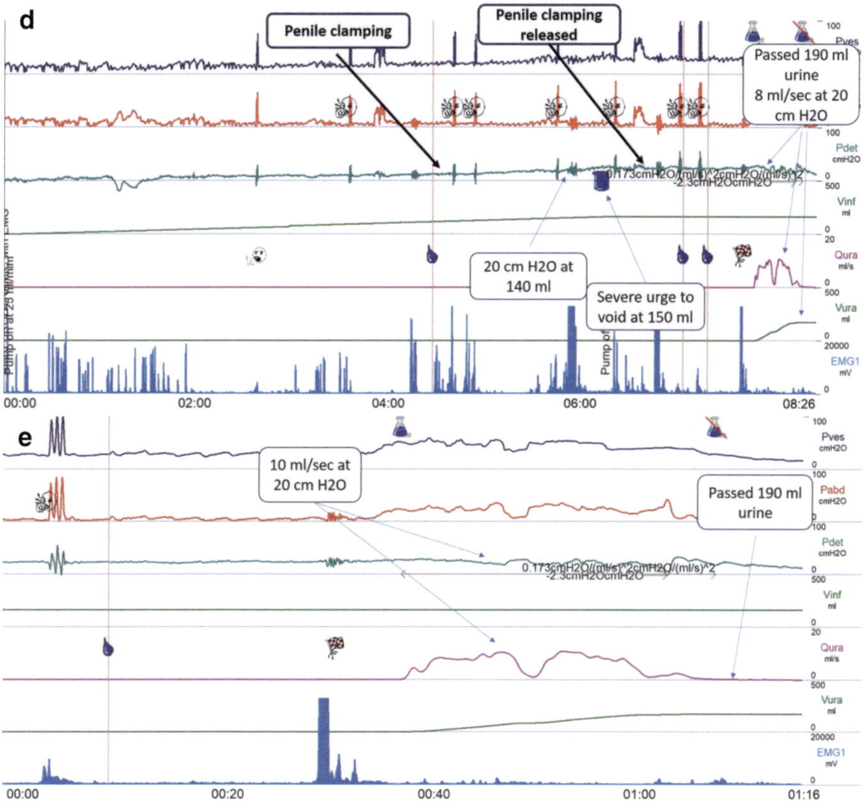

Fig. 19.23 (continued)

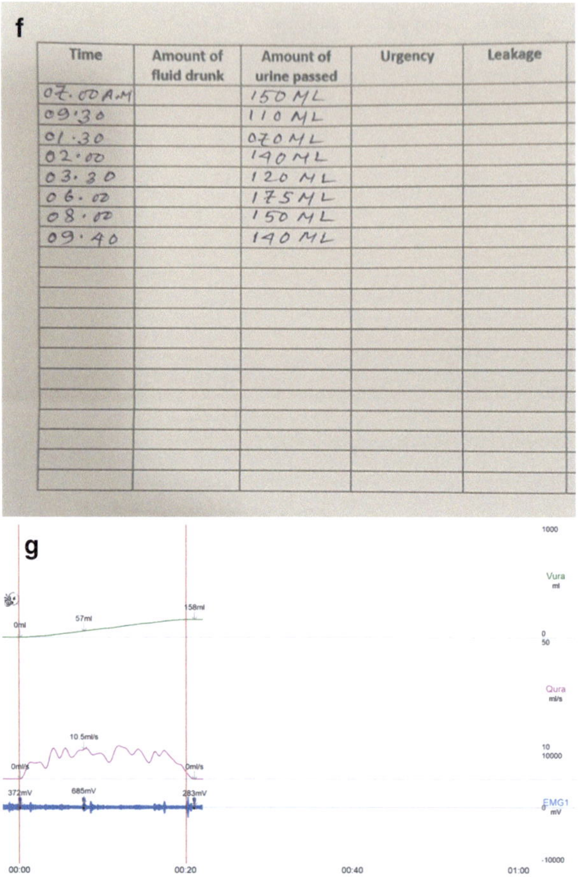

f

Time	Amount of fluid drunk	Amount of urine passed	Urgency	Leakage
07.00 A.M		150 ML		
09.30		110 ML		
01.30		070 ML		
02.00		140 ML		
03.30		120 ML		
06.02		175 ML		
08.02		150 ML		
09.40		140 ML		

Fig. 19.23 (continued)

Declarations

Competing Interests The author(s) has no competing interests to declare that are relevant to the content of this manuscript.

Ethics Approval The author(s) declares that this manuscript does not include primary research with human participants.

The author(s) declares that this manuscript does not include primary studies involving animals.

Suggested Reading

1. Androulakakis PA, Karamanolakis DK, Tsahouridis G, Stefanidis AA, Palaeodimos I. Myogenic bladder decompensation in boys with a history of posterior urethral valves is caused by secondary bladder neck obstruction? BJU Int. 2005; https://doi.org/10.1111/j.1464-410X.2005.05583.x.

2. Austin PF, Bauer SB, Bower W, Chase J, Franco I, Hoebeke P, Rittig S, Walle JV, von Gontard A, Wright A, Yang SS, Nevéus T. The standardization of terminology of lower urinary tract function in children and adolescents: Update report from the standardization committee of the International Children's Continence Society. Neurourol Urodyn. 2016;35(4):471–81. https://doi.org/10.1002/nau.22751. Epub 2015 Mar 14. PMID: 25772695.
3. Bael A, Lax H, de Jong TP, Hoebeke P, Nijman RJ, Sixt R, Verhulst J, Hirche H, van Gool JD; European Bladder Dysfunction Study (European Union BMH1-CT94-1006). The relevance of urodynamic studies for Urge syndrome and dysfunctional voiding: a multicenter controlled trial in children. J Urol. 2008;180(4):1486–93; discussion 1494-5. https://doi.org/10.1016/j.juro.2008.06.054. Epub 2008 Aug 16. PMID: 18710726.
4. Bhatt NR, Murchison L, Yardy G, Kulkarni M, Mathur AB. Bladder bowel dysfunction in children with Down's syndrome. Pediatr Surg Int. 2020;36(7):763–72. https://doi.org/10.1007/s00383-020-04682-4. Epub 2020 May 26. PMID: 32458130.
5. Binu V, Dash V, Bawa M, et al. Role of urodynamics in male patients of high-anorectal malformations: a prospective study. Pediatr Surg Int. 2021;37:461–8. https://doi.org/10.1007/s00383-020-04835-5.
6. Boemers TM, Beek FJ, van Gool JD, de Jong TP, Bax KM. Urologic problems in anorectal malformations. Part 1: urodynamic findings and significance of sacral anomalies. J Pediatr Surg. 1996;31(3):407–10. https://doi.org/10.1016/s0022-3468(96)90748-4. PMID: 8708913.
7. De Gennaro M, Capitanucci ML, Capozza N, Caione P, Mosiello G, Silveri M. Detrusor hypocontractility in children with posterior urethral valves arises before puberty. Br J Urol. 1998;81:81–5. https://doi.org/10.1046/j.1464-410x.1998.00014.x.
8. De Gennaro M, Capitanucci ML, Mosiello G, Caione P, Silveri M. The changing urodynamic pattern from infancy to adolescence in boys with posterior urethral valves. BJU Int. 2000;85(9):1104–8. https://doi.org/10.1046/j.1464-410x.2000.00700.x. PMID: 10848705.
9. Desai D. A review of urodynamic evaluation in children and its role in the management of boys with posterior urethral valves. Indian J Urol. 2007; https://doi.org/10.4103/0970-1591.36719.
10. Donohoe JM, Weinstein RP, Combs AJ, Misseri R, Horowitz M, Schulsinger D, et al. When can persistent hydroureteronephrosis in posterior urethral valve disease be considered residual stretching? J Urol. 2004;172:706–11. https://doi.org/10.1097/01.ju.0000129139.10189.3f.
11. Drzewiecki BA, Bauer SB. Urodynamic testing in children: indications, technique, interpretation and significance. J Urol. 2011;186(4):1190–7. https://doi.org/10.1016/j.juro.2011.02.2692. Epub 2011 Aug 16. PMID: 21849190.
12. Gomelsky A. Editorial Comment on "External Urethral Sphincter Botulinum Toxin Injection to Treat Pseudodyssynergia in Patients with Cerebral Palsy". Urology. 2024;186:53. https://doi.org/10.1016/j.urology.2024.01.016. Epub 2024 Feb 16. PMID: 38369196.
13. Haggart R, Loftus CJ, DeWitt-Foy M, Henry V, Grove S, Pariser J, Elliott S. External urethral sphincter botulinum toxin injection to treat pseudodysynergia in patients with cerebral palsy. Urology. 2024;186:48–52. https://doi.org/10.1016/j.urology.2023.11.037. Epub 2024 Feb 20. PMID: 38387511.
14. Harris KT, Wilcox DT. Management of the urological tract in children with anorectal malformations – a contemporary review. Ther Adv Urol. 2023;15:17562872231161468. https://doi.org/10.1177/17562872231161468. PMID: 36969498; PMCID: PMC10034273.
15. Hicks JA, Carson C, Malone PS. Is there an association between functional bladder outlet obstruction and Down's syndrome? J Pediatr Urol. 2007;3(5):369–74. https://doi.org/10.1016/j.jpurol.2007.02.003. Epub 2007 Apr 10. PMID: 18947775.
16. Hoebeke P, Van Laecke E, Van Camp C, Raes A, Van De Walle J. One thousand video-urodynamic studies in children with non-neurogenic bladder sphincter dysfunction. BJU Int. 2001;87(6):575–80. https://doi.org/10.1046/j.1464-410x.2001.00083.x. PMID: 11298061.
17. Holmdahl G, Sillen U, Bachelard M, Hansson E, Hermansson G, Hjalmas K, et al. The changing urodynamic pattern in valve bladders during infancy. J Urol. 1995; https://doi.org/10.1097/00005392-199502000-00058.
18. Inugala A. Neurovesical dysfunction in anorectal malformation. Int Surg J. 2020;7(12):4039–44. https://doi.org/10.18203/2349-2902.isj20205354.

19. Jiang YH, Chen SF, Kuo HC. Role of videourodynamic study in precision diagnosis and treatment for lower urinary tract dysfunction. Tzu Chi Med J. 2019;32(2):121–30. https://doi.org/10.4103/tcmj.tcmj_178_19. PMID: 32269943; PMCID: PMC7137365.
20. Jiang W, Sun H, Gu B, et al. Urodynamic study findings and related influential factors in pediatric spastic cerebral palsy. Sci Rep. 2022;12:6962. https://doi.org/10.1038/s41598-022-11057-3.
21. Kaufman MR, DeMarco RT, Pope JC 4th, Scarpero HM, Adams MC, Trusler LA, Brock JW 3rd. High yield of urodynamics performed for refractory nonneurogenic dysfunctional voiding in the pediatric population. J Urol. 2006;176(4 Pt 2):1835–7. https://doi.org/10.1016/j.juro.2006.03.125. PMID: 16945666.
22. Kitamura A, Kondoh T, Noguchi M, Hatada T, Tohbu S, Mori KI, Matsuo M, Kunitsugu I, Kanetake H, Moriuchi H. Assessment of lower urinary tract function in children with Down syndrome. Pediatr Int. 2014;56(6):902–8. https://doi.org/10.1111/ped.12367. Epub 2014 Oct 15. PMID: 24758352; PMCID: PMC4311436.
23. Kızılay F, İrer B, Özalp Kızılay D, Şimşir A, Kalemci S, Şen V, Altay B, Çoğulu Ö. Evaluation of lower urinary tract symptoms in children with Down syndrome: a prospective, case-controlled cohort study. Neurourol Urodyn. 2020;39(2):833–40. https://doi.org/10.1002/nau.24293. Epub 2020 Jan 23. PMID: 31971631.
24. Mirone V, Imbimbo C, Longo N, Fusco F. The Detrusor Muscle: An Innocent Victim of Bladder Outlet Obstruction{A figure is presented}. Eur Urol. 2007;51:57–66. https://doi.org/10.1016/j.eururo.2006.07.050.
25. Niemczyk J, von Gontard A, Equit M, Medoff D, Wagner C, Curfs L. Incontinence in persons with Down Syndrome. Neurourol Urodyn. 2017;36(6):1550–6. https://doi.org/10.1002/nau.23146. Epub 2016 Oct 4. PMID: 27701769.
26. Parekh DJ, Pope JC 4th, Adams MC, Brock JW 3rd. The use of radiography, urodynamic studies and cystoscopy in the evaluation of voiding dysfunction. J Urol. 2001;165(1):215–8. https://doi.org/10.1097/00005392-200101000-00061. PMID: 11125409.
27. Samijn B, Van Laecke E, Renson C, Hoebeke P, Plasschaert F, Vande Walle J, Van den Broeck C. Lower urinary tract symptoms and urodynamic findings in children and adults with cerebral palsy: a systematic review. Neurourol Urodyn. 2017;36(3):541–9. https://doi.org/10.1002/nau.22982. Epub 2016 Feb 19. PMID: 26894322.
28. Strine AC, VanderBrink BA, Alam Z, Schulte M, Noh PH, DeFoor WR Jr, Minevich E, Sheldon CA, Frischer JS, Reddy PP. Clinical and urodynamic outcomes in children with anorectal malformation subtype of recto-bladder neck fistula. J Pediatr Urol. 2017;13(4):376.e1–6. https://doi.org/10.1016/j.jpurol.2017.06.008. Epub 2017 Jul 10. PMID: 28733158.

Serial UDS in Dynamic Treatment Decisions

20

Poonam Guha Vaze

i-UDS proves to be an invaluable tool in several cases of bladder dysfunction as it gives useful insight into the further management strategy of the patient. In a select group of patients, UDS may have to be repeated when other investigations cannot provide the relevant details. Repeating UDS is especially easy in patients in neurogenic bladder as they usually have a non-sensate bladder. Repeat UDS may be required to identify the cause for recurrent UTIs or check whether the pressures of a hostile bladder have improved.

Here, we present four cases of varied aetiology wherein UDS was repeated 2–3 times and decision for further management was based on the UDS findings.

Case 1: NNNB in an Infant

A 2-month-old girl child had history of two episodes of febrile UTI with h/o straining at micturition. During the second episode, UTI was not responding to IV antibiotics and improved only after catheterisation. USG showed normal study.

MCU (Fig. 20.1a) showed a small capacity elongated bladder, bilateral VUR during voiding and evidence of dysfunctional voiding.

UDS (Fig. 20.1b) was performed at the age of 2 months with the baby in supine position. Voids/leaks have been marked with 'leak sign'. Baby was seen to void after every 5–10 ml fill with some prevoid detrusor overactivity and high-pressure voids.

P. G. Vaze (✉)
Neotia Bhagirathi Woman and Child Care Centre, Newtown, Kolkata, India

Department of Pediatric Surgery, Nilratan Sircar Medical College and Hospital, Kolkata, India

S. Saha, P. Guha Vaze (eds.), *Comprehensive Atlas of Practical Pediatric Urodynamics*, https://doi.org/10.1007/978-981-95-2709-0_20

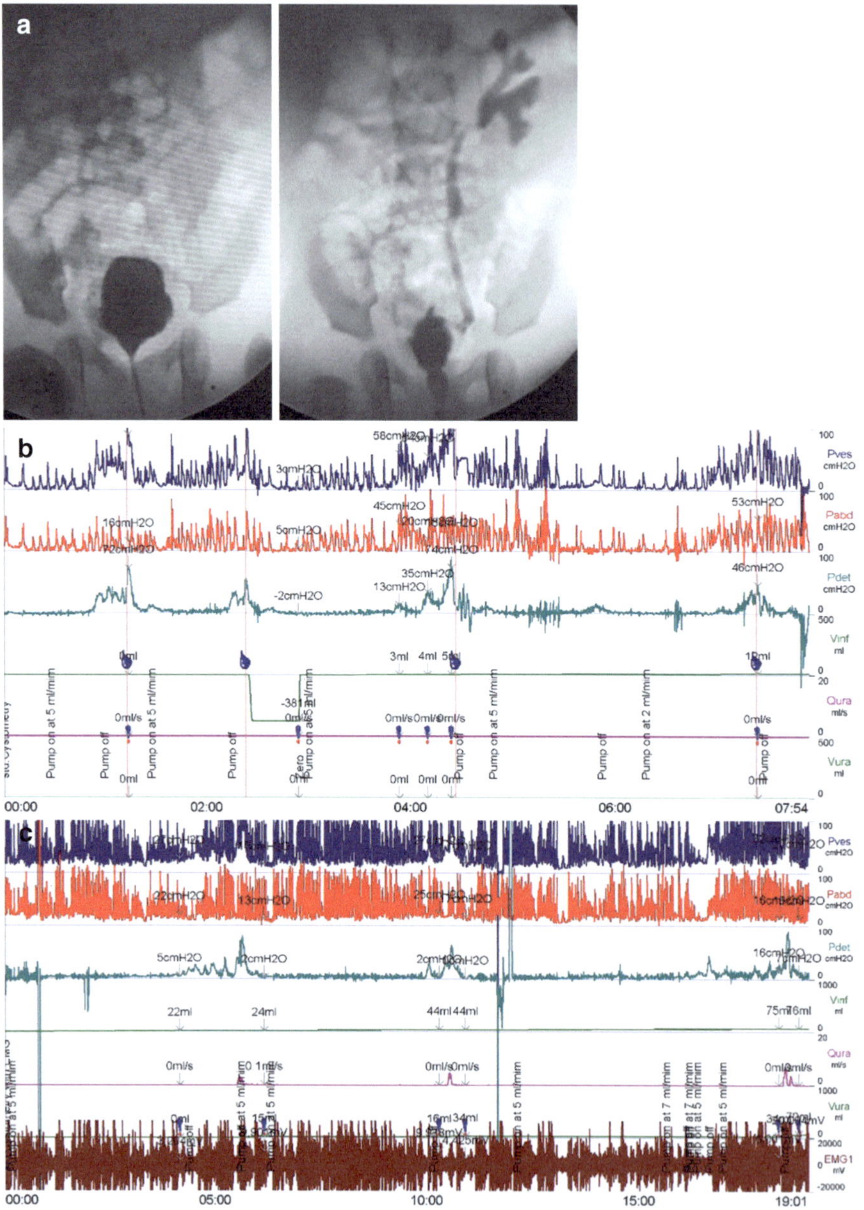

Fig. 20.1 (**a**) MCU image (2 months of age). (**b**) UDS tracing—2 months of age. (**c**) UDS tracing (10 months of age). (**d**) Voiding phase of the UDS tracing (10 months age) in an expanded form. (**e**) Portion of the UDS tracing (at 18 months of age) showing filling up to 50 ml. Episodes of detrusor overactivity are seen with leak/passage of some urine at 50 ml ('leak' sign). The study was done in supine position with fluoroscopic screening. (**f**) Voiding phase of the UDS curve (18 months of age) in Fig. 20.1e in an expanded form showing prolonged voiding detrusor contraction with interrupted void (points where flow started and ended are marked on the curve as annotations as the study was done in supine posture). (**g**) MCU images (18 months of age) showing smooth-walled rounded bladder with intermittent Grade I VUR on the left side (red arrow)

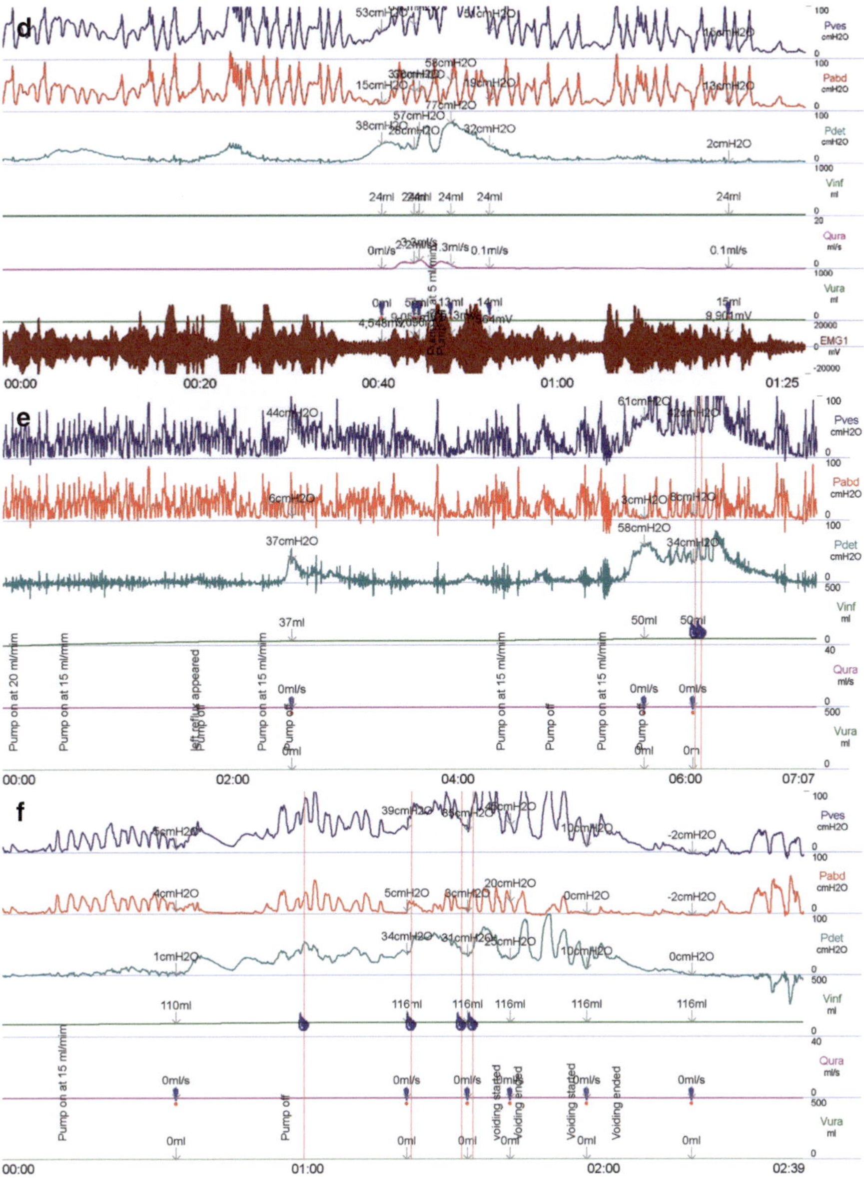

Fig. 20.1 (continued)

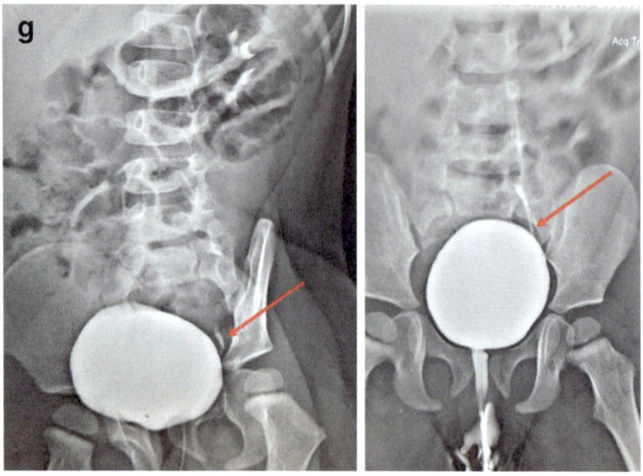

Fig. 20.1 (continued)

The UDS findings of detrusor overactivity and high-pressure voids are normal for this age, but when the findings were corroborated with the MCU findings of dysfunctional voiding and reflux appearing during voiding along with history of UTI, the UDS findings were considered significant and merited treatment.

She was started on anticholinergics/alpha-blockers and night-time catheter drainage.

She was well for the next 6 months after which she had two further episodes of UTI.

A repeat UDS (Fig. 20.1c) was done at 10 months of age which showed the bladder capacity to be 20–30 ml (which was still small for age, although better than before) with intermittent rise of detrusor pressure during voiding and cessation/ fluctuations in flow suggestive of dysfunctional voiding (Fig. 20.1d). There was a PVR of 8–10 ml after the voids.

Dose of anticholinergics and alpha-blockers were increased.

She continued to have one episode of UTI every 6 months. Repeat video UDS (Fig. 20.1e, f, g) at 18 months of age showed normal capacity bladder (110 ml) with significant DO and normal compliance. During voiding, the void was noted to be interrupted, dysfunctional void and left Gr II–III VUR during high detrusor pressures. Dose of anticholinergics were increased and she underwent left Dexell injection with Botox injection at the sphincter after which she has been infection free in the last 1 year.

Thus, this child had features suggestive of NNNB at infancy with intractable UTI. UDS was performed when deemed necessary based on clinical findings and management was based on the different UDS findings. A remarkable improvement was seen in bladder appearance and behaviour over time.

Case 2: Neurogenic Bladder Masquerading as PUV

A 6-month-old male child presented with recurrent episodes of complicated febrile UTI. He had history of poor urinary stream/dribbling while passing urine. USG showed left gross HDUN with thick-walled bladder. MCU (Fig. 20.2a) showed a small irregular bladder with gross left-sided VUR and abrupt cutoff of urethra at the

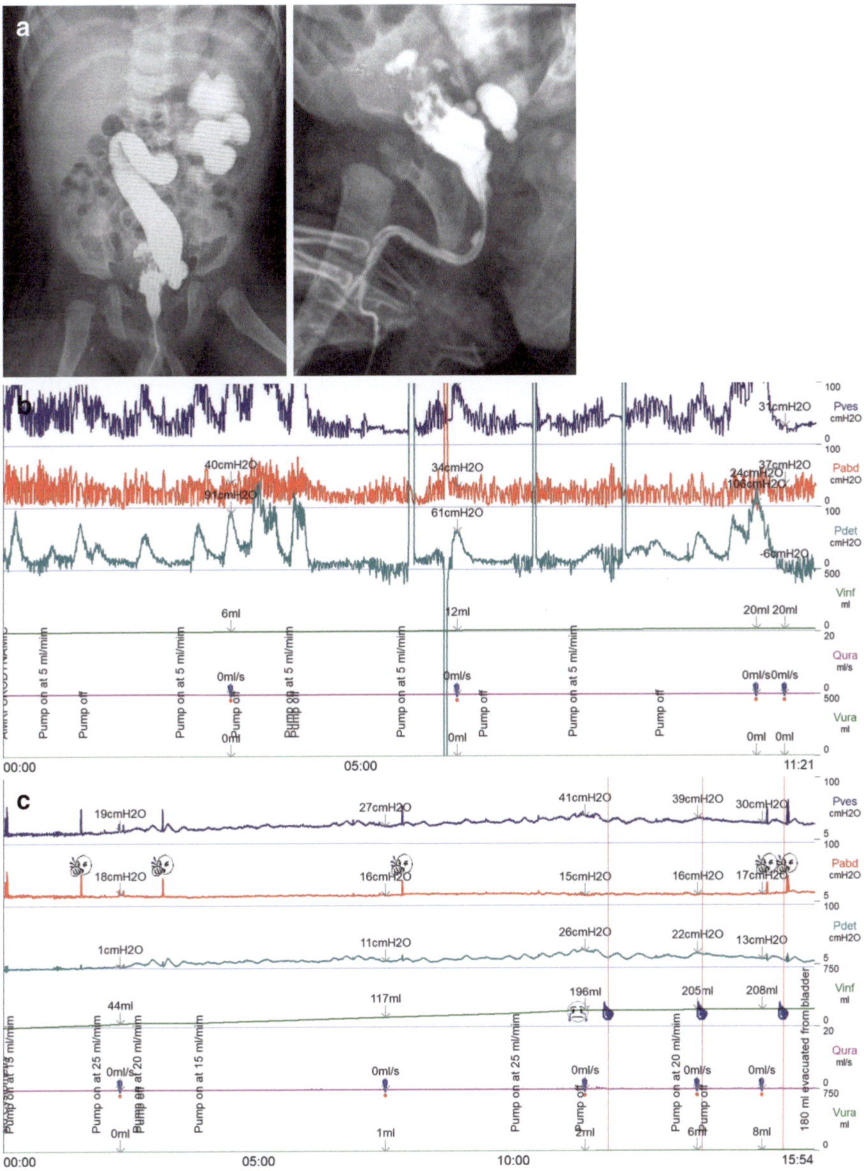

Fig. 20.2 (**a**) MCU images. (**b**) First UDS tracing (at 2 years of age). (**c**) Second UDS tracing (at 4 years of age)

level of membranous urethra raising suspicion of PUV. He underwent cystoscopy + fulguration of valves and left-sided loop ureterostomy at the age of 6 months.

He was re-evaluated at the age of 2 years. He had been well in the interim period with no further episode of UTI. He passed urine primarily through the stoma and dribbled per urethrally. USG showed bilateral normal upper tracts and normal bladder.

UDS (Fig. 20.2b) was performed by inserting the catheter per urethrally. Urine was seen to leak from the ureterostomy as soon as filling was started and it was kept occluded by digital pressure during the study. The study showed waves of strong detrusor contractions (60–110 cm H_2O) at volumes of 5–10 ml and the child became irritable so filling was stopped at 20 ml. Dribbling of small amounts of urine was noted per urethrally at detrusor pressures of 100 cm H_2O during episodes of DO.

The UDS findings were strongly suggestive of neurogenic bladder. An MRI spine was done which revealed partial sacral agenesis. He was started on anticholinergics and 3 hourly CIC perurethrally.

At 4 years age, he was passing urine every 2 - 3 hourly through CIC with no urine leak perurethrally. Output through the stoma had reduced significantly. UDS (Fig. 20.2c) was repeated at the age of 4 years when he was on tab oxybutynin 2.5 mg twice a day and mirabegron 25 mg once a day. Bladder could be filled up till 200 ml when the child complained of suprapubic discomfort; compliance was reduced (18 cm H_2O at 200 ml); mild overactivity was noted throughout the study with pressures increasing by 10 cm H_2O above baseline. No leak of urine was noted through the ureterostomy suggesting that the reflux had resolved. Leak of a few drops of urine was noted per urethrally at volumes of 200 ml when detrusor pressures were 20 cm H_2O. He could not void urine voluntarily during the study.

Thus, the diagnosis of neurogenic bladder, which was suspected during the earlier UDS, was substantiated. Bladder capacity had improved significantly and was now normal/large for age (200 ml; EBC, 150 ml) and reflux had disappeared. The CIC diary at this point showed CIC volumes of 200–300 ml, implying that although the capacity was 'adequate' for age, the compliance or end fill pressures at CIC volume was still high. So the dose of anticholinergics was increased further and overzealous fluid intake was asked to be limited.

Case 3: PUV

A 6-month-old male child presented after one episode of febrile UTI. He had no urinary complaints. USG showed mild left sided HDUN with a normal bladder. MCU (Fig. 20.3a) raised a suspicion of PUV and he was advised to undergo cystoscopy. The parents got the procedure done elsewhere where no PUV was detected. They reverted back after another episode of UTI at the age of 1 year when a repeat USG showed persistence of HDUN and mild thickening of bladder wall. The parents were advised for a repeat cystoscopy for which they were reluctant. UDS was offered to assess the bladder behaviour. The parents agreed that if the UDS suggested an abnormality, they would go ahead for cystoscopy.

UDS (Fig. 20.3b) was performed at 13 months of age. During UDS, the child voided spontaneously after every 30–40 ml fill (EBC 60 ml) suggesting a small

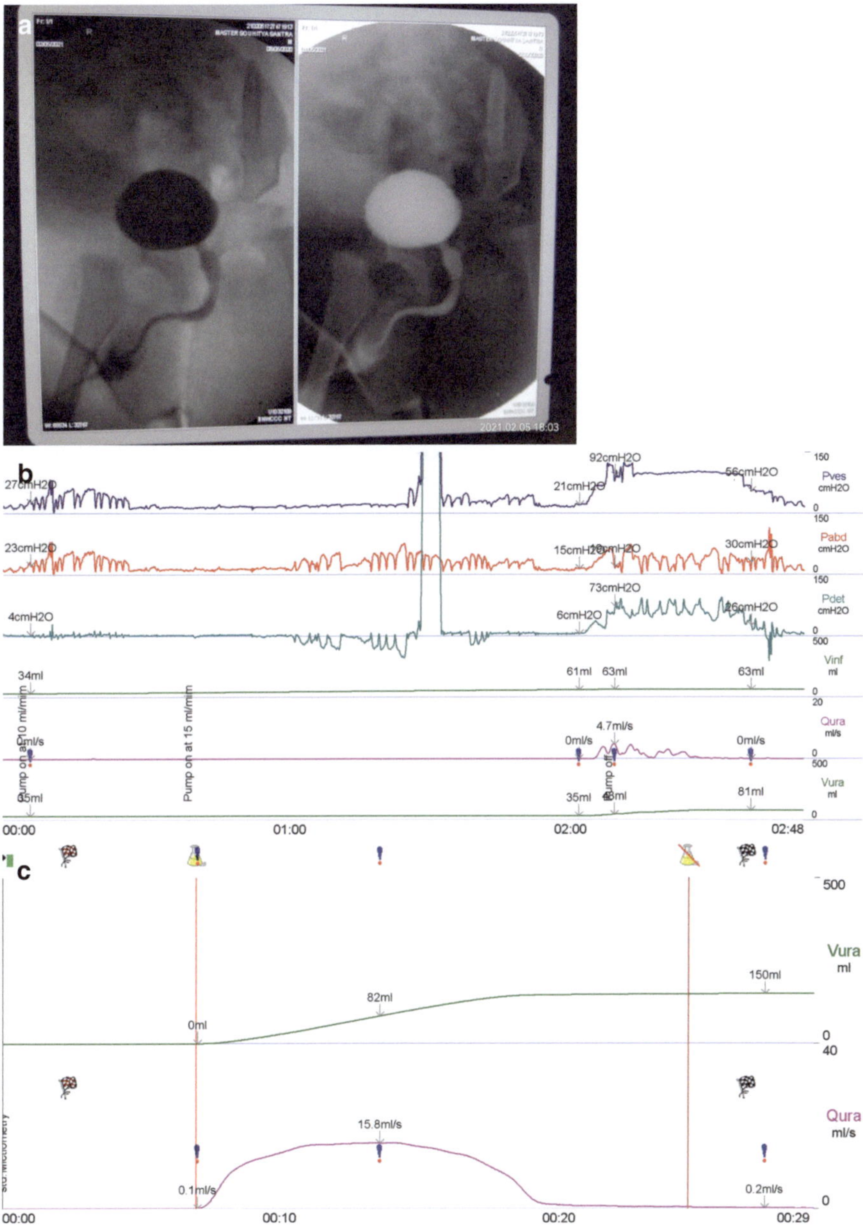

Fig. 20.3 (**a**) MCU images. (**b**) UDS tracing showing filling from 34 ml to 63 ml. He voided 45 ml after 30 ml fill with high voiding detrusor pressures. (**c**) Uroflowmetry curve. (**d**) UDS tracing (3 years of age). This curve was obtained with the child in supine position, so voiding parameters could not be assessed. (**e**) Voiding phase of the UDS tracing (3 years of age). The study was repeated in sitting position to assess the voiding parameters

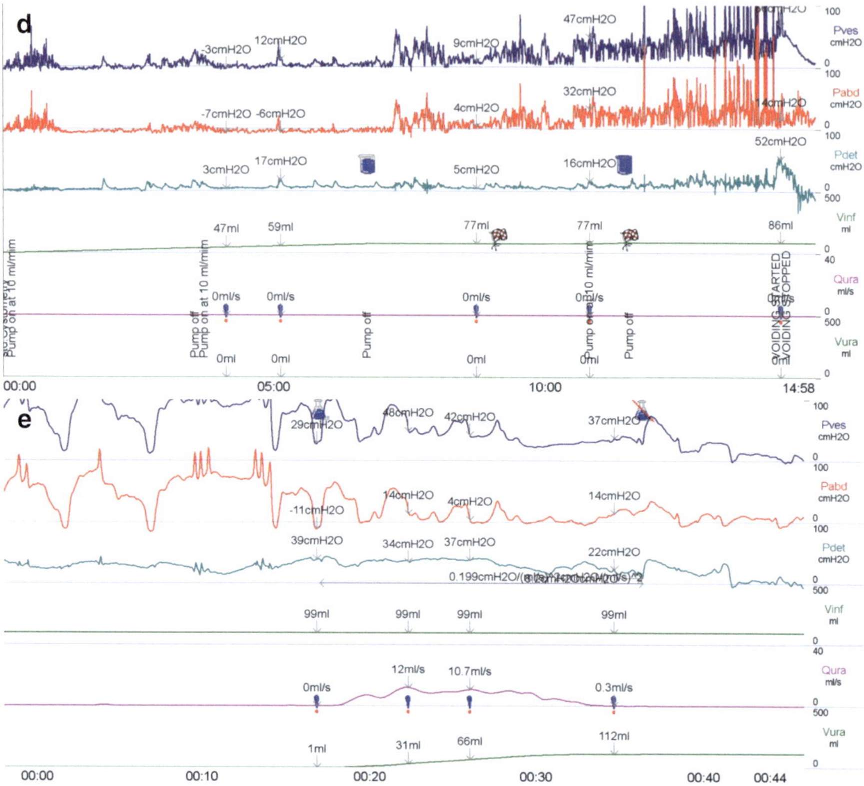

Fig. 20.3 (continued)

capacity bladder/probable DO. During voiding, PdetQmax was around 60–70 cm H_2O with flow rates of 4–5 ml/sec suggesting probable BOO.

The child was taken up for cystoscopy and was detected as having PUV, which was missed in the earlier cystoscopy, which was fulgurated.

He underwent another check cystoscopy after 3 months when no residual valves were detected. His stream improved and bladder wall thickness improved.

At 3 years of age, he had another episode of febrile UTI. Voiding diary showed that he voided 9–10 times/day, usual volumes being around 60–80 ml; max daytime volume was 120 ml. Uroflowmetry (Fig. 20.3c) showed good flow rates with adequate voided volumes. He was suspected as having overactive bladder, but UDS was performed to rule out any residual/recurrent BOO before starting anticholinergics.

UDS (Fig. 20.3d) showed small capacity bladder (100 ml) with significant detrusor overactivity after 90 ml fill and normal compliance. PdetQmax was 34 cm H_2O at flow rates of 12 ml/sec (Fig. 20.3e). Thus, there was no evidence of BOO, but the child had DO. So he was started on anticholinergics.

Case 4: Neurogenic Bladder with Gross VUR

A 4-year-old female child, follow-up case of LSMMC repair in neonatal period, had history of urinary dribbling and fecal soiling. She presented with complicated UTI with AKI with a creatinine of 2.4 mg/dl. USG showed bilateral mild pelvic fullness with a thick-walled UB. After she was catheterised and UTI was treated, her creatinine dropped to 0.4 mg/dl. She underwent MCU and UDS. MCU (Fig. 20.4a) showed a very small capacity bladder, typical of neurogenic bladder with bilateral VUR. During UDS (Fig. 20.4b), the pressures increased to 70 cm H_2O at volumes of 17 ml denoting a very small capacity and poorly compliant bladder.

The patient was considered for diversion because of the poor bladder dynamics and an episode of acute kidney injury, but the parents did not want diversion. So she was started on anticholinergics and CIC. At 3 months follow-up, her creatinine was stable and she was dry in between CICs. CIC volumes were around 100–120 ml. Video UDS was repeated to check whether storage capacity increased due to increase in reflux or increase in bladder size. MCU (Fig. 20.4c) showed a significant improvement in bladder capacity and disappearance of reflux on one side. UDS (Fig. 20.4d) showed considerable improvement in compliance with pressures reaching 40 cm H_2O at 60 ml.

Dose of anticholinergics was increased to reduce the bladder pressures further. DMSA scan showed a small scarred right kidney with 30% function.

The patient was lost to follow-up. They continued the CIC but stopped all medications. The child was well for 3 years in between. She presented at the age of 7 years with recent onset recurrent UTI. She was on 3–4 hourly CIC, night-time catheter drainage and rectal washouts for constipation. She was off all medications. She could feel the urge to pass urine several times in between the CICs and she passed urine in the toilet. She had urgency but could control the urge for some time. She did not require diapers.

USG showed bilateral gross HDUN with thick-walled UB. DMSA scan showed right non-functioning kidney.

Her voiding diary (Fig. 20.4e) showed that she emptied 130–150 ml of urine each time with CIC, and self-void volumes were around 40–50 ml several times in between CICs.

Video UDS was performed to identify the state of VUR and assess the bladder pressures.

MCU (Fig. 20.4f) images showed a highly irregular, elongated bladder with gross right-sided VUR. UB and the right renal pelvis appeared similar in size.

UDS (Fig. 20.4g) showed significant overactivity and poor compliance. She reported urge to pass urine whenever the detrusor pressures were >30 cm H_2O. No leak was documented during the study. She could not pass urine voluntarily during the study. It could be inferred from the study that whenever the child felt urge to void and voided on her own, i.e., self-void, the detrusor pressures were >30 cm H_2O.

She was restarted on anticholinergics; CIC was continued and her CIC/self-void volumes were monitored on follow-up. Doses of anticholinergics were escalated till her self-voids reduced to nil.

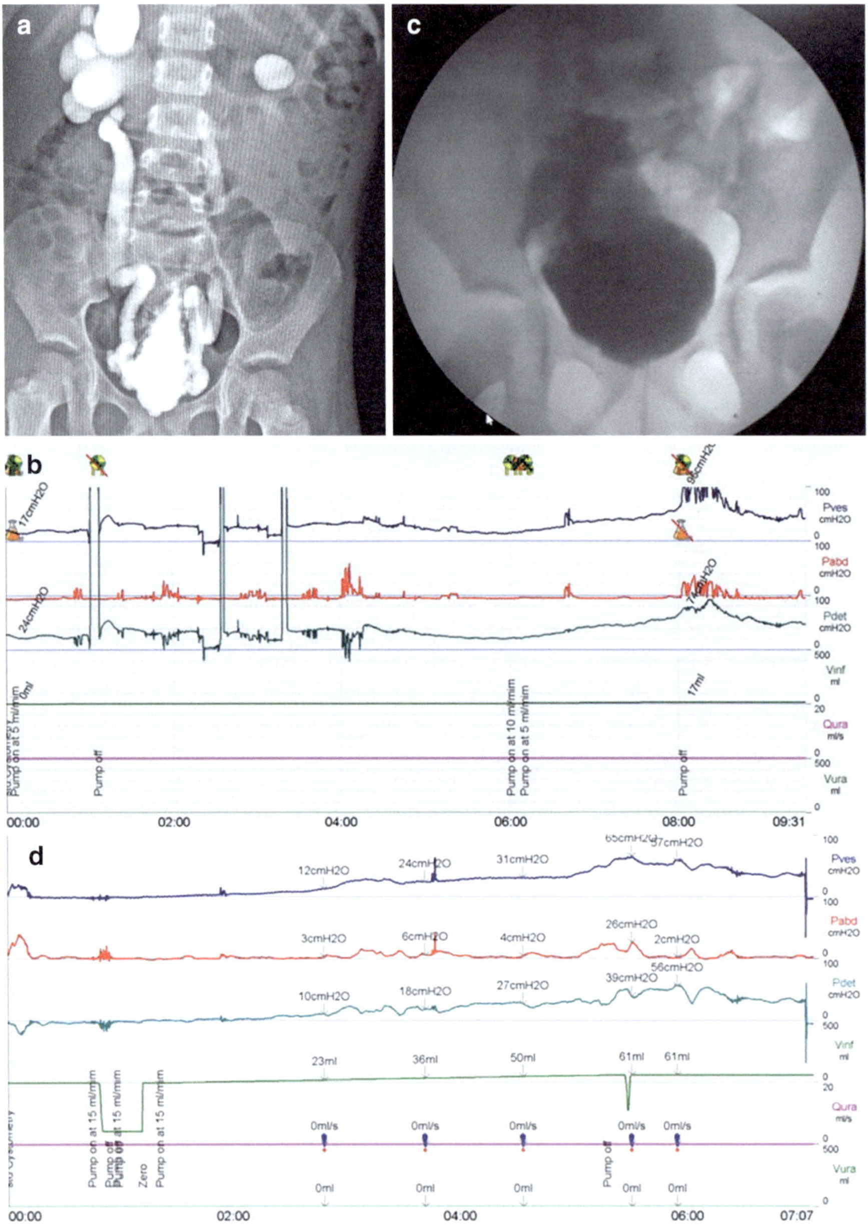

Fig. 20.4 (**a**) MCU image at baseline. (**b**) UDS tracing at baseline. (**c**) MCU image after 3 months. (**d**) UDS tracing. (**e**) First voiding diary. Voids highlighted in yellow are self-voids; those in blue are CIC voids. (**f**) Third MCU image. (**g**) Third UDS tracing. 'Blue beaker' signs indicate the points where patient reported urgency to pass urine. (**h**) Second voiding diary. (**i**) Fourth MCU. (**j**) Fourth UDS. (**k**) Fifth UDS

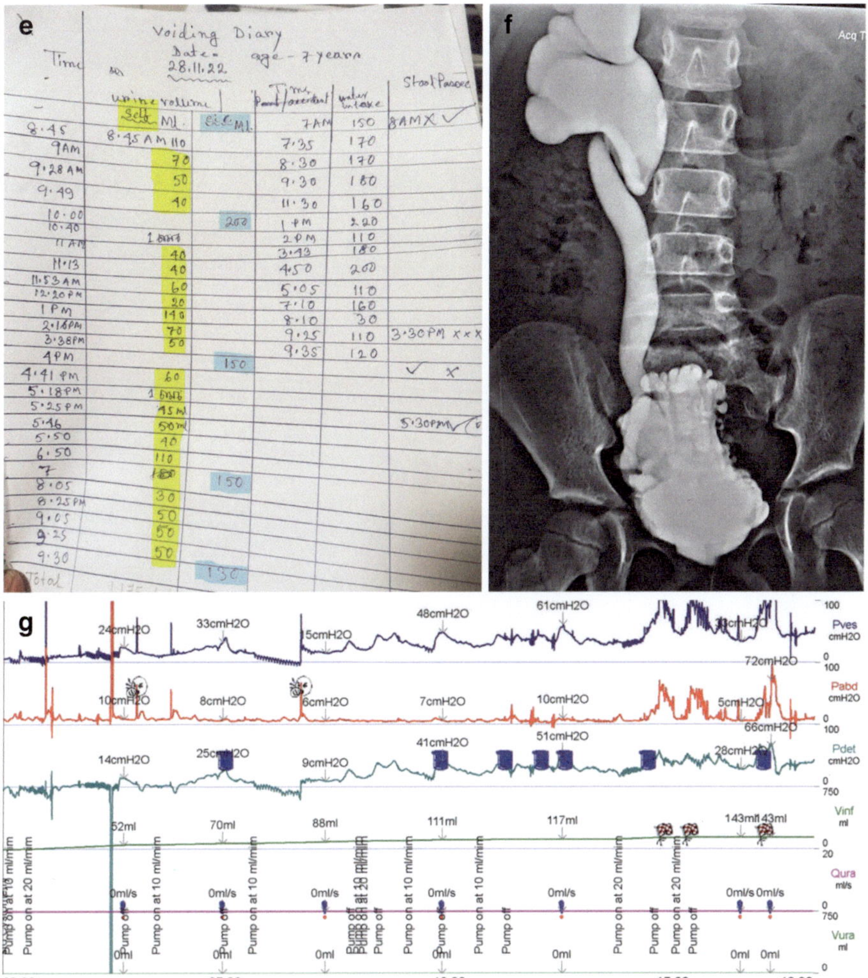

Fig. 20.4 (continued)

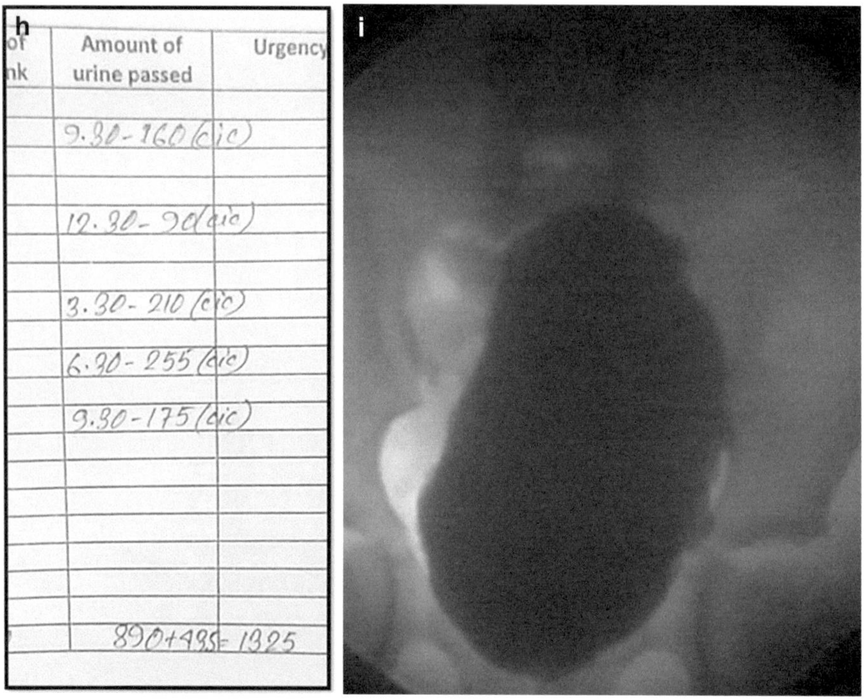

Fig. 20.4 (continued)

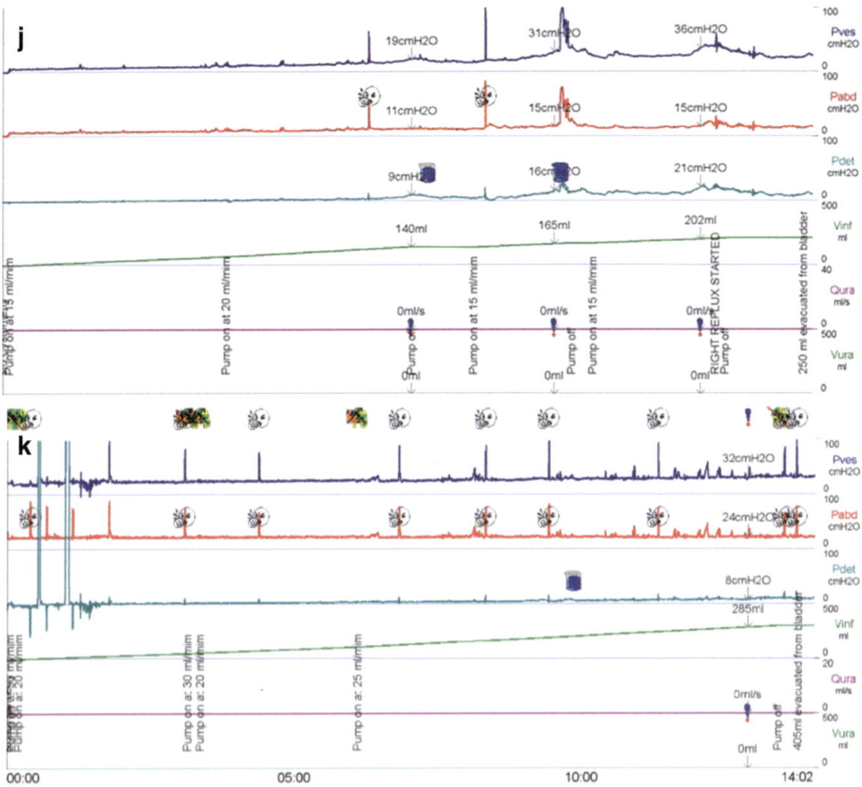

Fig. 20.4 (continued)

After 6 months, her CIC volumes (Fig. 20.4h) were around 100–250 ml, and she had no voids in between. A video UDS was repeated to check whether exacerbation of reflux had caused the bladder capacity to increase or the bladder had actually increased in size.

MCU (Fig. 20.4i) images showed that the bladder had significantly improved in appearance and capacity.

On UDS (Fig. 20.4j), bladder capacity was normal (250 ml), compliance was normal, but there was mild overactivity.

There was no reflux till 200 ml capacity when the pressures were <20 cm H_2O. Right VUR appeared when the detrusor pressures reached 20 cm H_2O.

Dose of anticholinergics were adjusted further. She was on oxybutynin 10 mg/day and mirabegron 50 mg per day. She passed urine only with CIC and did not have any self-voids. Repeat UDS after 6 months (Fig. 20.4k) showed a normal capacity bladder with normal compliance. USG showed significant reduction in bilateral upper tract dilatation.

MCU was not needed any further as her 'reflux' point pressure was 20 cm H_2O and we could manage to reduce the detrusor pressures to <20 cm H_2O.

Declarations

Competing Interests The author(s) has no competing interests to declare that are relevant to the content of this manuscript.

Ethics Approval The author(s) declares that this manuscript does not include primary research with human participants.

The author(s) declares that this manuscript does not include primary studies involving animals.

Atlas of Artefacts and Troubleshooting 21

Poonam Guha Vaze and Shirish Yande

Artefacts in Uroflowmetry

1. Changing the limits in the graph
2. Time frame shown in the graph
3. Effect of voided volume
4. Miscellaneous
    (a) Sudden peak
    (b) Staccato curve
    (c) Sudden dip

Artefacts in EMG

Wetting of electrode

P. G. Vaze (✉)
Neotia Bhagirathi Woman and Child Care Centre, Newtown, Kolkata, India

Department of Pediatric Surgery, Nilratan Sircar Medical College and Hospital, Kolkata, India

S. Yande
Ruby Hall Clinic, Pune, Maharashtra, India

Crystal Centre for Urinary Incontinence and Neurourology, MMF- Ratna Memorial Hospital, Pune, Maharashtra, India

S. Saha, P. Guha Vaze (eds.), *Comprehensive Atlas of Practical Pediatric Urodynamics*, https://doi.org/10.1007/978-981-95-2709-0_21

Artefacts in Invasive Urodynamics

1. No deflection
2. Reduced/damped deflection
3. Drifting of tracing
4. Negative deflection in Pdet
5. Catheter slipping out
6. Transducer malfunction
7. Time lag between pressure and flow sensing

Artefacts in Uroflowmetry

Changing the Limits in the Graph

The software gives us the option of changing the 'limits' of flow rate (Qura) from 10 ml/sec to 100 ml/sec. The height of the flow curve changes with the limit set—the lower the limit, the higher the height. Thus, the same curve may appear tower shaped if the limit is set at 10 ml/sec and plateau shaped if the limit is set as 50 ml/sec (Fig. 21.1a–c, d and e).

If the limit to set at 40 ml/sec, the graph height obtained is appropriate.

Changing the Time Frame Shown in the Graph

Some UDS software allow us to set the time frame which is supposed to be displayed when a uroflowmetry curve is printed. If the time frame displayed is small, the curve tends to get stretched and may appear like a plateau, whereas if a longer time frame is displayed, the curve tends to get collapsed and may appear like a tower (Fig. 21.2). The stretch of the graph is normal if 1 minute frame is displayed in the print.

Role of Voided Volume on the Shape of Curve

Appropriate uroflowmetry curve should always have adequate voided volumes; otherwise, the shape of curve may be erroneously interpreted.

Figure 21.3a and b show the uroflowmetry curve of a 5-year-old boy who is a follow-up case of PUV (EBC 180 ml; functional bladder capacity 110 ml). Uroflowmetry with a 52 ml void gives a bell-shaped curve, wherein flow rate is proportionate to the voided volume, whereas a voided volume of 100 ml unmasks that the boy's maximum flow rate has a ceiling of 7 ml/sec and generates a plateau-shaped curve, suggesting outflow tract obstruction.

Figure 21.3c and d show the uroflowmetry curve of a 6-year-old girl with bladder-bowel dysfunction (EBC 210 ml, functional capacity 180 ml). When she voids

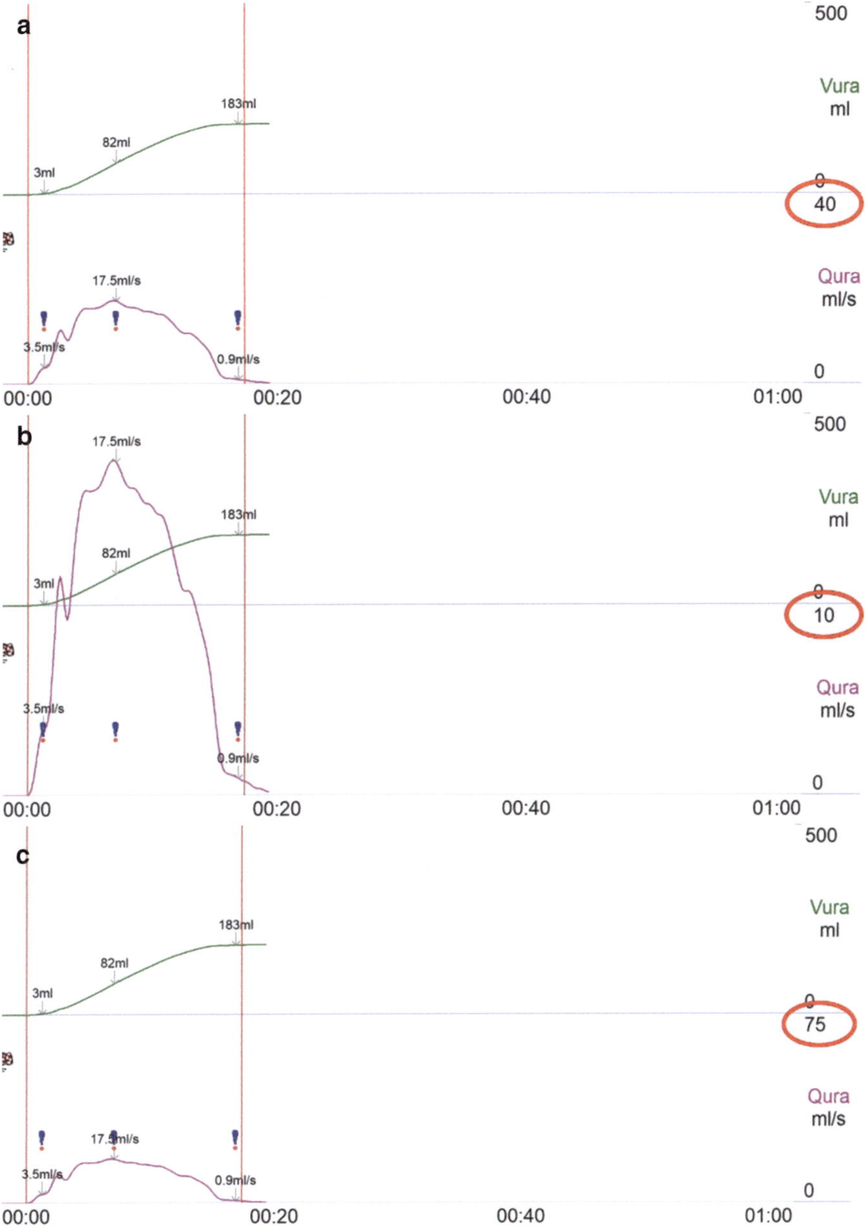

Fig. 21.1 (**a**) Uroflow curve of an 8-year-old boy showing a bell-shaped curve with appropriate flow rates. (**b**) The same curve as in (**a**) appears to be towed shaped if the maximum limit of flow rate is set at 10 ml/sec. (**c**) The same curve as in (**a**) appears flat, almost plateau shaped if the maximum limit for flow rate is set at 75 ml/sec. (**d**) Uroflowmetry curve. Note that the limit of Qmax upper limit is set as 20 ml/sec instead of the usual 40 ml/sec (marked by red oval) and lower limit is set as 10 ml/sec instead of 0 (marked by green oval). Thus, the height of the curve is apparently quadrupled. Also, the time frame showed is 1.25 minutes rather than 1 minute (marked by blue oval). So the curve is also horizontally squeezed. Hence, the curve which should be flat due to suboptimal flow rates appears tower shaped. (**e**) Corrected image of (c) showing true flattened out curve

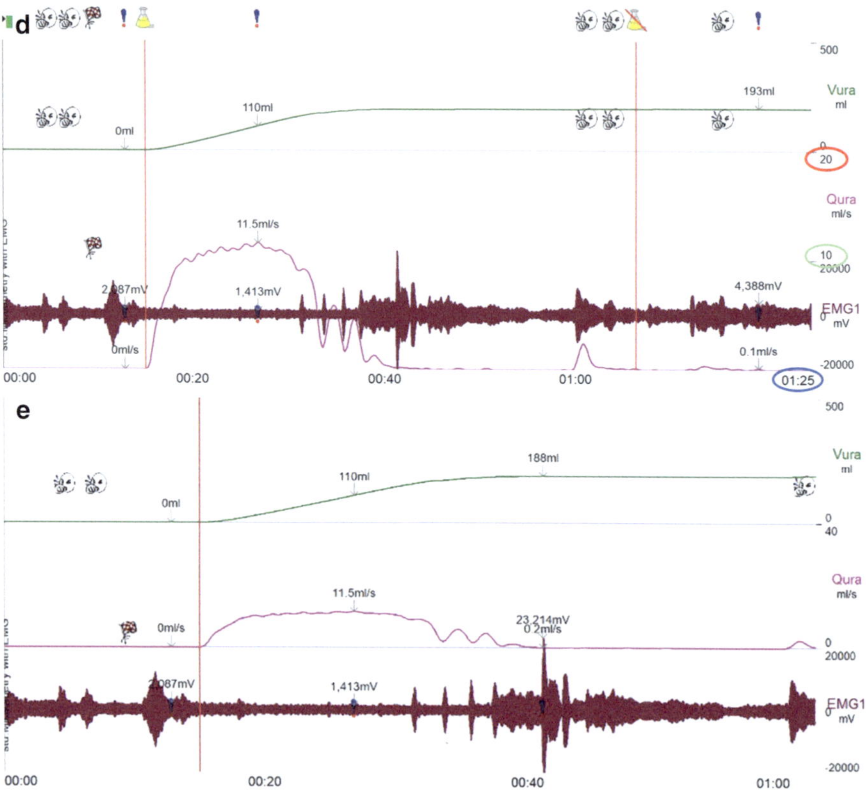

Fig. 21.1 (continued)

a volume of 173 ml, she generates a bell-shaped curve, whereas when she voids 370 ml, the curve becomes flattened due to the age-appropriate ceiling of flow rate at 25 ml/sec and a plateau-shaped curve is generated.

Miscellaneous

Sudden peak

An inadvertent kick to the uroflow jar during the study can cause sudden deflection in the flow curve (Fig. 21.4a, b) The characteristic associated finding is that the voided volume stays down to baseline/zero at the end of such a deflection, showing that no urine was passed during the deflection.

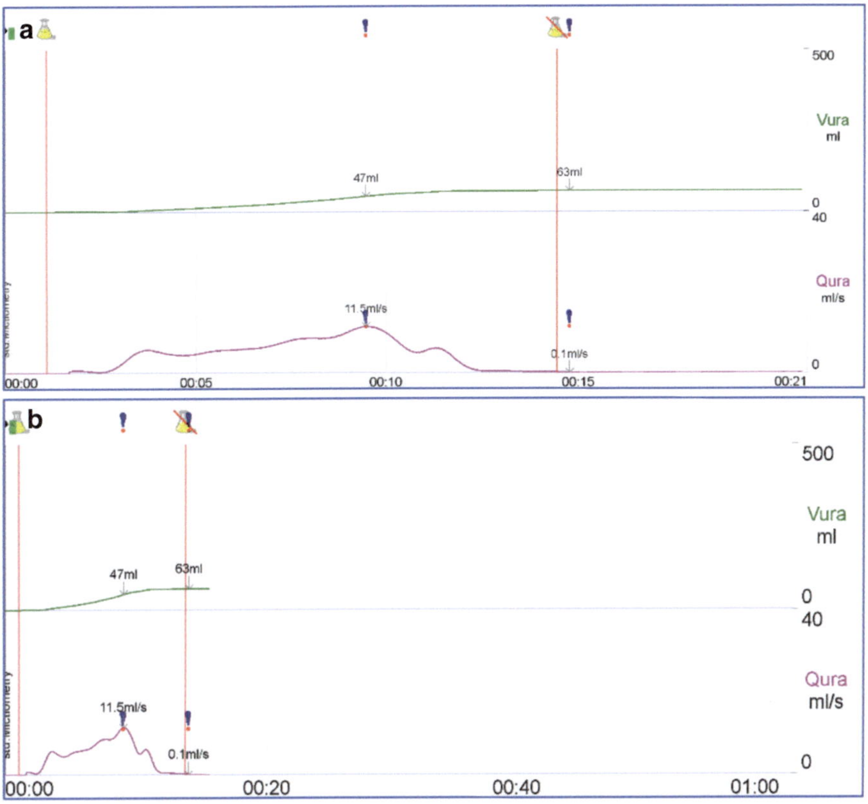

Fig. 21.2 (**a**) Small volume void with good flow rates, but the curve appears plateau shaped. Note that only 21 seconds time frame is shown in the tracing, thus stretching the curve. (**b**) Corrected curve of (**a**) with 1-minute time frame shown in the graph. (**c**) Apparent tower-shaped curve. Note that time frame shows recording of 2 minutes and 30 seconds implying that the curve width is actually squeezed. (Image courtesy: Dr. Jyoti Sharma, Consultant Pediatric Nephrologist, KEM Hospital, Mumbai). (**d**) Corrected curve of (**c**) wherein 1-minute time frame is shown in the curve. Tower changes to bell shape. (Image courtesy: Dr. Jyoti Sharma, Consultant Pediatric Nephrologist, KEM Hospital, Mumbai)

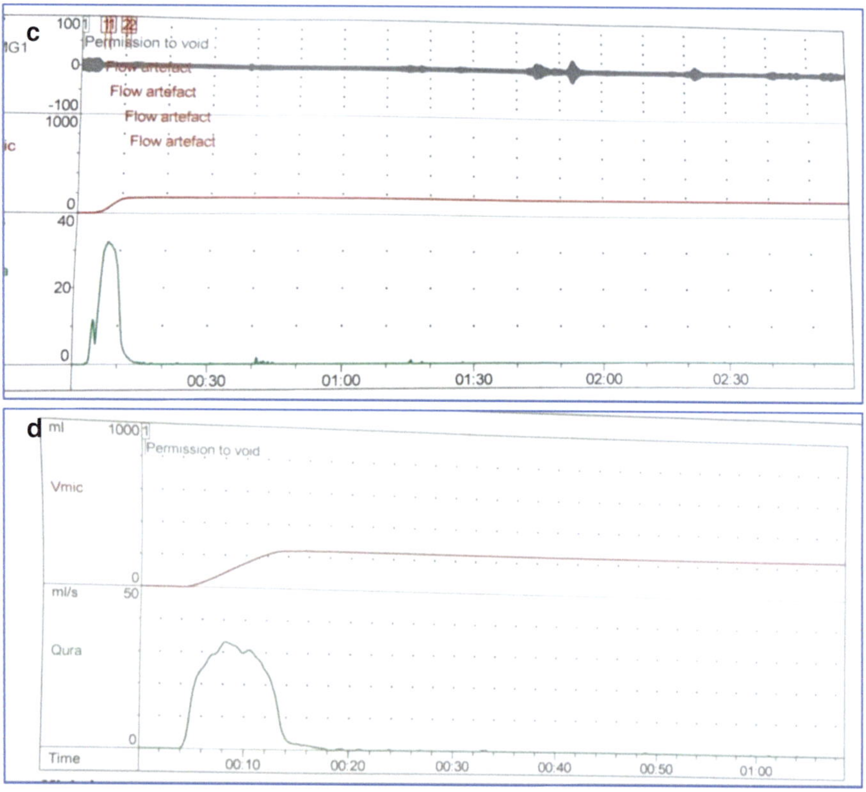

Fig. 21.2 (continued)

Staccato

Urine falling on different parts of the funnel can create a spurious staccato curve (Fig. 21.4c). It can only be detected by the person performing the test and needs to be mentioned in the report. If there are sharp undulations in the flow rate, either due to urine stream falling on different parts of the flowmeter or due to straining while voiding, it may lead to false estimation of Qmax (Fig. 21.4d). The flow curve needs to be smoothed out manually before estimation of Qmax (Fig. 21.4e).

Sudden Dip in Flow Rate

If the flow of urine is good, some part of the flow may overshoot the funnel and may fall outside the jar causing a sudden dip in flow rate (Fig. 21.4f). A vigilant observer can detect this and the test needs to be repeated.

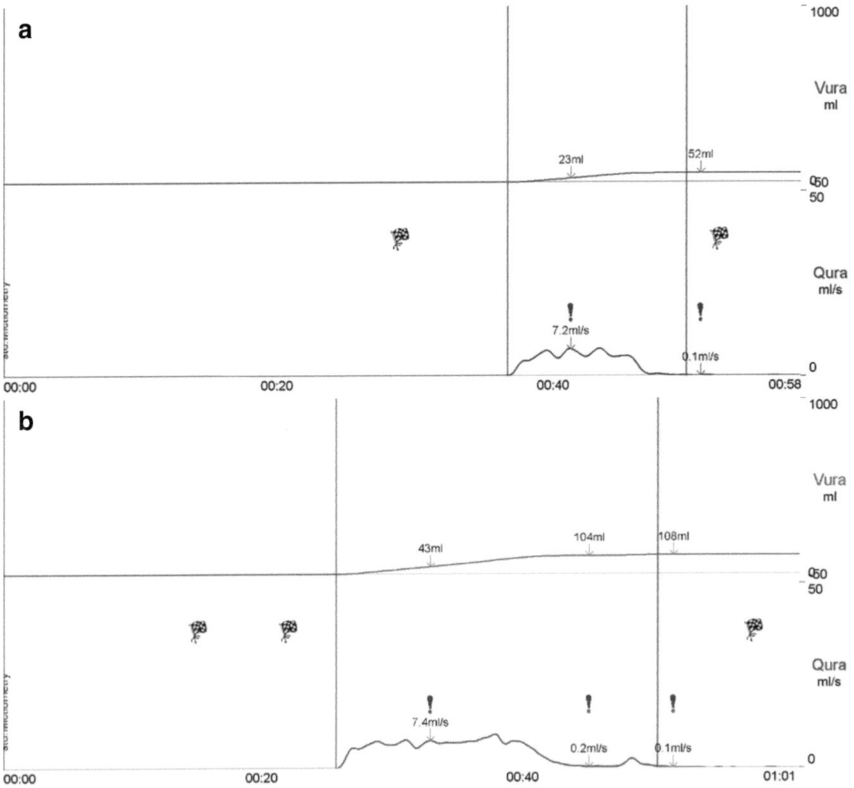

Fig. 21.3 (**a** and **b**) show the uroflowmetry curve of a 5-year-old boy who is a follow-up case of PUV (EBC—180 ml; functional bladder capacity—110 ml). (**c** and **d**) show the uroflowmetry curve of a 6-year-old girl with bladder-bowel dysfunction

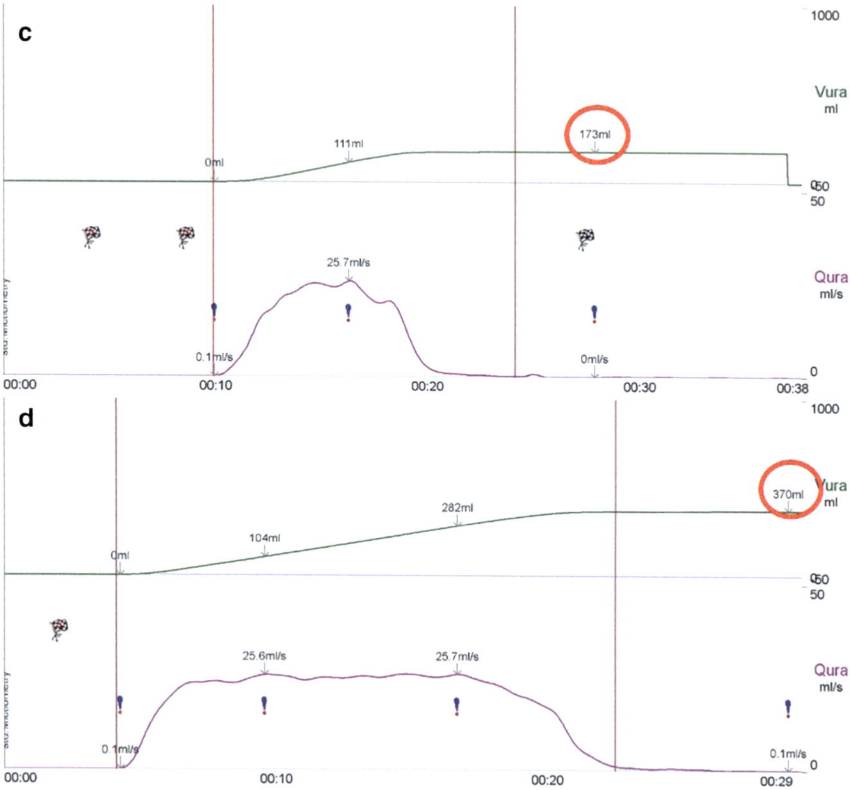

Fig. 21.3 (continued)

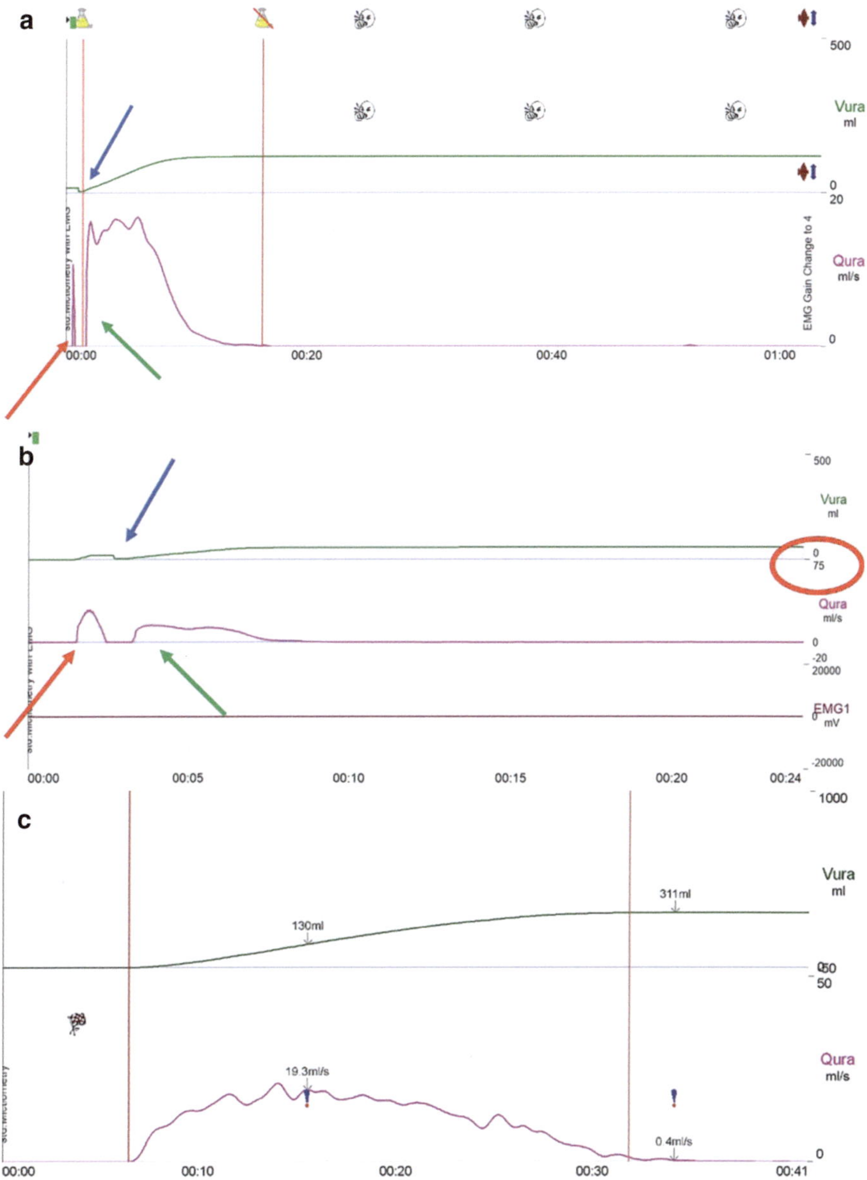

Fig. 21.4 (**a**) Uroflowmetry tracing showing an initial sharp deflection (red arrow) at the end of which the volume tracing returns to 'zero' (blue arrow) signifying that the deflection was due to inadvertent 'kick' to the uroflowmetry jar when the patient stands in front of the uroflowmeter. Green arrow shows the true flow. (**b**) Similar to the figure in 5a, this tracing shows 'kick' to the uroflowmeter, but in a blunted manner. Note that the limit of flow rate is set at 75 resulting in reduction in height of the traces and 20 sec time frame is shown resulting in the curves getting stretched. (**c**) Mild undulations in the tracing because of urine falling in different parts of the jar. The highest point on the curve cannot be marked as Qmax as it lasts for <2 seconds. (**d**) Sharp undulations in flow curve due to straining while passing urine—Qmax recorded as 20 ml/sec. (**e**) Same uroflow curve as in (**d**) with manual smoothening of the curve—true Qmax of 14 ml/sec. (**f**) The uroflow curve appears to be staccato with a significant dip in the flow. But the observer during the study noted that at that point, the urine stream overshot the jar and fell outside. The test thus is not reliable and needs to be repeated

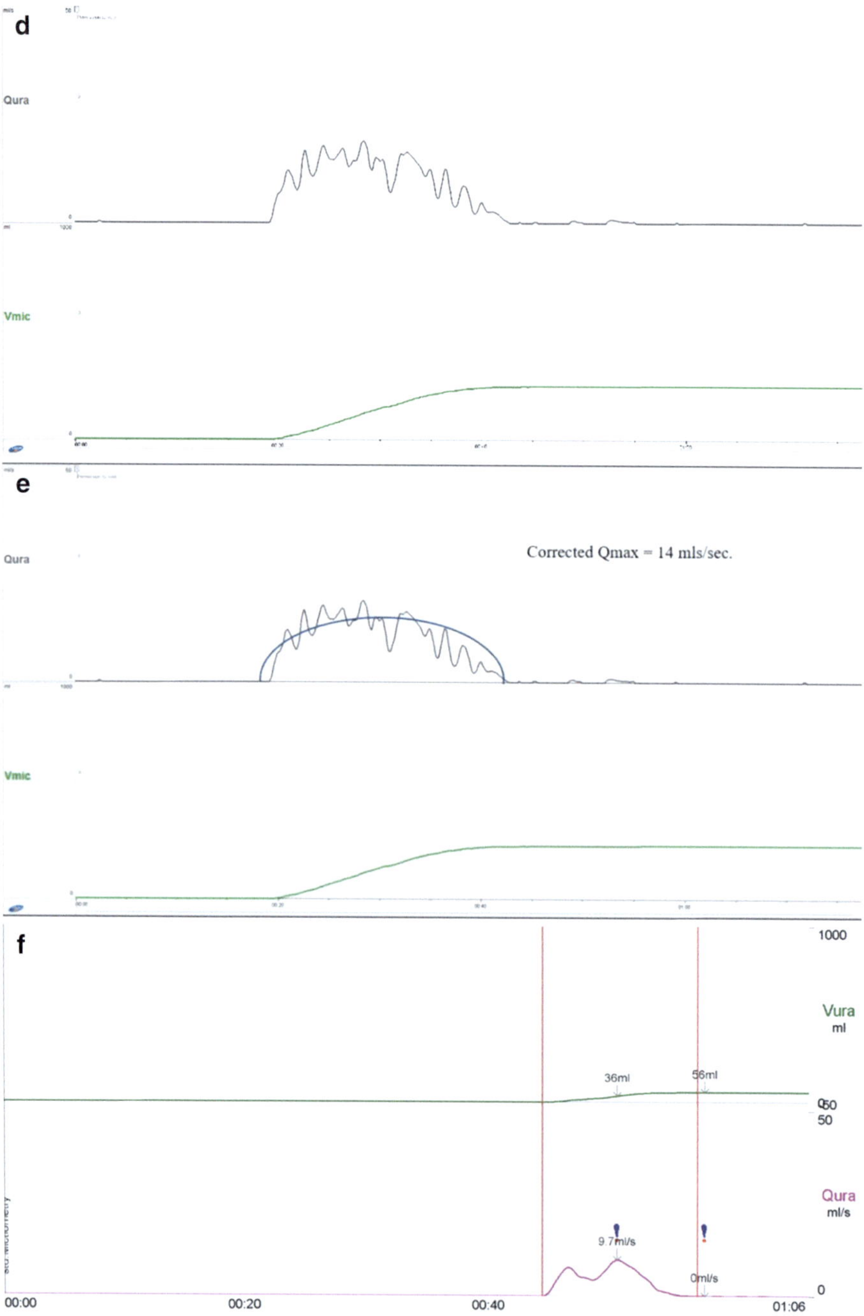

Fig. 21.4 (continued)

Artefacts in EMG

Wetting of Electrode

The EMG electrodes give abnormal readings whenever they get wet by electrolyte-rich urine and the recordings become unreliable (Fig. 21.5a, b). Covering the electrodes by a waterproof adhesive dressing usually solves the problem.

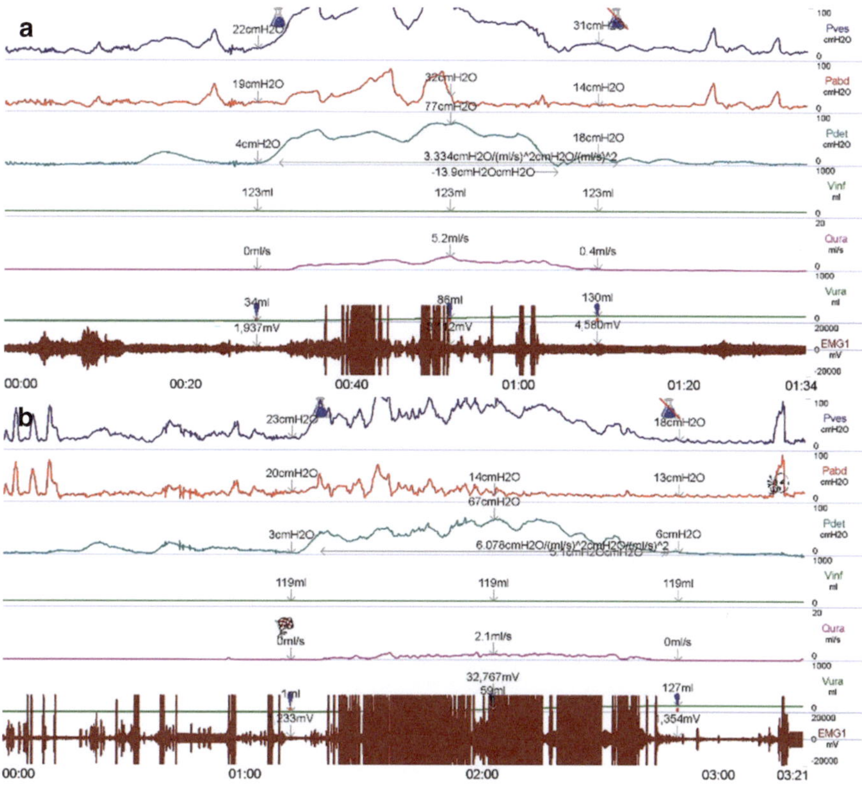

Fig. 21.5 (**a**) Voiding phase of a UDS performed with EMG electrodes. This is the first void which shows poor flow rates with definite increase in EMG activity during voiding. EMG activity also shows some artefactual increase intermittently which is usually seen due to wetting of electrodes. (**b**) Second void of the same child in (**a**) shows wetting artefact throughout the void and no meaningful activity can be discerned

Artefacts in Invasive UDS

To be able to identify and then rectify artefacts in invasive UDS, it is important to have a clear concept of the basics of the tracings

- Pdet = Pves – Pabd
- To interpret Pdet always keep watch on Pves and Pabd.
- Abnormal/unwanted deflection in *either* will produce an ARTEFACT in Pdet tracing.
- Deflections in Pabd lead to inverse deflection in Pdet.
- It is important to remember to flush the tubes after connecting to the patient to remove any air bubbles.
- The observer should be present throughout the study to detect any abnormal deflections and correct them instantaneously. Cough response should be checked at repeated intervals to assess that both the tubes are working properly (Fig. 21.6).

No Deflection

It may be caused if the tubes are blocked or kinked. Flushing the tubes, checking the tubes for any physical kink and checking the connections to see whether the three-way tap is closed and then rechecking for cough response solves the problem.

If the catheter is introduced into the bladder for more than required length, the catheter gets kinked inside the bladder when the bladder is empty in the early part of the study and does not read. As soon as the bladder distends, the catheter straightens and starts reading well (Fig. 21.7).

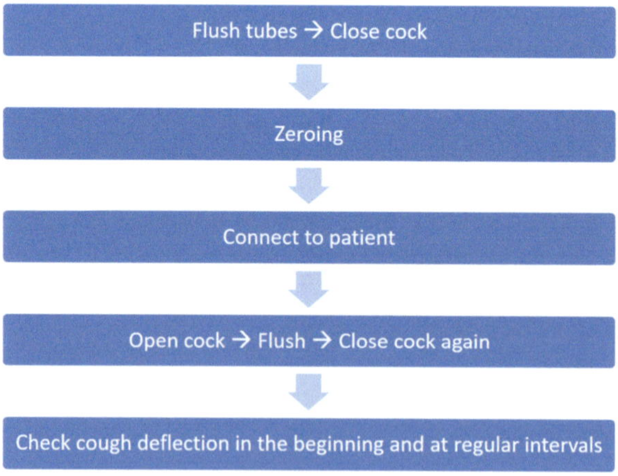

Fig. 21.6 Routine steps to ensure proper working of the two catheters

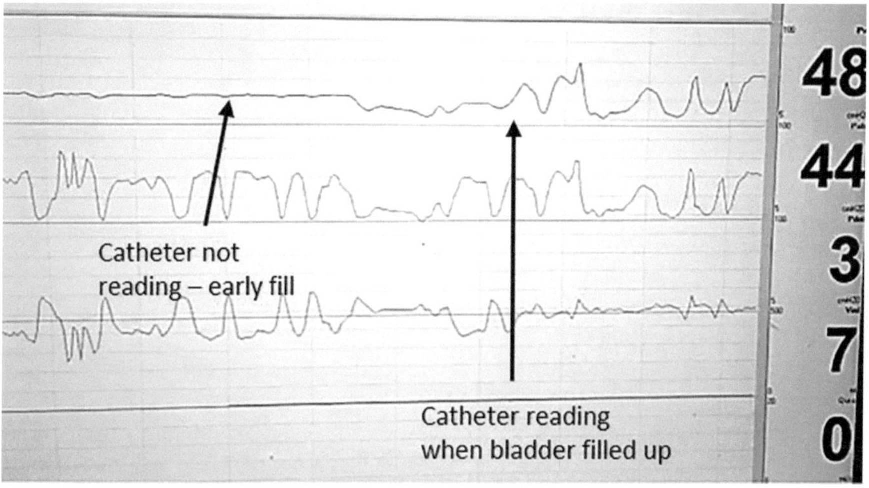

Fig. 21.7 As soon as the bladder distends, the catheter straightens and starts reading well

Fig. 21.8 Tiny air bubbles in the tubings can cause the deflections to get damped

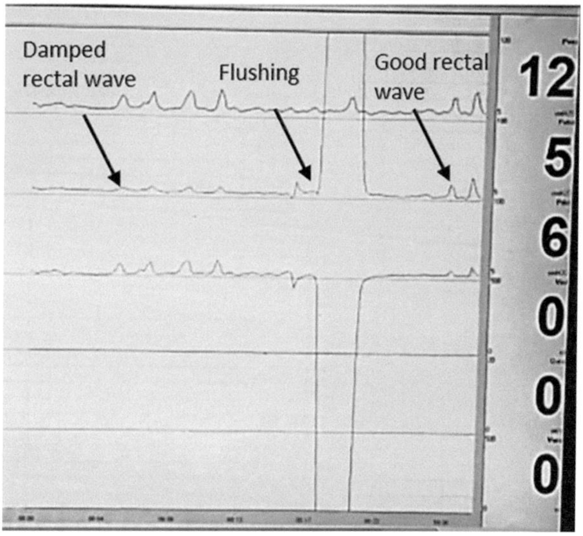

Damped Deflection

Tiny air bubbles in the tubings can cause the deflections to get damped (Fig. 21.8). Checking cough responses every 50 ml fill can detect such artefacts, and flushing the tube free of air bubbles can correct the problem.

Drifting of Either Trace

Either trace may slowly drift downwards if there is a slow leak of fluid from the channel (Fig. 21.9) or some of the connection is loose. Tightening the connections or changing the tubes may be necessary.

Negative Deflections in Pdet

Any positive deflection in rectal pressure tracing will cause a negative deflection to appear in the Pdet tracing (Fig. 21.10).

These deflections are usually seen due to rectal contractions in loaded rectum.

Repeated negative deflections in the Pdet tracing due to rectal contractions make interpretation of Pdet difficult – in such cases with severe rectal contractions, analysing the Pves tracing rather than the Pdet tracing is more reliable and informative.

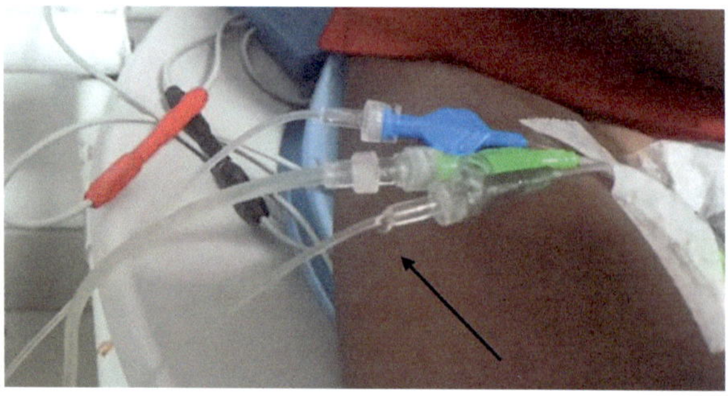

Fig. 21.9 Leak of fluid from a pressure tubing, due to a crack, leads to downward drift in pressure tracing

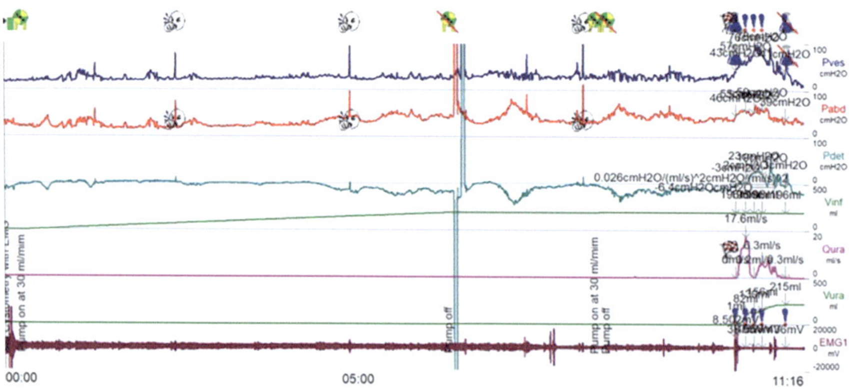

Fig. 21.10 Any positive deflection in rectal pressure tracing will cause a negative deflection to appear in the Pdet tracing

Catheter Slipping out

During the study, one or both the catheters may slip out if the adhesive has become loose after being wet of if the child strains significantly. This causes a sudden and persistent dip in the respective pressure tracing and then it fails to show any deflections with coughing/crying (Fig. 21.11a, b) The catheter needs to be repositioned and refixed. In children with anorectal malformation of neurogenic bladder, where anal tone is abnormally low, the rectal catheter tends to slip out repeatedly and inserting a nasogastric tube for assessment of abdominal pressure helps.

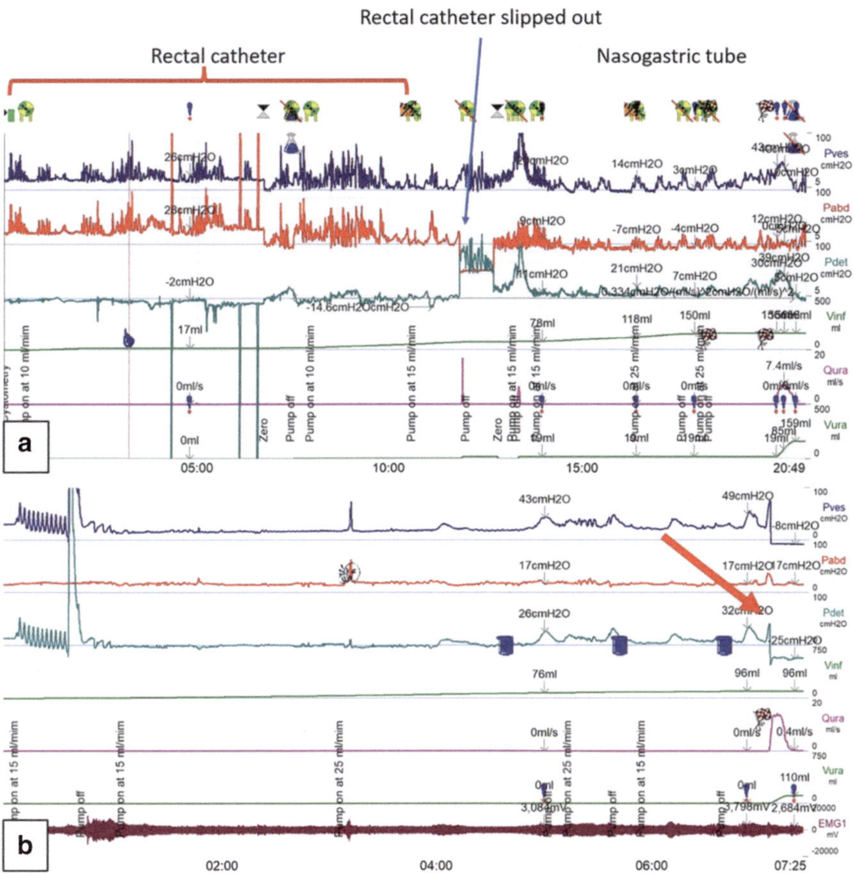

Fig. 21.11 (**a**) UDS tracing using a rectal catheter which slipped out during the study. Blue arrow points to the sudden drop in rectal pressure tracing at the point when the catheter slipped out. It was replaced by a nasogastric tube after which the study was completed. (**b**) Red arrow points to the sudden drop in vesical and detrusor pressure tracing after 96 ml fill when the vesical catheter slips out

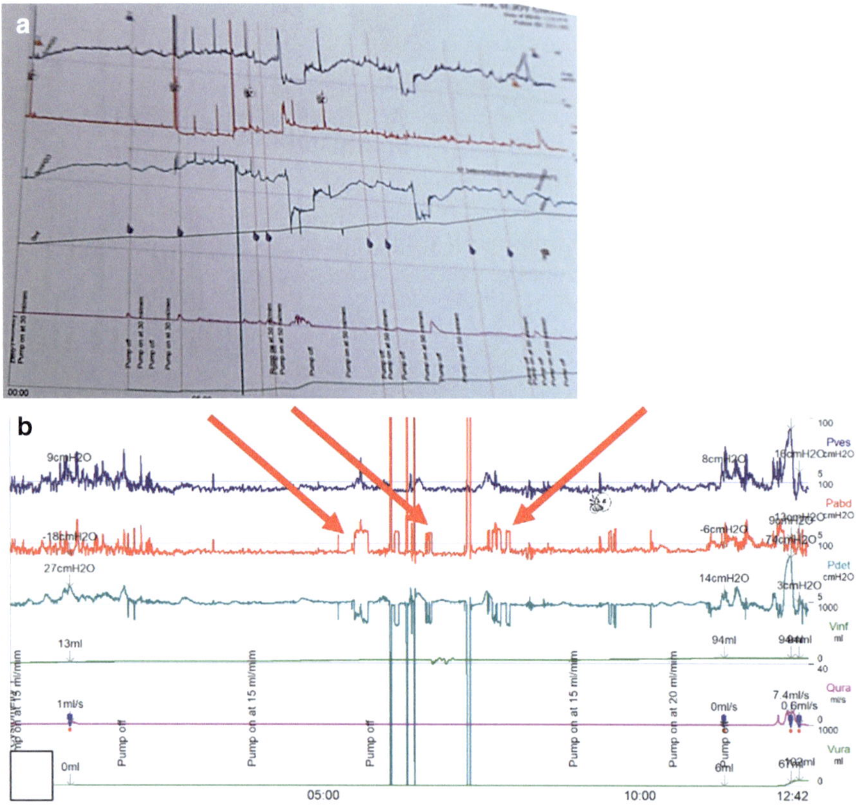

Fig. 21.12 (**a**) The vesical pressure tracing shows sudden dips when it stops reading and then it starts reading again. The vesical pressure transducer had malfunctioned and needed to be replaced. (**b**) Rectal tracing shows sudden upward deflections which returns to the baseline after a short while (red arrow). This causes corresponding negative deflections in detrusor tracing. Some dirt had accumulated on the diaphragm of the abdominal pressure transducer which was cleaned and the problem was rectified

Transducer Malfunction

Rarely, the transducer itself may have been damaged and not recording pressures appropriately (Fig. 21.12a, b) In this case, the transducer needs to be changed.

Time Lag Between Pressure and Flow Sensing

During voiding, detrusor contraction pushes out the urine. The machine senses the detrusor pressure change and the corresponding flow rate. The detrusor pressure is

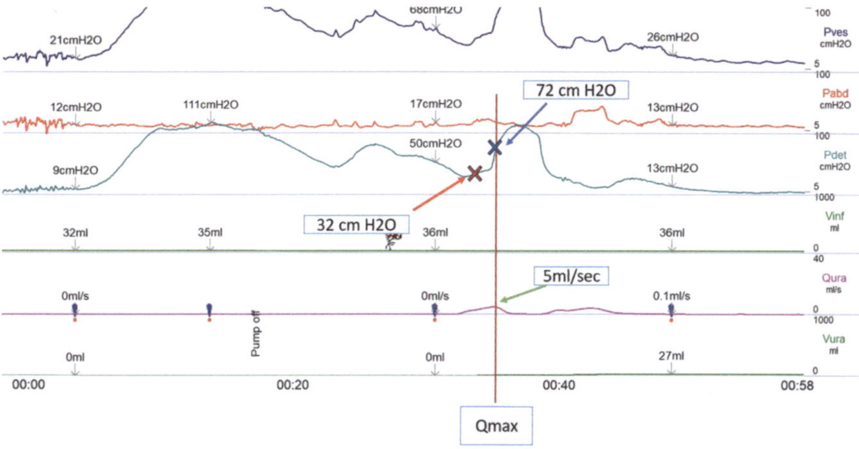

Fig. 21.13 Voiding phase of the UDS of a 2.7-year-old male child showing intermittently high detrusor pressures and a weak flow pattern with waxing-waning flow rates due to dysfunctional voiding. During periods of sphincteric contraction, flow rate diminishes and the detrusor pressure rises. Note that the maroon line is drawn through the point corresponding with Qmax. So the Pdet at Qmax should theoretically be 72 cm H_2O (blue cross and blue arrow). But the detrusor contraction which has pushed out the urine at 5 ml/sec occurs a few seconds before the urine hits the flowmeter. Thus, the actual Pdet at Qmax should be around 32 cm H_2O* (**This phenomenon of delay in registering in the peak flow applies to almost all pressure flow traces. Careful interpretations must be performed, therefore considering the distance between the urethra and the uroflowmeter and the way the stream of voided fluid finds to reach the uroflowmeter.)*

read instantaneously, whereas the urine stream takes a few seconds to reach the flowmeter depending on the height of the patient from the flowmeter. Thus, the detrusor pressure at a particular point of time actually corroborates with the flow rate of a few seconds later (Fig. 21.13).

Declarations

Competing Interests The author(s) has no competing interests to declare that are relevant to the content of this manuscript.

Ethics Approval The author(s) declares that this manuscript does not include primary research with human participants.

The author(s) declares that this manuscript does not include primary studies involving animals.

MIX
Papier aus verantwortungsvollen Quellen
Paper from responsible sources
FSC® C105338

If you have any concerns about our products,
you can contact us on
ProductSafety@springernature.com

In case Publisher is established outside the EU,
the EU authorized representative is:
Springer Nature Customer Service Center GmbH
Europaplatz 3, 69115 Heidelberg, Germany

Printed by Libri Plureos GmbH
in Hamburg, Germany